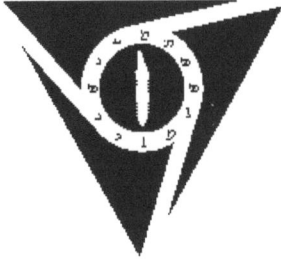

A Clinical Guide to Dental Implant Treatment, How to Do It Right.

Shahram Namjoy Nik

BDS (University of Central Lancashire, UK), DDS,

MSc (Oral Surgery, The University of Manchester, UK),

PhD (Dental Implantology and Bone Grafting

in the Speciality of Oral and Maxillofacial Surgery, The University of Manchester, UK)

Published by: Book Publishing Pros

Available at: Amazon, Waterstones, and Barnes & Noble

Printed in USA

ISBN-13: 978-1-917667-70-8

ISBN-10: 1-917667-70-8

This page is intentionally left blank

Foreword / Introduction

It is important to emphasise some fundamental principles that apply to all aspects of patient care. Remember the principle 'First, not harm.' All protocols must support this.

Dental implant treatment algorithms are of fundamental importance, and it is the responsibility of the head of the implant team to ensure that these algorithms are strictly adhered to.

As one might expect, the emphasis on different aspects of dental implant treatment has changed over time. The current focus is on immediate loading and one-piece dental implants.

This book may not answer all your questions, but I hope the tips and techniques can help you help your patients. More than 140 illustrations and 500 references were used with original, unpublished research.

The subject of anatomy was not introduced in a separate chapter, but the application of anatomy in dental implant surgery has been discussed.

All practices amalgamate ongoing research and experienced enterprise combined with settled conclusions and evidence -based principles.

The author believes it is wrong to believe that purchasing only expensive equipment will replace science and discipline.

Invariably, the dentist must bear in mind that increasing the cost will put patient safety in danger even though, from the surface, it is protecting the patient. However, it protects a small percentage of society, but the most vulnerable group cannot use the technology as it is too expensive. If the dentist can achieve the same evidence-based quality treatment as the conventional dental implant technique, it should do so and not get trapped in the companies' adventures.

There is no carte blanche of technique or magic wand of an instrument to be used in dental implant treatment.

Even though the GDC guidelines are limited to the UK, I must admit they are what each dental practitioner should believe and implement. This is how we want our loved ones to be cared for, and I hope it improves yearly.

We should remember Dr Burwell's speech as a Dean of Harvard Medical School in the 1940s: "Half of what we are going to teach you will be wrong, and half of it is right; our problem is we do not know which half is which."

This page is intentionally left blank

Afterword:

One of a person's fortunes is meeting people who can help improve their lives.

I had the fortunes of my family support, my father and sons, and to meet Dr Quayle as my PhD supervisor and Mr. Eldridge and Smith, the restorative consultants of the University Dental Hospital of Manchester, to teach me the science of dental implants. Foremost, I owe a debt of gratitude to my late father, Dr Kh Namjoy Nik, an accomplished endodontist specialist and a guiding light in my professional development. From him, I learned the importance of exploring all treatment options before considering dental implants as a primary solution. His insights continue to resonate with me, underscoring the value of conservative approaches in oral care.

I am grateful for my late paternal uncle, Professor MA Onsory, an esteemed ENT specialist whose advanced oral surgery expertise has profoundly influenced my career. His medical and ENT surgery education in Germany deepened my grasp of German language techniques and literature in oral surgery, pushing me to explore innovative approaches in this field.

I also had the privilege of the acquaintance of Mr. Stanley Freedman, who supported me through editing the book.

A retired dentist edited the book, Mr. Stanley Freedman (LDS-RCS, BDS, London, UK), and a recent graduate, Mr. Iman Namjoy Nik, my elder son, BSc (Hons), BSc (Oral science), BChD, MChD (Leeds University, UK) and postgraduate student at the University of Central Lancashire (UK), working toward an MSc in Periodontology.

Additionally, my younger son, Amin Namjoy Nik (BSc), is in the final year of the undergraduate dental course and integrated MDSc (the University of Dundee, UK), whose contributions are noteworthy. Two generations unfamiliar with dental implant science provided valuable feedback by identifying and highlighting any complex sentences, ambiguities, or areas needing further explanation. This feedback allowed me to refine the content and structure of the book, making it more reader-friendly and comprehensible, especially for young dentists entering the field.

Special thanks are extended to my wife for her patience and encouragement while writing this book.

I thank my colleagues, undergraduate and postgraduate students who, with their brilliant questions, guided me to write a better book.

Dental nurses each participated in taking photos and helped me to treat the patients with care. Mr Zakarya provided the animated illustrations.

The dental implant team must always focus on precision and will see to the end. We hope you enjoyed the book. Tell us what you think so that the next edition may prove even more useful.

TABLE OF CONTENTS

CHAPTER ONE:

BIOLOGY RELATED TO THE DENTAL IMPLANT SCIENCE

1. BIOLOGY RELATED TO THE DENTAL IMPLANT SCIENCE

Aim:

To explore the fundamental biological principles underlying dental implantology, providing insights into the interaction between implants and living tissues for a comprehensive understanding of the field.

Necessary Knowledge:

At this stage, you are assumed to have a general knowledge of bone biology, biophysics, oral anatomy, and physiology.

Learning Outcome:

After completing this module, the reader will learn basic about the tactile function of dental implants and the reaction of bone and mucosa to the implants. You will have gained an insight into the all-important relationship between systemic health and oral function.

> Osseointegration is not the result of an advantageous biological tissue response but rather the lack of a negative tissue response under loading (mastication) to the surface of the non-vital component.
>
> Do not wash the prepared cavity with saline prior to implant placement.
>
> Primary mechanical stability of a dental implant is a key factor for success.

1.1 The Relationship between Systemic Health and Oral Function

The Maintaining adequate oral function by preserving a functional dentition is crucial for systemic health. Research indicates that individuals with a full set of teeth or well-maintained prosthetics exhibit better nutritional intake and overall health. Loss of teeth, lack of replacement, and reduction of occlusal contact lead to impaired mastication, often resulting in lower consumption of essential nutrients and higher intake of processed, high-calorie foods. This dietary shift can exacerbate conditions such as obesity, cardiovascular disease, and metabolic syndrome. The reduction of occlusal contact, as seen in individuals with complete dentures, leads to reduced occlusal forces, decreased masticatory performance, and diminished salivary flow. Consequently, patients may turn to soft foods like potatoes or rice, which can enhance the risk of diabetes. People with a reduced functional dentition also tend to have a significantly lower intake of fibrous foods such as carrots and salads, leading to lower serum levels of beta-carotene, folate, and vitamin C [1,2]. Efficient chewing stimulates salivary flow, which is vital for digestion and oral health, and properly masticated food improves nutrient absorption in the gastrointestinal tract, supporting better systemic health. Therefore, ensuring patients retain their teeth or have functional dental prostheses is essential for preventing nutrition-related systemic diseases and maintaining overall health.

1.2. Physiology of the Tactile Function of Dental Implants

The oral function is dependent on the sensory inputs. The periodontal ligaments are richly innervated. They carry refined mechanoreceptors that function through contacts between collagen fibres and Ruffini-like endings, slowly adapting, encapsulated receptors that detect skin stretch, joint activity, and warmth (Figure 1.1).

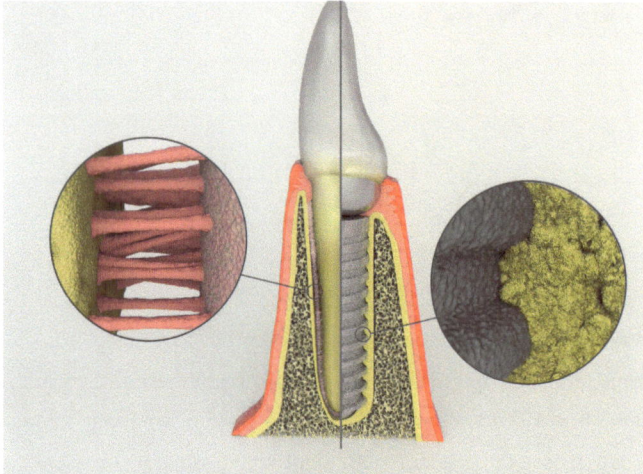

Figure 1.1 The implant lacks PDL and has a direct bone interface. The left magnification demonstrates the Periodontal dental ligament (PDL) between the cementum and bone, and on the right side, magnification demonstrates direct contact between the titanium surface and bone.

Forces transferred to the periodontal ligament and subsequently to the Ruffini receptors. By afferent sensory impulses, the mechanoreceptors in the PDL relay information to the CNS, and the efferent response provides the jaws' muscular activity.

Dental implants do not have periodontal ligaments, but other pathways will mimic the PDL reflex function [8]. After implant placement, the tactile sensitivity improves by the other receptors[3,4,5,8]. The mechanoreception in the absence of a functional periodontal mechanoreceptor input called Osseoperception is obtained from TMJ, muscles, cutaneous, mucosal and periosteal and the remnant of the PDL after the extraction, which contact between the dental implant prosthesis.

Golgi tendon organs are found at the Musculo-tendon junction, activated by muscle contraction in biting [7].

The TMJ receptors have a low threshold and a protective role by positioning the TMJ.

The mucosal mechanoreceptors that have been identified are Ruffini-like endings, free nerve endings, Merkle cells, glomerular endings, and Meissner corpuscles. This group of receptors is involved in the perception of complete denture patients [4].

The periosteal mechanoreceptors have been identified. The nerve-free endings are activated by pressure and stretching

of the periosteum by contraction of the muscles and skin and deformation of the bone during mastication by dental implant prosthesis [9] (figure 1.2).

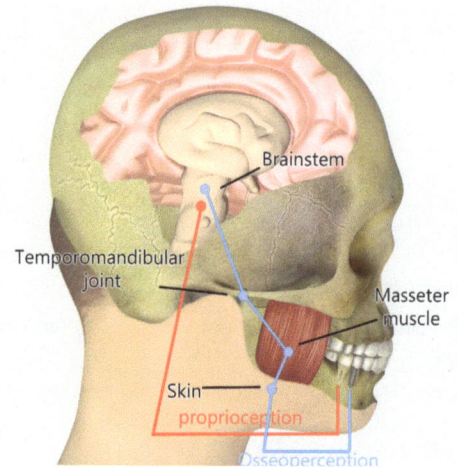

Figure 1.2 Summary of proprioception and osseoperception reflex.

The osseoperception may also occur by the nerve fibres in peri-implant tissue and inside the Haversian canals of the osteonal bone [10].

The oral tactile sensibility is the patient's ability to analyse the minimum pressure during mastication, expressed by the thinnest foreign body with a 10-70 um thickness [11].

The tactile perception of vital and non-vital teeth is similar, with an active detection threshold of 20um, while the implant-supported prosthesis has 50um and a removable prosthesis 150um. Dental implants require more force than the natural tooth to perceive the touch. The dental implant prosthesis perceives mechanical stimuli and functions well. It can be improved three months after replacing the removable denture with a fixed dental prosthesis [7].

The phantom feeling can also play a role in the physiological integration of an implant-borne prosthesis, as in the sensory-motor perception of a phantom limb after amputation.

The initially inadequate exteroceptive feedback of the new implant may present an early risk of overloading both the prosthesis and implant. However, the feedback pathway to the sensory cortex is partially restored after a few months through a hypothetical representation of the prosthesis in the sensory cortex, leading to more natural function and an improved ability to avoid overload [12] (figure 1.2). The patients will adapt well to perform masticatory functions, but during non-habitual functions such as maximal occluding force, there is less coordinated muscular activity that induces eccentric function and, if not managed, can lead to implant failure.

Oral stereognostic ability is defined as the ability to recognise and discriminate between different shapes, and a bilateral mandibular block reduces sterognostic ability by 20% [13]. There is no significant difference between implant-supported fixed or removable prostheses.

The tip of the tongue has an essential role in the stereognosis of objects inserted into the mouth, as has the palate and, to a lesser extent, the periodontal ligaments [14]. The physiological integration of a dental prosthesis on a dental implant can be beneficial and may lead to greater acceptance and improved psychological integration.

1.3. Bone in Direct Opposition to Implants

There are several books and papers which discuss the subject of bone healing and osseointegration, but what are the basic principles that a clinician needs to follow in order to achieve this in practice?

Since compact bone is essential to mechanical and biological stability, we must first revise its structure.

Compact bone is composed of osteons, which are tubular structures resembling leeks in form. (figure 1.3). Each tube is constructed of the protein collagen, and Hydroxyapatite mineralizes this collagen.

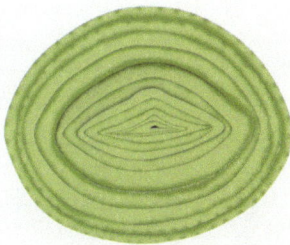

Figure 1.3 Cross-section of leek.

Each outer tube of osteon has an inner tube that lines its inner wall, which, in turn, has another even smaller inner tube lining its inner wall. The most miniature tube has a central canal running through it, carrying the blood supply for that osteon (Fig. 1.4).

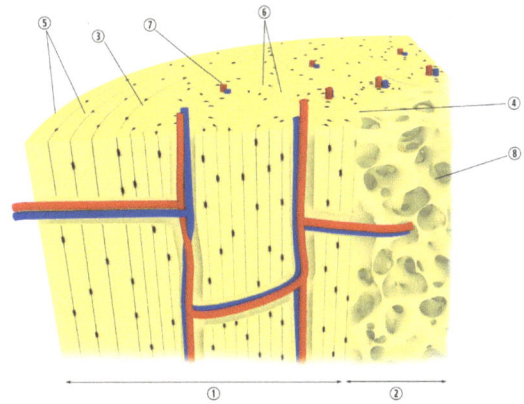

Figure 1.4 The cross-section of cortical bone and spongy bone. 1. Compact bone, 2; spongy bone, 3. Interstitial lamellae, 4. inner circumferential lamellae, 5. outer circumferential lamellae, 6. concentric lamellae, 7. blood vessels in the central canal, 8. trabecule.

Now imagine a bunch of leeks in cross-section (osteons). Each osteon's outer tube is cemented to its neighbouring osteon's outer tube, with the contact points occurring at intervals around the periphery.

Arresting the propagation of cracks through the very presence of the concentric lamellar structure of the osteons constitutes one line of defence.

A spider's web of canaliculi runs throughout the structure, transporting nutrients and oxygen to all parts. The entire structure is both solid and resilient.

While there are many challenges in dental implant placement, one of the most important is providing an environment that promotes bone attachment to the implant surface. A synopsis of the biology of bone healing is needed to understand this phenomenon.

Many biological factors that influence bone healing have been identified. One of them is microcracks. While microcracks are associated with bone resorption, they can also promote intracortical remodelling. Accumulated microdamage due to repetitive load can result in fatigue, and the resulting microcracks in the bone act as part of the repair process. Microcracks may be a direct and significant stimulus of osteonal remodelling.

Greater bone remodelling occurs in the monkey who eats a hard rather than a soft diet, with a more significant percentage of secondary osteonal bone growth being stimulated in the

4

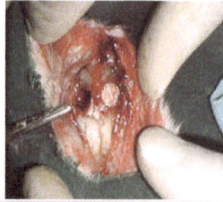

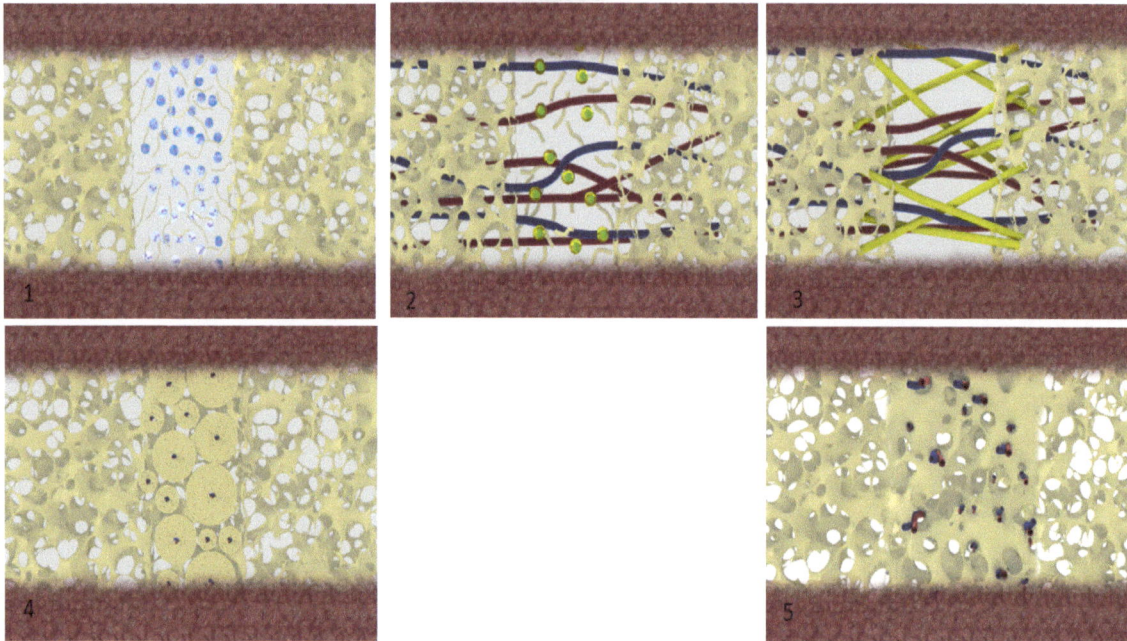

Figure 1.5 Stages of bone healing were studied using the parietal bone of rabbits, a standard procedure to study bone healing and bone substitute materials in dentistry as they heal by intramembranous ossification, such as bones of the skull. In other cases, mesenchymal cells differentiate into cartilage and are then replaced by bone, called endochondral ossification:
1. Fibrinous exudate contains fibrin, polymorphonuclear, leukocytes and macrophages 2. Granulation tissue: blood vessels, early fibroblast, range of thin collagen fibres 3. Pretrabecular scaffold: dense, thick and oriented collagen 4. Mixed woven and lamellar bone 5. Bicortical bridge.

greatest fatigue area [15].

This adaptive repair mechanism for fatigued mandibular bone is stimulated by the higher strain imposed and the increase in the number of strain cycles – up to a limit.

The bone temperature must be below 47 °C during drilling to avoid thermal osteonecrosis [16,17]. Even below 47°C, friction between the drill and bone increases the temperature, and in consequence, osteocytic death may extend to 0.5-1 mm, but this layer is eventually replaced by cutting/filling cones, both derived from the endosteal surface (figure 1.6). Note: the temperature rise during screw or cylindrical implant placement has not been accurately determined.

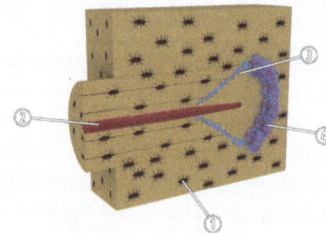

Figure 1.6 Cutting/filling cones. The osteoblasts create osteons, the osteoclasts are at the tip, and the lamellar bone is laid down. 1. Osteon, 2. the central vessel, 3. Osteoblast, 4. Osteoclast (cutter cone).

Finally, woven bone is formed, but its mechanical competence is lower than that of lamellar bone due to the random orientation of its collagen fibres. Woven and trabecular bone fills the initial gap at the implant-bone interface. The early peri-implant trabecular bone formation and biological fixation begin 10-14 days after surgery. This provides a type of stability different from the primary mechanical stability obtained during implant placement. Woven bone is progressively remodelled and replaced by lamellar bone. At three months, a mixed bone texture of woven and lamellar matrix can be found on titanium implants.

Bone debris, either from the implant drill preparation or implant insertion, envelopes the implant and helps to form peri-implant trabecular bone. It continues to be involved in trabecular bone formation during the early weeks - thus, it is not advisable to wash the prepared cavity with saline prior to implant placement [18,19].

The last stage of implant integration is continuous, localized remodelling, which repairs fatigue damage within interfacial and supporting bone - and it takes more than 12 months [18].

Bone-implant interface

The newly formed network of bone trabeculae ensures the biological fixation of the implant and surrounds marrow spaces containing many mesenchymal cells and wide blood vessels. A thin layer of calcified and osteoid tissue is deposited by osteoblasts directly onto the implant surface. Blood vessels and mesenchymal cells fill the spaces where no calcified tissue is present (figure 1.7).

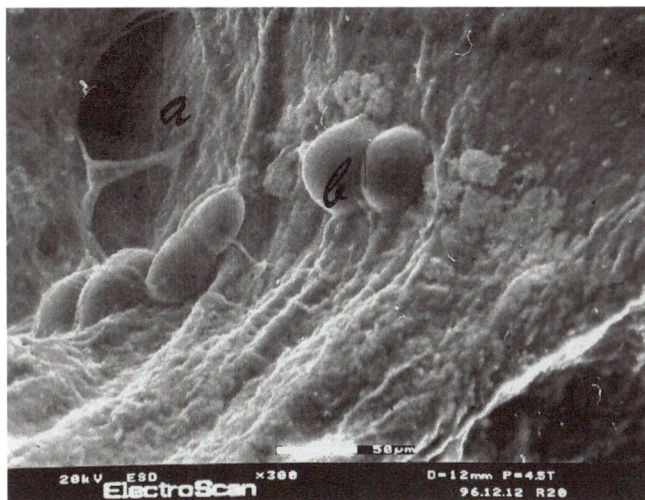

Fig 1.7 Fresh frozen section. Environmental SEM demonstrates the blood vessels, mineralized collagen fibres, vessels (a) and young osteoblasts (b) on the titanium surface of the dental implant.

Light microscopy and morphometry studies on ground sections showed that the significant parts of retrieved threaded implants after 1-16 years were occupied by mineralized bone by 79-95%. A large percentage of 56-85% of the implant surface was in direct contact with mineralized bone without any intervening fibrous tissue. In some cases, the tissue was detached from the implant. This was seen as an empty zone or contained red blood cells [20] (figure 1.8).

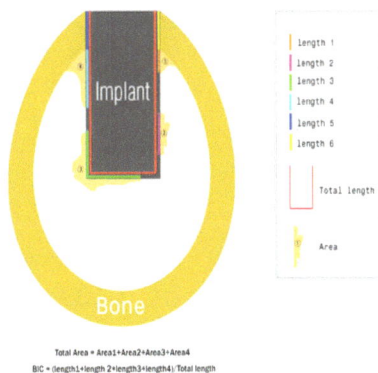

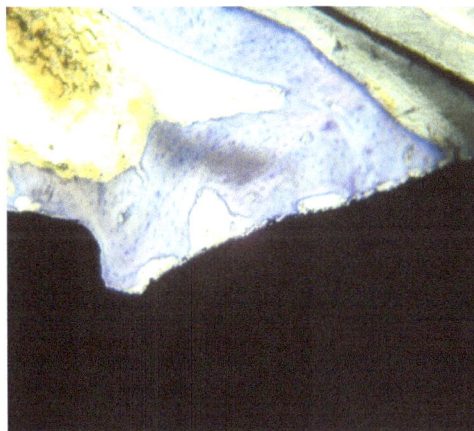

Figure 1.8 Left: Measuring Bone Implant Contact (BIC) by histomorphometry. Right: undecalcified resin section, toluidine blue staining. The micro-architecture of bone is evident: lamellar and woven bone attached to the titanium surface. There is no 100% bone-titanium attachment.

The SEM study demonstrates a 100-400 nm-thick layer of amorphous or fine granular material between the mineralized bone and the implant surface (figure 1.9).

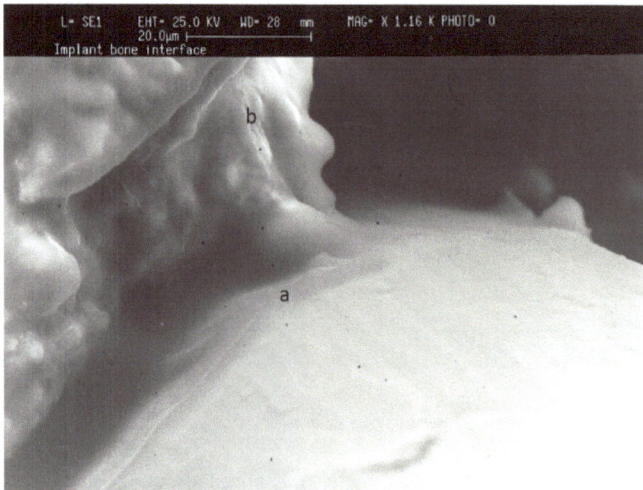

Fig 1.9 Fresh frozen section: In the environmental SEM, the titanium with the oxide layer (a) is attached to the foam structure (b), called the amorphous layer.

In general, mineralized bone bordered on the amorphous layer, but unmineralized tissue was also present close to the implant surface, either as a 0.5-1 um wide zone containing collagen fibrils or as a deeper pocket containing osteocytes or vessels. Collagen fibrils do not appear to be in direct contact with the implant. Osteocytes were found close to the implant surface but never observed located directly on it. Osteocyte canaliculi could be seen reaching the surface of the mineralized bone and ending in the amorphous layer.

The factors that will jeopardise osseointegration need to be identified and prevented, which are as follows:

• TRAUMATIC SURGERY

Traumatic surgery in implantology is caused by excessive heat. Different failings of attention usually cause excessive heat. These can be considered under one of two heads – overuse of the drill or poor irrigation.

Overuse of the drill:

Ignoring the manufacturer's instructions: each manufacturer can have different requirements. Inadequate training, poor surgical technique, and cavalier disregard for protocols.

Poor irrigation:

Equipment malfunction.
The team's error in failing to spot the emptying saline bag.
The dentist failed to spot the wobbly removable cannula clip set.
The team failed to note that the dentist wears gloves that are too big, which hinders continuous irrigation (whose fault?).
Stopping drills can reduce the quantity of irrigation at the drill-bone surfaces in the last few millimetres, which is needed the most (figure 1.10).

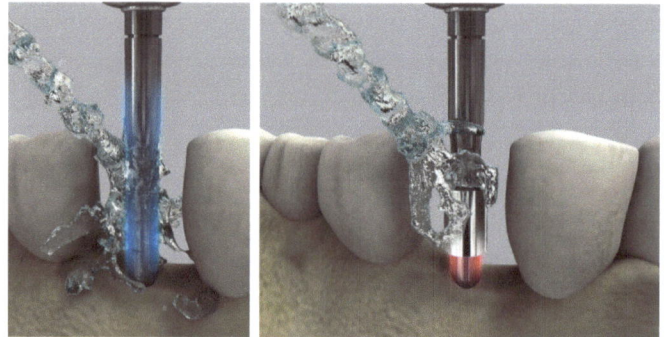

Figure 1.10 Left: irrigation cools the drill during bone preparation. Right: the extension drill application may jeopardize the irrigation.

Avoiding traumatic surgery

During drilling, the team must ensure that the irrigate reaches the drill and cools it continuously. Be vigilant.

When the bone is hard to drill, and with a surgical bur which is not newly sharp but still usable, there is a tendency to use increased hand pressure to compensate. This will increase the friction and the temperature. Be careful.

What is the correct hand pressure for dental implant drilling?

Wide disagreement exists on an acceptable drill speed, and the amount of force to be applied, and since bone-drilling thrust varies with the surgeon, it has been difficult to arrive at a consensus. Therefore, until proven otherwise, low hand pressure that usually falls in the range of 2 kg should be applied for bone preparation to generate less heat. This seems to be as close as we can currently get to an optimal feed rate, with a force that is not excessive and a drilling time as short as possible to minimise the duration of the friction between the drill and bone [21]. It has been taught that a push and pull movement needs to be applied during drilling to reduce the drill-bone contact and give a more cooling effect, but the precision of the bone cavity can be compromised. The author believes that non-spiral drills, which are more like an engineering reamer with a minimum of 2 flutes, can be applied with a push-drilling-only technique to provide a more accurate bone cavity. This means cleaner cavity dimensions without clinical side effects. (Most dentists reading this will be slightly confused by the above because their reamers are spiral where engineers are not, and that is because dentistry has adopted the engineering term 'reaming' without the precision of its original meaning).

• IMPLANT MOVEMENTS

Prolonged implant mobility can disturb cell differentiation [22]. Loading a dental implant before a sufficient amount of bone has stabilised jeopardises such differentiation and its long-term stability – unless it has been designed for immediate restoration or loading.

• OVERLOADING

The weakest part of the osseointegrated bone-to-implant complex is the bone tissue itself. Branemark et al. [23] measured the forces necessary for unscrewing an

experimental osseointegrated implant from the canine jaw. They found that when applying forces around 100-kilogram force, the anchoring bone tissue fractured, while the bone-to-implant interface and the implant

remained intact.

• POOR IMPLANT BIOCOMPATIBILITY

The surface properties of titanium are, to an extent,

determined by the surface oxide that covers the metal (fig 1.9). It is this oxide layer that the biomolecules meet when the implant is placed into bone. The conditions during oxidation (temperature, type and concentration of oxide layer, presence of contaminants) strongly influence the physical and chemical properties of oxide layer [22].

Analysing the surface layers on Ti implants, which had been implanted in humans for periods of up to 10 years or more, showed that the oxide thickness had grown from the original 5nm to over 200nm. In addition, Ca and P ions had become incorporated in the oxide layer on the implant [24].

The covering oxide layer consisted mainly of TiO_2. Divalent

and trivalent states of titanium were also detected, showing that TiO and Ti_2O_3 layers occurred [24]. It is essential that inorganic contaminants be avoided on this surface because they can possibly provoke the dissolution of titanium [25].

Titanium particles have been detected in Haversian canals at the implant-bone interface, and the titanium particles are deposited at the implant-bone interface and ultimately transported to lymph nodes and distant parenchymal organs [25,26].

The ideal roughness of an implant concerning long-term function remains to be described.

The ideal implant surface would minimise the immune response without impeding the normal immune response to pathogens.

Factors Affecting Reduction of the bone-implant Interface and Implant Failure:

• QUANTITY AND QUALITY OF BONE:

Jaffin and Berman classified bone quality into four groups based on the radiological assessment of cortical thickness and density of the trabecular bone. The group with the thinnest cortices and the least trabecular density

(class IV) had the lowest implant success rate. The cortical bone may cover as much as 90% of the implant surface, whereas considerably less contact is found in medullary space [27,28]. This author believes this classification cannot

cover all scenarios and does not guide the dentist on how to alter any osteotomy approach appropriately during surgery. Furthermore, differentiation between classes II and III is challenging. Another classification is recommended in this chapter.

The quality and potential of healing of the recipient's bone cannot be diagnosed unless we study it under a light microscope. The author believes prolonged untreated or apical periodontitis can affect the healing potential. That could be one of the reasons why there is a lower success rate of implants in patients suffering from periodontal disease. Some dentists do not remove granulation tissue after tooth extraction, as they used to; if they do, it will be incomplete removal. Usually, the remaining granulation tissue is resorbed, and as much bigger parts remain, there is a chance that some parts will remain after some resorption. The border between granulation tissue and sound bone is unclear, especially when the quality of the trabecular bone is poor. The only tools the dentist has are softness and heavy bleeding in the bone, which will not help in this scenario. Degranulation burs have been introduced in the market, but how replacing a sharp bone curette will help the dentist is unclear.

• AGE

It has been demonstrated that the mineral content of mandibular bone is related to age; the higher the age, the lower the bone mineral content. A correlation was also reported for the bone mineral content of the mandible and the forearm. Kribbs did not find age-related changes in mandibular bone mass or density, but he did find that cortical thickness at the gonion decreased with age, and the mandibular bone mass and cortical thickness of the gonion were related to skeletal bone mass [19,20,29].

• OSTEOPOROSIS

There is a debate about whether senile and post-menopausal osteoporosis affects mechanical and biological factors in bone healing and whether reduced trabecular bone volume affects the rate of fracture healing. Bone cell numbers, activity and proliferation are reduced by osteoporosis [21-24]. Stem cell therapy offers great promise in dental implantology and improves bone quality [25,26].

It has been suggested that osteoporosis may be associated with extensive residual ridge resorption as well as reduced mandibular bone mass and density. A thinner cortex at the gonion was observed in an osteoporotic group compared to the normal group [30,31].

A large number of meta-analysis studies, with more than 40,000 dental implants placed (but excluding patients with life-threatening conditions), concluded that the influence of osteoporosis on the risk of dental implant failure was direct but not significant and that there is no relationship between osteoporosis and the risk of implant failure [32].

• SMOKING

Studies covered patients surgically treated for wrist, tibial shaft, spine, foot and ankle injuries. Of these patients, almost all of the non-smokers healed completely, while a significantly reduced number of smokers healed completely. The average time until complete healing was over two months longer in smokers.

Numerous other studies on patients with different injuries have shown a similar effect. The delay in the union is more apparent in those cases requiring bone grafts, as there is an increased risk of de-vascularising the graft. Smokers have a 40% delayed time to union and a 40% increased chance of non-union compared with non-smokers [33].

Bones are nourished by blood much like other organs and tissues in our body. Nutrients, minerals, and oxygen are all supplied to the bones via the blood stream. Smoking elevates the levels of nicotine in the blood, and this causes the blood vessels to constrict. Nicotine constricts blood vessels by approximately 25% of their average diameter. Because of the constriction of the vessels, decreased levels of nutrients are supplied to the bones. It is thought this is the reason for the effect on bone healing [33,34]. Smoking cessation advice should be offered to smokers before elective procedures are undertaken, along with warnings of potential failure[35,36]. In the meta-analysis study, a direct relationship between smoking and dental implant failure has been observed [37]. Dentists need to be warned of the possibility of implant failure in smokers and the need for an extended healing period.

On the matter of e-cigarettes and their effect on the osseointegration of dental implants, there seems to be too little research with accompanying disagreements. The short-term and long-term side effects have yet to be determined.

Inhalation of the vapour aerosol is not as safe as advertised. The composition of the electronic liquid is variable, and it may contain propylene glycol, glycerine, and nicotine. Aldehydes, carbonates, and carcinogenic heavy metals have been identified, and glycol may cause respiratory and ocular complications [38].

The potential DNA damage needs to be emphasised. A significant reduction in the growth of the osteoblast culture has been observed [39]. Worse, as there is the belief that it is harmless, they smoke heavier.

Studies on animals have confirmed the effect of nicotine on Haversian canals and the potential for reduced bone healing.

An epidemiological study in a Finnish city revealed that eleven per cent of the patients over 65 were regular smokers. The bone quality was estimated to be less suitable for implantation in 21% of the cases. The effect of smoking on initial dental implant failure before functional loading with fixed prosthetic restorations was studied and showed [29,33,36,37]; even though bone quality in both groups was comparable, the failure rate before loading was statistically significantly higher in smokers [40,41].

The author has observed that there is a difference between one-piece and multiple-piece conventional dental implant use. The hypothesis behind it is the need to eliminate the space between the dental implant and the abutment since this connection has a micro gap, which may become a breeding ground for bacteria (figure 1.12).

Even though there are controversies, like many other issues, it seems that placing a three-piece dental implant not at the alveolar crest level but 0.5 mm countersunk can benefit the patient[42]. Choosing a conical shape of implant-abutment connection is logical to minimise mechanical and biological complications. This connection has the best bacterial seal and the best mechanical stability currently available [43,44].

A conometric connection of less than 2° assures a valid bacteria-sealing implant-abutment interface [45].

The size of PolyMorphoNuclear (PMN) is 12-15 um, the gap between the abutment and the implant is a minimum of 4 um, and the size of bacteria is less than 4 um, e.g. gram-negative bacillus is 0.5-0.8 um. and A. actinomycetemcomitans which is found in severe infections, is 0.4-1um. It should be evident that there is a greater chance of successful bacterial growth where the dimensions are 0.4-1 um unless the gap between the abutment and the implant is less than 0.4um, which can only be observed with conical attachments.

Factors to maximise the bone-implant interface and osseointegration:

Different materials, shapes, lengths, diameters, implant surface treatments and coatings have been proposed in order to enhance clinical performance. The surface preparation processes are numerous, and the parameters defining each process (e.g. temperature, pressure, time, type and size of blasting particles, types and concentrations of etching acids) are extensive, and the numbers are unlimited. They are difficult to group.

There are three theories on how altered implant topography has succeeded in increasing bone-to-implant contact and could improve this still further:

1. Biomechanical
2. Osteogenetic
3. Surface signaling

It is difficult to compare the topography of different implant surfaces, and no accepted standardisation method is available. Titanium is widely used, and its advantages include high biocompatibility, increased resistance to corrosion, a lack of toxicity on macrophages and fibroblasts, and diminished inflammatory response in peri-implant tissues. Its surface is composed of an oxide layer that has the ability to repair itself by reoxidation when damaged.

Modifications of metal surfaces are often employed as a means of controlling tissue-titanium interactions and shortening the time of bone fixation. Surface treatments, such as titanium plasma-spraying, grit-blasting, acid-etching, anodization or calcium phosphate coatings, and their surface morphologies are commercially available and have proven clinical efficacy (>95% over five years). The precise role of surface chemistry and topography in the early stages of implant osseointegration remains poorly understood. In addition, comparative clinical studies of different implant surfaces are rarely performed. These therapeutic strategies should ultimately enhance osseointegration [46]. At the macro (visible) level, osseointegration is related to implant geometry. When we say 'geometry,' we refer to all aspects of the shape of the implant, which can mean the overall shape of the implant itself and the shape of the surface, i.e., roughness. Thus a threaded screw and a macroporous surface treatment that produces a surface roughness of more than 10um will improve primary stability and osseointegration. However, the surface roughness level must be carefully gauged because a surface that is too rough can increase the risk of subsequent peri-implantitis. Why? Because gingival recession is inevitable, and if the level of roughness is too high, the chances of subsequent plaque adhesion to the now-revealed metal surface are greater, hence peri-implantitis.

Numerous reports have shown that both early fixation and the long-term mechanical stability of the prosthesis can be improved by a high roughness profile rather than a smooth surface [47]. The high roughness may lead to an increase in peri-implantitis as well as an increase in ionic leakage [48]. A moderate roughness of 1–2 um may limit these two parameters [48].

The micro-topographic profile of dental implants is defined, for surface roughness, as being in the range of 1–10um. This range of roughness maximises the interlocking between mineralized bone and the implant's surface. A theoretical approach suggests that the ideal surface should be covered with hemispherical pits approximately 1.5um in depth and 3-5 um in diameter [49]. These might stabilise the fibrin clot and stabilise the fragile extracellular matrix scaffold, thus stimulating the adherent behaviour of osteoblasts. Grit blasting and acid-etching the surface preparation at the micron level can promote rapid bone formation.

However, the Cochrane Collaboration has not found clinical evidence demonstrating the superiority of any implant surface [50].

Primary Stability

For successful fracture healing, it is crucial to immobilise the fragments of a fractured long bone after alignment to prevent any movement between them [51].

The primary mechanical stability of the implant is essential to obtain implant osseointegration, especially in one-piece implant surgical procedures.

Primary stability limits the micro-motion of the implant in the early phases of tissue healing and favours successful osseointegration. Primary mechanical stability consists of rigid fixation between the implant and the host bone cavity, with no micro-motion of the implant or even minimal distortional strains. Excessive implant motion or poor implant stability results in tensile and shear motions, stimulating fibrous membrane formation around the implant and causing displacement at the bone-implant interface. Poor primary stability inhibits osseointegration and leads to aseptic loosening and failure of the implant [52].

Primary stability depends on the surgical technique, implant design, and implantation site. Cortical bone allows a higher mechanical anchorage for the implant than cancellous bone.

We do not know whether bone condensation improves bone healing or not, but it does improve primary stability, which is an essential factor in dental implant healing, and even more so for one-piece dental implants or immediate load three-piece dental implants.

Early implant failure is thought to be due to excessive mechanical load applied to the implant and lower stability at implant placement. In contrast, by reducing micro-motion to within the critical threshold, it is possible to apply mechanical load to the implant with a reduced healing period [52].

Mechanical stress and implant micro-motion are associated with implant osseointegration or failure. In a study, 20-30 microns of oscillating displacement was compatible with stable bone ingrowth with high interface stiffness, whereas 40 and 150

microns of motion were not [53].

Different types of bioactive barriers, such as hydroxyapatite nanoparticles, have been introduced to reduce the release of metallic ions [54,55].

As noted above, surface roughness can increase the primary stability of the implant, but the effectiveness of different types and profiles of roughness has not been established. [56].

Applying osteotomy and an undersized preparation technique improved the early fixation of dental implants with a pronounced effect [57].

Implant loading leads to micro-motion at the bone-implant interface. Some degree of micro-motion is tolerated. Within certain limits, mechanical loading stimulates bone formation.

Micro-motion at the interface generally influences tissue differentiation, but excessive micro-motion compromises implant osseointegration. The magnitude of micromotion at the interface significantly influences tissue differentiation around immediately loaded implants.

Tolerated micromotion affects the healing sequence, leading to bone ingrowth into porous implants or directly affecting implant bone anchorage [58].

Implant mobility can be divided into macromobility (> 0.5mm), which the naked eye can observe; micromobility (01.-0.5 mm); micron-mobility (< 0.1mm), which can not be checked by most specific instruments, and when the mobility is less than 100um, is called fretting [59]. Fretting refers to a particular wear process at the contact area between two materials under load, observed at the bone-implant interface and other interior interfaces in any dental implant complex. The biomechanical effect caused by fretting is the damage to the bone tissue and the resultant stimulation of the cell signal pathway that produces a positive biological effect. The full effects of fretting on bone cells remain to be discovered [60].

Branemark stated that a stress-free environment during the healing period was mandatory to achieve osseointegration and suggested that the micromotion produced by early loading would induce fibrous tissue encapsulation [61, 62].

However, further studies demonstrated that micromotion-stimulated soft tissue encapsulation and early-loaded implants can achieve osseointegration [63].

For implants with a bio-inert surface, the critical threshold lies somewhere between 50 and 150 μm and 100 μm may be the threshold level, as proposed by Brunski as a rule of thumb. However, the surface and implant design affect the threshold. Nevertheless, it was suggested that this threshold should be determined according to the surface topography and implant design [64,65].

The cortical-cancellous ratio is essential for mechanical primary stability. The implant length has a weak correlation with stability, and cortical bone thickness has greater importance than the length of the dental implant.

Cortical bone thickness is also a key factor for primary stability in type IV bone. The stress concentration regions may be located at the implant neck between the cortical and cancellous bone [66].

Space is needed between the bone and the implant to make room for osteogenic cells, which migrate towards the implant surface. It is these cells that will ensure osseointegration. Poor bone formation, or even bone resorption, has been observed when the space is tight. Conversely, when the space is too large, with gaps exceeding 500 um, this reduces the quality of the newly-formed bone and delays the rate of gap filling.

Increasing the temperature during drilling will produce 100-500 um bone cell necrosis [67-70]. While some bone necrosis is inevitable, this level of necrosis – 500um - must not be exceeded.

The clinical strategies that can maximize implant/bone contact area include placing longer and wider implants, increasing the number of implants, and bone compression. The other means are vague and have not been proven clinically. It might be by titanium surface treatment (surface charge, nanotubular titanium, HA coating, with or without other means like zinc at the nano-level, and using ceramics and Zirconium).

Placing HA-coated or Zirconia implants has a controversial long-term success rate; however, if the dental implant will be placed close to wire (e.g. after orthognathic surgery), HA-coated or Zirconia dental implant is the material of choice.

Placing bone substitute particles in prepared bone cavities prior to dental implant placement has also been recommended.

Nano-technology has influenced dental implant surface treatment. For instance:

1. Compaction of nanoparticles of Ti2O3 has been used to protect the chemistry of the implant's surface.

2. Self-assembled monolayers (SAMs): Nanotechnology has increased biological activity and facilitated osseointegration. This is done by imprinting the monolayers on the surface of the biomaterials. SAMs have an amphiphilic layer at one end and a functional layer at the other. The functional group layer improves the hydrophilic and hydrophobic properties of the substrate. The functional end group can be osteoinductive, a cell-adhesive molecule, or a self-adhesive peptide, which is applied to the titanium implant surface [71].

Chemical treatment of the implant surface is to expose the reactive group. This is more popular during the implant manufacturing process. Nanotopography influences cell adhesion, proliferation, and differentiation and may promote an ideal future healing process [72].

1.4. Soft Tissue Reaction to Dental Implants

Soft Tissue Reaction to Immediate Restoration and Loading of Dental Implants.

The recognition that soft tissue healing around dental implants is essential for successful osseointegration led to the agreement that the establishing/confirmation of successful soft tissue integration should be included in the definition of osseointegration [73].

This is how we go about achieving this. These are the factors which influence the establishment of successful soft tissue healing as follows: keratinized vs non-keratinized soft oral mucosa, biologic width, abutment-implant interface, type of oral mucosa surgical technique, type of dental prosthesis (figure 1.11).

The implant/soft tissue interface is similar to natural teeth with epithelium, sulcular epithelium, junctional epithelium and underlying connective tissue [74] (figure1-11).

The cuff-like barrier of keratinized oral epithelium with its fibroblast-rich layer resembles that around natural teeth except that the collagen fibres with similar diameters are parallel with the transmucosal abutment and provide a protective barrier between the oral cavity and the internal environment [75].

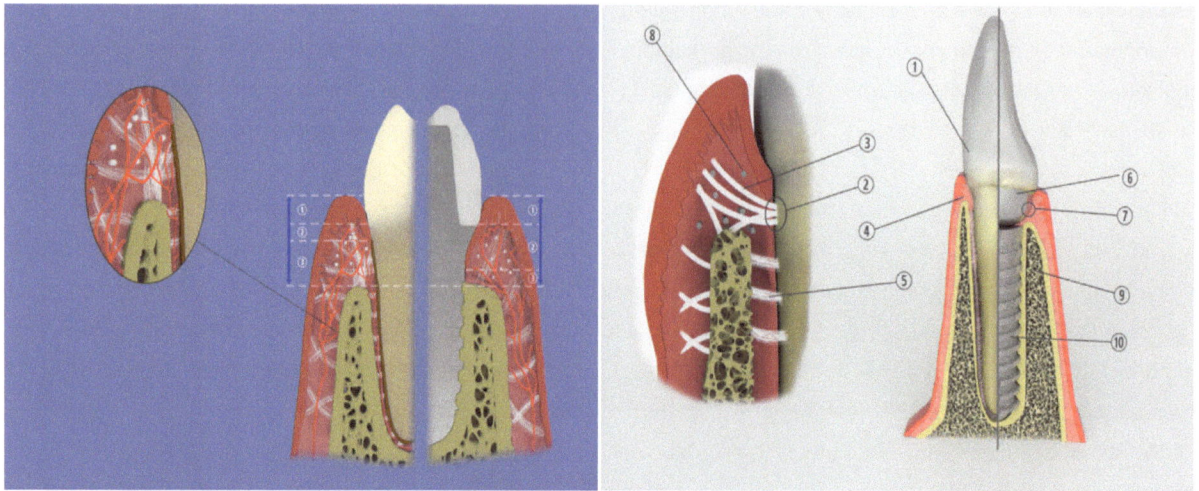

Figure 1.11 here are cross sections of the tooth with attached gingiva and implant with attached gingiva. The aim is to replicate the natural relationship as much as possible.

Left: Connection of soft tissue to natural tooth vs titanium dental implant. 1. Gingival sulcus, 2. Junctional epithelium, 3. Gingival fibre group. The implant has a longer junctional epithelium than the natural tooth.

Right: 1. Enamel, 2. Fibres attached to the root surface, 3. Dentogingival fibres, 4. Attached gingivae, 5. Periodontal ligament, 6. Abutment (platform switch), 7. Junctional epithelium 8. Circumferential fibres, 9. Alveolar bone, 10. Titanium dental implant.

Similarly, the non-keratinized sulcular epithelium has dense circular fibres close to the implant surface [76]. The soft tissue adjacent to the implant consists of the free gingival margin composed of collagenous stroma covered by stratified squamous epithelium. The lack of a vascular supply indicates an impaired defence system, and plaque formation allows the growth of inflammatory cells adjacent to pocket epithelium [77]. These small stud-like structures (hemidesmosomes) are a part of the inner basal surface of keratinocytes and were observed when oral epithelial cells grew on the films of titanium-coating epoxy resin. With epithelial attachment of 2mm and a connective tissue attachment of 1 mm around the dental implant abutment, there is disagreement over whether a countersunk-implant relationship with bone would maintain its biological width, consonant with the theory that bone will resorb to a level of approximately 2mm from the micro-gap [81] (figure 1-12).

Increased width of keratinized mucosa around implants is associated with lower mean alveolar bone loss and improved indices of soft tissue health. Implants with a narrow zone of keratinized mucosa were also more likely to bleed upon probing, even after plaque removal [82]. Significant independent correlation was found between the width of keratinized mucosa and bone loss. When there was less than 2mm of keratinized mucosa, there was radiographic bone loss [78].

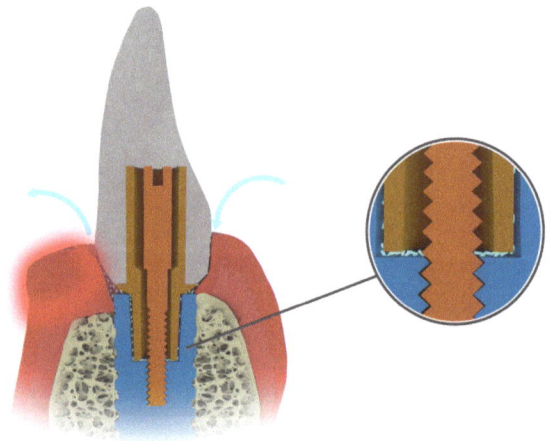

Figure 1.12 The dental implant complex has a microbe reservoir. Saliva, sugars and oral flora penetrate the space, and bacterial exudate is pumped out of the reservoir, which helps to develop periimplantitis.

Evidence analysis shows that present knowledge about biologic width around implants is mainly derived from animal studies and that, to date, clinically controlled human studies have proved inconclusive [83].

Most soft tissue recession was found during the first six months on the lingual sites, and this was found more often in women than men and more often in the mandible than the maxillae [84]. The degree of soft tissue recession is similar for both a single-stage and a 2-stage approach [85]. As most recession occurs during the first three months post-surgery, it is recommended that one wait a minimum of 3 months post-surgery before definitive impressions are taken [86]. The soft tissue width of 3-3.4 mm is needed to cover the crestal bone between implants [87,88]. The clinical attachment is the distance from the CEJ, a fixed point to the depth of the gingival sulcus. The clinical attachment level is a reliable indicator of bone level, and probing around dental implants does not harm the protective soft tissue seal. However, periodontal indices have limited value in indicating the status of the bone that supports implants [89]. Several factors influence peri-implant soft tissue reactions but are not well understood yet.

For instance:

Do different abutment surface textures alter the healing pattern of adjacent soft tissues?

Do fixed or removable prostheses have differing effects on soft tissue healing?

Does surgical technique influence soft tissue healing?

To investigate the first question, the following three studies (two were histological and the third clinical) were conducted.

In Study #1, human epithelial cells, which had been growing on different titanium implants, were extracted and studied. They were found to have spread on all the titanium surfaces but to differing degrees. The most excellent spread was found on the polished surfaces, and the smallest spread was found on the plasma-sprayed surfaces [90].

In Study #2, using gingival keratinocytes, cell attachment and spread were only observed on polished and plasma-sprayed surfaces but not on sandblasted surfaces [90].

Study #3, the clinical study, demonstrated that the attachment between the peri-implant mucosa and titanium abutments, whether with a turned or an acid-etched surface, was similar, both quantitatively and qualitatively. The soft tissue attachment that formed next to titanium dental implants was not influenced by the roughness of the titanium surface [91].

Clinical studies have also investigated the soft tissue reaction to fixed and removable prostheses to investigate the second question. They indicate that the prosthesis does not influence the histological features of the connective tissue around long-term loaded titanium abutments. No histological differences were found between tissue sampled around implants supporting a fixed restoration or those anchoring an overdenture [92].

Research has also been conducted on the influence of different surgical techniques on soft tissue healing. They found that surgical technique can indeed influence subsequent soft tissue healing. The supracrestal connective tissue lateral to the implant was found to be more richly vascularised in the flapless group than in the flapped group, and it was concluded that the flapless procedure might increase the vascularity of the peri-implant mucosa [93].

Other comparative studies were conducted to evaluate soft tissue healing following three different surgical procedures:

The first study compared the soft tissue healing around the final restoration on a submerged implant with the soft tissue healing around the immediately loaded implant.

In the second case, a standard three-piece implant was placed, with the abutment placed after three days.

In the third case, a one-piece implant was placed. After nine months, histomorphometric measurements of the sulcular epithelium and junctional epithelium were made. The percentage of connective tissue contact of the soft tissues around the test and control implants was similar. In a few cases, sulcular epithelium and a long junctional-like epithelium with moderate inflammatory cells were observed. No statistically significant differences were present in test and control implants.

Thus, neither immediate loading nor early abutment placement produced a change in the dimensions of the peri-implant soft tissues [78].

Soft tissue healing around one-piece and three-piece dental implants compared.

[Clinical observation] The Biologic Width of one-piece implants where the rough/smooth border was located at the bone crest level was significantly more coronal when compared to that of three-piece implants where the microgap (interface) was located at or below the crest of the bone.

[Histological study observation] Histological study shows that with one-piece implants, the tip of the gingival margin was located significantly more coronally (P<0.005) compared to three-piece implants, just as it is with the natural tooth [94].

The inflammatory response adjacent to dental implants has been investigated. [In the following study] Three implant designs were placed in the mandibles of dogs. Three-piece implants were placed at the alveolar crest, and abutments connected either at initial surgery (non-submerged) or three months later (submerged). The third implant was one piece. Adjacent interstitial tissues were analyzed. Both three-piece implants resulted in a peak of inflammatory cells approximately 0.50 mm coronal to the micro gap, and these consisted primarily of neutrophilic polymorphonuclear leukocytes. No such peak was observed for one-piece implants. Also, significantly greater bone loss was observed for both three-piece implants compared with the one-piece implant.

For the one-piece implant, the designed absence of an implant-abutment interface (therefore no micro gap) at the bone crest was associated with reduced peri-implant inflammatory cell accumulation and minimal bone loss [95].

Pro-inflammatory cytokines have revealed less inflammation around dental implants when the final abutment is delivered at the second stage of surgery, as opposed to when the standard procedure is adopted of placing the gingival former with its associated extension of treatment time and the attendant opportunity for peri-implantitis [96].

In other words, the three-piece implant and its microgap inevitably produce a level of peri-implantitis. The initiation of peri-implant neutrophil accumulation suggests that a bacterial chemotactic stimulus originates at or near the microgap of three-piece implants. This induces and sustains the recruitment of inflammatory cells. The microbes attracted by the microgap proliferate within the internal aspects of the implant. The phenomenon of microbial and/or fluid leakage through the implant-abutment interface has been documented [97, 98].

The micro gap, however, is too small to allow access to host defence mechanisms, and this can perpetuate an acute inflammatory process, which can be further exacerbated by limited access to effective oral hygiene. The three-piece implant design may create a reservoir of bacteria and possibly facilitate the development of peri-implant inflammation (Figures 1-12).

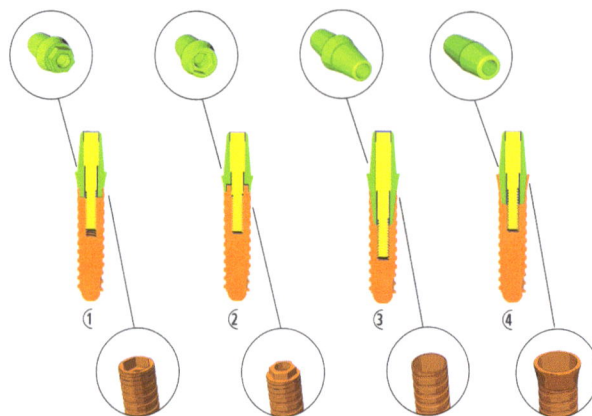

Figure 1.13 Different implant-abutment connections,1. External butt-joint, 2, Internal butt-joint, 3. Platform-switched, 4. No-interface (tissue-level).

It is unknown whether different implant-abutment connections, such as an internal cone, would yield a different distribution or intensity of inflammatory cell recruitment as compared with the flat, butt-joint interface. The microleakage is unavoidable among current implant systems, regardless of the connection type or interface size. One can expect a similar inflammatory response for any interface located at the alveolar bone level. Different tightening torques do not statistically affect the microleakage in the implant-abutment external hexagon [99].

The presence of an intense inflammatory process accompanied by significantly greater bone loss has been observed around three-piece implants as compared with one-piece implants. A relationship between inflammatory events and bone loss seems likely.

The micromovement between the abutment and implant can develop bone loss. The study compared the effect of welding the abutment to the implant in order to eliminate potential micromovements between the abutment and implant and compared the results to those found when the abutment was screwed into the implant with no welding carried out. The results showed that even though the micro gap still existed between the weld points, there was a significant reduction in bone loss where welding was carried out [100]. Soft tissue reaction to cutaneous-mucosal diseases such as Epidermolysis bullosa is another challenge in the dental implant era, which is usually treated as a fixed prosthesis retained by dental implants [101].

15

Attempts to control plaque by polishing the Titanium surface produced another controversy. Blasting small alumina particles at the titanium surface reduced adhesion for S.sanguinis and L.salvarius. This indicates that a slightly rough surface best inhibits dental plaque formation. They recommended a roughness of 2-4 um.

So far, The discussion has focused on the optimal surgical approach that can best produce healthy soft tissue around implants. We cannot forget the patient's responsibility for aftercare. This, in turn, depends on the surgeon's foresight in designing prostheses that can be effectively cleaned.

Unbelievably, there are no specific guidelines for the amount of space needed for a patient to clean beneath a fixed implant-supported prosthesis. Nor are there recommendations for dealing with the changing soft tissue condition that will occur at intervals over time.

1.5. Patient Selection and Management of the Medical Compromised Patients.

Regarding this subject, some countries have guidelines, and the author recommends that dentists apply the local guidelines, even though there are discrepancies between countries and continents. In the UK, SDCEP and NICE guidelines are applied. The information below should be used only as general knowledge.

Logically, only patients with ASA (American Society of Anaesthesiologists) grade I or II status should be selected for elective surgery, and the surgical risks should be weighed against the benefits of such treatment.

Explanation of ASA I/II and where the medical condition has dictated an alternative treatment plan point out the patient's right to choose from the available possibilities.

The ASA classification system is a system for assessing the physical status and fitness of the patient. ASA I status indicates an average healthy patient. ASA II status is applied where there is a moderate but definite degree of systemic disturbance.

If the dentist diagnoses the patient as belonging to ASA II, then clearly, the treatment plan will be affected. After the patient has heard the short- and long-term risks that now apply, s/he will be better able to choose the preferred treatment.

The dentist must identify any controlled or uncontrolled diseases, especially diabetes, bleeding disorder, weakened immune system, cognitive impairment, epilepsy, risk of osteoradionecrosis, previous myocardial infarction, osteoporosis, smoking habit, HIV+, hypothyroidism, Crohn's disease, alcoholism, history of cerebrovascular accidents, previous or proposed transplant or valvular prosthetic surgery, active treatment of malignancy, drug abuse, or psychiatric illness.

Anaemia is a reduced level of circulating haemoglobin which the aetiology is reduced production (due to drugs, radiation, infection, malabsorption, reduced marrow stimulation), blood loss (chronic bleeding) and haemolytic (drug interaction, Malaria, RBC defects, Sickle cell and Thalassemias).

Common types are Microcytic anaemia (MCV <80) due to Iron deficiency and Thalassemia, Normocytic anaemia (MCV 80-100) due to chronic disease, Sickle cell and Macrocytic anaemia (MCV > 100) due to Vitamin B12 or acid folic deficiencies or alcoholism.

Clinical features include fatigue, heart failure, angina, pallor, and spoon-shaped nails. Oral manifestations are mucosal pallor, dry mouth, recurrent ulcers, oral lichen planus, numbness, burning sensation, abnormal taste and dry mouth.

Thalassemia reduces bone mineral density but is not a direct risk factor for periodontitis [102].

Oral mucosal lesions such as ulcers or atrophy may be detected, which needs to delay the implant surgery.

Bleeding can be of local or systemic origin. If any bleeding has a systemic origin, it can exacerbate any concurrent bleeding of local origin (e.g. local inflammation exacerbated by high blood pressure).

Old patients may have increased high blood pressure, which can induce heart stroke.

Upper airway obstruction has been reported as arising from mandibular lingual cortical perforation, invasion of the mouth's floor, and rupturing of the lingual artery and vein.

Vascular, platelets and coagulation defects characterize bleeding disorders. Vascular defects include easy bruising syndrome, which is vascular fragility in females, senile purpura and scurvy. Platelet defects are the clinical signs that arise when the unit level is below 50 *109 litres. Abnormal platelets are observed in renal disease, where urea impairs its function. Drugs like Furosemide, NSAID, Penicillin, Quinidine, Ranitidine, Sulfonamide and gold can induce thrombocytopenic purpura.

The most common coagulation disorder is Von Willebrand's factor disease, which affects factor VIII and platelets. Haemophilia

A (factor VIII deficiency), in which only males develop symptoms, with an increase in APTT and B (factor IX deficiency), which are inherited disorders. Impairment of liver function impacts bleeding due to Vitamin K and folic acid deficiency and reduces the synthesis of coagulation factors.

Alcoholics can suffer from bleeding due to liver disease and reduced folate and Vitamin B due to malnutrition and osteoporosis [103].

Medication which impairs blood clotting is classified into three groups: Anticoagulants such as Warfarin, Vitamin K antagonists such as (Acenocoumarol and phenindione), and anti-factor X (Apixaban). Antiplatelet as Aspirin, Dipyridamole, Clopidogrel, Abciximab. Heparin is short-acting and inhibits the formation of prothrombin to thrombin 2a, which, with factor 13a, inhibits the formation of fibrin that should stabilise the hemostatic plug.

A high success rate of dental implant treatment in haemophiliac patients was reported. It is generally considered that the placement of one dental implant can be expected to produce as much bleeding as the extraction of three teeth. However, the author believes that properly executed implant placement should produce bleeding equivalent to that expected from the extraction of only one tooth. Most of the bleeding is from the soft tissue incision and reflection of the flap instead of the bone perforation. A meticulous atraumatic incision and the design of the flap play an essential role during the surgery, as well as postoperative bleeding, which will be addressed.

Patients on anticoagulant therapy need to be identified. Such patients may be subject to atrial fibrillation, have artificial heart valves in situ, and be recovering from deep vein thrombosis, myocardial infarction or pulmonary embolisms. The attending physician may recommend different treatment strategies. These can include suspending oral anticoagulants for several days, suspending the current anticoagulant (Warfarin / Lovenox) but administering heparin before dental treatment, reducing the drug dose, or maintaining the current treatment while applying local haemostatic measures at the surgical site. Consultation with the doctor in charge of the patient's treatment is mandatory [104-6].

Staging extensive or complex procedures should not interrupt antiplatelet drugs such as Aspirin, Clopidogrel, and Dipyridamole. Bear in mind that a mixture of Aspirin and Clopidogrel compared with a mixture of Aspirin and Dipyridamole has more bleeding tendency.

Direct Oral Anticoagulants (DOAC) such as Apixaban, Rivaroxaban (anticoagulant factor X), and Dabigatran (anticoagulant Factor II, thrombin) miss or delay morning dose before treatment as a dental implant, especially with simultaneous extraction or bone grafts which will need a larger area of soft tissue flap reflection.

Vitamin K antagonist (Warfarin, Acenucomanol or Phenindione) Check the last 24 hours INR and if the patient is stable up to the last 72 hours, and it should be between 2-4.

Injectable anticoagulant (Dalteparin, Enozapron, Tinzaparin): if the dose is high or there is uncertainty, consult with the GP and recommend staging an extensive or complex procedure.

Consulting with the GP is necessary if the patient has a combination of different anticoagulants and antiplatelet medications. If the patient has other relevant medical complications, consult with the patient's GP.

Generally, patients' anticoagulant or antiplatelet should not be interrupted if the patient has prosthetic metal heart valve coronary stents or suffers from pulmonary embolism or deep vein thrombosis in the last three months and or the patient is cardiac. The adverse effect of hyperlipidaemia on bone metabolism is documented. Even though the adverse effect on bone graft healing and the use of atorvastatin contribute to bone healing observed, the impact on bone formation around the dental implant in the clinic is uncertain [107].

There is an excellent tendency to maintain direct oral anticoagulant therapy where it is in place. Platelet aggression inhibitors (PAI), which are Vitamin-K inhibitors, New/direct oral anticoagulants (NOACs/ DOACs), direct thrombin inhibitors Dabigatran (Pradaxa) and factor Xa inhibitors Rivaroxaban (Xarelto) and Apixaban (Eliquis) prior to dental surgery should not be discontinued for dental procedures [108-9].

It is hypothesised that the cessation of Vitamin-K inhibitors and bridging with low-molecular-weight heparin (LMWH) is associated with a greater risk of postoperative bleeding and probably a higher risk of thromboembolic complications [110].

Altering or discontinuing heparin carries an increased risk of thromboembolism, which far outweighs the alternative low risk of haemorrhage [111].

Patients with an INR of less than 2-4 who are on Warfarin and Acenocoumarol do not need to alter the anticoagulant as they do not have a high risk of bleeding [112].

The postoperative bleeding risk after single tooth implant surgery without bone grafting procedures is shallow for patients continuing their OAT.

The dentist needs to study the guidelines of the country in which he/she is practising.

It is necessary to acquire specialist advice, but generally, it is recommended to avoid NSAIDS and inferior dental block, use local anaesthetic with vasoconstrictor, apply minor flaps and start with one implant placement. Do not do the surgeries when there is poor access to specialists, on weekends, holidays, or evenings.

Cardiovascular disease does not affect the success rate of dental implant treatment.

Antihypertensive drugs may induce postural hypotension and transient loss of consciousness when the patient gets up quickly from lying to a standing position. For all the patients, the author recommends putting the patients in 2 stages of chair movement while putting the chair back in the sitting position and, between each stage, 1-minute rest.

Severe blood loss in excess of 2 litres (40% of the total volume), which is 5 litres, will result in irreversible shock, and if blood transfusion is not given within the golden hour (first hour of trauma), multiorgan failure will result.

Hypertension is a chronic and consistently raised blood pressure of more than three months, systolic more than 140 and diastolic more than 90. Hypertension is a risk factor for renal failure, ischaemic heart disease and cerebrovascular accidents. The cause of 95% of hypertension is unknown, which is called essential hypertension. However, the rest is due to renal dysfunction and endocrine disease. It is essential that the blood pressure is taken on the consultation day and also before the surgery.

Hypertensive crises are elevations of blood pressure higher than 180/120 mmHg that are complicated and need urgent attention. Failure to successfully manage the different complications among older individuals is associated with significant morbidity and mortality [113].

In general, elective oral surgery should be avoided after a recent myocardial infarction, stroke or cardiovascular surgery.

A condition called isolated diastolic hypertension needs to be addressed. Patients having low diastolic pressure, even when their systolic pressure is normal, could be dangerous for the heart as the heart muscles will not get enough oxygenated blood and can lead to diastolic heart failure. Alpha-blocker med-

ications, too much salt in our diet, and the ageing process in which we lose the elasticity of the arteries can exacerbate the scenario. Over-treatment of blood pressure, bradycardia and dehydration needs to be added. Thus, referral to medics is essential if the diastolic blood pressure is 60 or below. Frequent falls, dizziness, fainting, tiredness, nausea, and blurred vision are the common symptoms.

The oral side effects of the drugs prescribed for cardiovascular disease should be considered. Dry mouth has been influenced by B blockers (Atenolol), alfa blockers (Alfuzocin), and ACE inhibitors (Rampril). Lichenoid reactions may induced by B blockers and ACE inhibitors. The drug interaction of statins (Atorvastatin), azole antifungal, and macrolide antibiotics (erythromycin) needs to be considered.

Patients with a history of Rheumatic fever are likely to damage the heart valve. Antibiotic prophylaxis is not recommended anymore. Foci of infection due to any oral disease, such as peri-implantitis, must be eradicated, especially in patients suffering from CV disease and Rheumatic. Patients at risk of infective endocarditis may be on anticoagulants.

> The three key words which the dentist need to bear in mind, artificial, previous and cyanotic.

Dyspneic patients should be treated with the patient sitting upright, and local anaesthetic without vasoconstrictor is preferred even though two cartridges are safe.

Antibiotic prophylaxis is routinely not required for patients at risk of infective endocarditis; however, consultation with the patient's cardiology consultant or surgeon is necessary for invasive procedures. Artificial material in any tissue in the heart, previous infective endocarditis, and cyanotic

Chronic heart disease (CHD) need special consideration. Prosthetic materials treat CHD for up to 6 months; however, if residual shunt or valvular regurgitation remains, long life needs to be given special consideration. Consultation with a cardiology consultant, cardiac surgeon or specialist is mandatory for this group of patients.

The patient must be reminded that hypersensitivity, anaphylaxis, colitis (diarrhoea) and antibiotic resistance are the side effects, and the antibiotic is preferred to the patient in the surgery, one hour before the surgery. If Amoxicillin or Clindamycin are unsuitable, the dentist should contact an expert, such as a consultant microbiologist or pharmacist, to alter the drug.

Antibiotics used: Amoxicillin capsules, 3 grams (some countries recommend 2 grams); Clindamycin Capsule, 600 mg. Amoxicillin may alter the effect of Warfarin, and the patient's INR should be considered. The author recommends dental implant surgery in a hospital environment as all medical specialities are available [114].

While intravenous sedation stabilises haemodynamics and prevents increased blood pressure, it does not prevent myocardial arrhythmias. It should not be used as a tool to justify elective surgery, and the patient must be referred back to the doctor. It is mandatory to have medical advice before undertaking surgery. One year of delay after Myocardial infarction is recommended. Short appointments are necessary, and mornings should be avoided due to high levels of endogenous adrenaline. It is essential to reduce the discomfort and anxiety of the patients. Prophylactic GTN has been recommended.

A high relationship has been observed between periodontitis and coronary heart and cardiovascular disease [115].

The author recommends the same reaction should be taken to peri-implantitis as the pathogenic species associated with periodontitis (e.g., Fusobacterium ssp, A. actinomycetemcomitans, P. gingivalis) are also associated with peri-implantitis[116].

The repeated exposure to the bacteria and the endotoxins and metabolites induces endothelial dysfunction, platelet aggregation in the wall of the vessel, and enhanced low-density lipoprotein and cholesterol [117].

Disease of the respiratory system with principal symptoms of cough, dyspnoea and wheezing has become common. Upper tract infections include cold, sinusitis, pharyngitis and tonsilitis. Dental implant surgery is an elective surgery, and the author recommends postponing the surgery until the disease is treated as the patients suffer from chronic obstructive pulmonary disease (COPD), which is caused by more than three months per year for three months of bronchitis and emphysema. Smoking is the prime cause, and the patient is under steroid therapy. The use of a spirometer of the patient is recommended before the surgery. The patient is asked to expire air as quickly as possible during the test—the amount of exhaled air in the 1st-second call FEV1.

FEV less than 80% demonstrate COPD, and between 50-80% diagnosed as middle COPD.

Asthma is reversible bronchoconstriction with the signs of wheezing and dyspnoea. Usually, there is an allergen involved. NSAIDS precipitate the signs and symptoms, and allergy to aspirin and penicillin is common. The patient should bring his inhaler to the surgery.

Amoxicillin and Ampicillin should be avoided as the glandular fever mimics the signs and symptoms and will produce a severe rash.

The patient is at risk of oropharyngeal candidiasis due to inhalation of corticosteroids. Treating the patient sitting upright is recommended to assist in their breathing. The mouth breathing may cause xerostomia and double the increase of risk caries.

The dental team should be protected by a mask and efficient aspiration of saliva and water coolant by the dental nurse to reduce the probability of inhalation of particles which are less than 2.5 um and can pass to the alveoli.

Stress during treatment can induce asthma attacks. Call for help, and till the ambulance arrives, administer an inhaled B2-adrenergic agonist like Salbutamol (blue Ventolin) with four puffs initially and two puffs every 2 minutes up to 10 puffs. Also, oxygen should be administered at 15 litres/per minute, and the SPO2 should be between 94-98%. The pulse oximeter is essential in dental surgery, especially with the COVID-19 pandemic. It is expensive but low-cost, as Contec CMS50DL and Beijing Choice C20 met the ISO criteria for accuracy [118].

Patients suffering from gastrointestinal disease affect dental implant treatment as the side effects of the disease could be anaemia and malabsorption. The patient may be under steroid or immunosuppressant therapy.

The renal disorder is the damage of nephrons, which the serum creatinine and urea can analyse the function. The aetiology consists of diabetes mellitus and hypertension.

Patients suffering from renal disorders may have an increased tendency to bleed due to uraemia, cardiovascular complications due to thrombus formation and infection, which may be exacerbated by immunosuppression. Hypertension does cause chronic kidney disease, but the disease also exacerbates hypertension.

Renal disorder side effects could be pale mucosa, nausea and, subsequently, teeth erosion, reduced number of bone trabeculae and thinning of the cortical border of the mandible.

Patients suffering from chronic kidney disease may have retrograde parotitis, chronic periodontal disease and the ammoniacal odour of their breath. However, the caries rate is reduced, possibly due to the raised salivary urea.

Oral ulcers, white patches, and gingival enlargement could be due to the prescribed Ciclosporin or calcium channel blockers like Digoxin.

Potential carriage of HIV or Hepatitis B. Drug excretion can be affected. Local bone lesions of the jaws due to renal osteodystrophy or secondary hyperparathyroidism should be mentioned. Infections should be treated aggressively. Treatment should be performed immediately after dialysis. Doses of drugs should be reduced, and some are contra-indicated. Liaise with the patient's specialist before treatment planning. When the serum albumin is reduced, the number of free drugs increases, and the potential for toxicity increases. Non-steroid anti-inflammatory drugs such as Ibuprofen, Diclofenac, Naproxen, and Indomethacin are contra-indicated. Avoid systemic Fluoride treatment. Angiotensin-converting enzyme inhibitors (ACE-inhibitors) diuretics, which increase potassium and potassium supplements, are contra-indicated due to increased serum potassium, and as a result, arrhythmia or myocardial infarction appears despite controlling the blood pressure. Tetracycline, Neomycin, Kanamycin, and Amphotericin should be avoided. Acyclovir should be prescribed in reduced doses. Lidocaine is safe as it is metabolised in the liver. Amoxicillin and Paracetamol are safe.

Cholecalciferol is made in the skin by ultraviolet B, which changes in the liver to 25-hydroxycalciferol, which binds to protein and then by albumin as a transporter in the kidney changes to 1.25 dihydroxycholecalciferol, which promotes calcium uptake in intestine. Leakage of protein into the urine promotes the reduction of Vitamin D3 in the serum, and the metabolism of 25-hydroxy calciferol to active 1.25 dihydroxycholecalciferol is reduced in chronic kidney disease that affects the bone.

There is a high chance of dialysis patients suffering from hepatitis C and, consequently, Cirrhosis. The patient may be prescribed nucleoside analogue drugs like Entecavir. The kidney produces erythropoietin, which regulates the production of red blood cells in the bone marrow, which the disease causes anaemia. The anaemia aggravates if the patient has diabetes.

Endocrine disease is complex, and we try to address the main issues related to dental practice and oral surgery, which is reflected in dental implant surgery.

The reproductive hormones are oestrogen, follicle-stimulating hormone, inhibin, progesterone and luteinizing hormone. The main component of oral contraceptives is oestrogen, and oestrogen replacement therapy is prescribed for peri-menopause and post-menopause women. The male reproductive hormones are luteinizing hormone, testosterone, gonadotropin-releasing hormone, follicle-stimulating hormone, and inhibin. Testosterone is produced by Leydig cells and some from the adrenal cortex. Reduced testosterone due to age decreases muscle volume and bone density. Gastrointestinal hormones do not directly affect dental implant treatment, so we pass on this subject.

The Parathyroid hormone affects the kidney and increases renal calcium reabsorption and phosphate excretion. 1.25 hydroxyvitamin D3 has been discussed. Bone resorption has been observed in menopause due to increased expression of RANKL in bone marrow cells. Primary hyperparathyroidism stimulates osteoclastic activity to increase serum calcium. This can be observed in the lateral cephalometric x-rays, such as salt and pepper appearance, demonstrating the trabecular bone resorption. Hypoparathyroidism is usually secondary to thyroid surgery. Serum can be reduced, and tetany appears. Chvostek signs are diagnosed by tapping over the facial nerve, which is the spasm that appears in the facial muscles.

The adrenal glands lie above the kidneys, where the catecholamines synthesize in the medulla and are steroids from the cortex. The deficiency of cortisol is called Addison and the excess Cushing syndrome. The systemic effects of Addison's disease are muscle weakness, weight loss, low blood pressure and hypoglycaemia. The systemic effects of Cushing's syndrome are muscle weakness, weight gain, hypertension, hyperglycaemia and diabetes. Patients under corticosteroid therapy should be considered for supplementation using the guidelines of the country where the dentist practices.

The thyroid gland is filled with thyroglobulin, which converts to thyroxine and triiodothyronine. Also, the parafollicular cells synthesize calcitonin, which inhibits osteoclastic bone resorption. Thyroxine regulates the body's metabolic rate. The systemic effects of hyperthyroidism are increased metabolic rate, cardiac output, bulging of eyes and muscular atrophy, but hypothyroidism, which is intolerant to the cold, reduces cardiac output and tongue enlargement. Thyroid disorders can indirectly affect bone health, healing processes, and overall systemic health, which may influence the success of dental implant procedures as they affect bone density and quality, delay wound healing, and affect the patient's ability to tolerate surgical procedures.

The hypothalamus stimulates the anterior pituitary gland to release growth hormone, which affects the liver. The liver produces insulin-like growth factor, which causes growth. Excess of the growth hormone causes the continuous enlargement of the head, neck and feet, frontal bossing, spacing of the teeth, prognathic mandible, hypertension, and insulin resistance. Growth hormone plays a significant role in bone metabolism, collagen synthesis, wound healing, and overall systemic health, all of which can indirectly influence the success and outcome of dental implant procedures as it has a vital role in bone metabolism by stimulating osteoblasts and promotes the synthesis of collagen which affects bone and soft tissue healing and affect cell proliferation and wound healing.

The immunocompromised patients need special attention. The two main effects are increasing susceptibility to infection and the cross-infection control of AIDS.

Any change in the host environment is a favour for opportunistic pathogens and could be fatal. Patients use immunosuppressant drugs like corticosteroids, ciclosporin, and azathioprine. Aggressive antimicrobial prophylaxis is needed. Acquired immunodeficiency includes autoimmune disease (SLE, rheumatoid arthritis), chronic kidney disease, anaemia, diabetes mellitus, and viral infection (AIDS).

CD4 T lymphocyte defect leads to opportunistic infection. The HIV antibody is a valuable marker of infectivity; its absence does not guarantee any infection. Highly Active Antiretroviral Therapy (HAART) is required for the treatment of AIDS and to reduce the morbidity of the patients, but the effect on bone healing has not been conclusive [119].

The strong association of the oral manifestation of AIDS includes candidiasis, bilateral hairy leucoplakia, severe gingivitis, necrotizing ulcerative gingivitis, Kaposi sarcoma and non-Hodgkin sarcoma.

Bone and bone healing - the effects of diseases and drugs
There are a few data for patients suffering bone diseases such as osteogenesis imperfecta, polyarthritis, or ankylosing spondylitis. Patients who have rheumatoid arthritis with pronounced bone resorption and bleeding have been studied, but only when it was with concomitant connective tissue diseases like Sjogren's Syndrome [120,121].

No direct connection has been established between systemic bone mineral density (BMD) and mandibular BMD. Mandibular bone quality assessment should be studied through tomography.

In the UK, 20% of the population suffers from vitamin D deficiency. Vitamin D deficiency has many side effects, including obesity, diabetes, insulin resistance, heart disease, PMS in women, urinary tract infection, IBS, eczema, asthma, Alopecia, multiple sclerosis, cancer, osteoporosis, tooth decay and periodontitis.

Bisphosphonates (BPs) such as Alendronate are used for the treatment of metabolic and oncologic pathologies involving the skeletal system. The molecule attaches to bone, disrupts osteoclastic function and induces apoptosis. It helps to maintain bone density but negatively affects bone healing by reducing bone turnover. While some research indicates that prolonged use of oral bisphosphonates might affect the integration and stability of dental implants, the evidence remains inconclusive. It is vital for patients undergoing bisphosphonate therapy to be carefully monitored during implant placement and subsequent follow-up appointments to evaluate healing and implant stability.

There are drugs associated with Medication-Related Osteonecrosis of the Jaw (MRONJ). There are three types: Bisphosphonates (e.g. Alendronic acid), RANKL inhibitors (e.g. Denosumab), and Anti-angiogenic (e.g. Sunitinib). There are risks for invasive dental treatments affecting the bone. It is classified into three groups: no, low, and high. The high-risk cases are as follows: previous MRONJ, patients treated with anti-resorptive or anti-angiogenic for cancer, taking Denosumab for the last nine months classified or using bisphosphonate less than five years is low risk. If the patient has taken Denosumab for the last nine months and simultaneously takes glucocorticoid or bisphosphonate for less than five years, it is high risk. If the patient has been taking bisphosphonate for more than five years, he is a high-risk patient.

The FDA has issued a warning that patients who are being treated with bisphosphonates with a history of concomitant risk factors such as cancer, chemotherapy, radiotherapy, corticosteroids, and who also have poor oral hygiene, pre-existing dental disease or infection, anaemia, or coagulopathy, should not undergo invasive dental procedures if possible. For patients requiring dental procedures, there is no data available to indicate whether discontinuance reduces the risk of ONJ.

The most important issue for osteoporotic patients is the

administration of bisphosphonates prior to dental surgical intervention. This can induce osteonecrosis in the jaws. This is more likely to occur in the posterior regions [122].

The real issue is with IV-administered treatment as opposed to orally administered medication.

The American Association of Oral and Maxillofacial Surgeons guidelines recommend carefully timed surgical intervention. Great caution should be exercised immediately after stopping treatment and for the succeeding three years.

It should be noted that patients undergoing Bisphosphonate medication and being considered for dental implant treatment can be risk-assessed using the serum CTX test [123]. See below under "Prevention".

Radiotherapy may induce endarteritis obliterans, and this can predispose the patient to osteoradionecrosis of the jaw. The problems begin with radiotherapy's effect on the salivary glands. Salivary flow may be reduced, and saliva's protective antimicrobial effects are reduced if this happens. This allows increased local microbial proliferation, and the combination of reduced salivary flow plus the resultant microbial proliferation induces bone resorption followed by mucosal recession [124].

It is recommended that dental implants be placed not less than 21 days before radiotherapy is started. The total radiation dose should be less than 66 Gy to minimise the risk of osteoradionecrosis and less than 50 Gy to reduce osseointegration failure. If it is more, hyperbaric oxygen is recommended, but the effect is not well documented. Implant placement should be carried out nine months after radiotherapy has been completed. Immediate loading is not advised [125].

Even though a limited number of papers have been published about chemotherapy, it can be conjectured that it does not affect the success rate of dental implants. Implant placement must take place either 60 days before or 60 days after chemotherapy. Corticosteroids reduce bone density and increase epithelial fragility. They can increase immunosuppression and hinder osseointegration. Systemic use of corticosteroids causes suppression of the hypothalamic-pituitary-adrenal axis, and the standard recommendations that apply prior to any oral surgical procedure should be followed.

The dentist should know why the patient is on these drugs and consider the underlying disease.

Patients prescribed a daily dose of 10mg prednisolone are advised against altering the dosage. However, if corticotherapy has been administered for a period exceeding three weeks, it is recommended to consider prescribing increased corticosteroids.

It was concluded that patients taking a minimum of 5 mg prednisolone for at least one month might be at risk of adrenal crisis and require steroid coverage.

It was recently recommended that for minor surgery, an extra-oral dose be taken one hour before and after the surgery, but it has not been specified for dental treatment [126].

However, there are references which recommend otherwise. Dentists must follow the local regulations.

However, it is also recommended that a single 50 mg intramuscular injection of Hydrocortisone 30 minutes before a minor oral surgery procedure is needed. In the more advanced or traumatic surgeries, double the dose on the day of surgery, the day after the average dose plus 50%, the next day standard dose and 25% and finally, the next day, return to the regular dose[127]. Cohort studies reveal no adverse influence of properly controlled diabetes on successful implant treatment. Poorly controlled diabetes, however, has adverse effects on osseointegration because of impaired immunity, microvascular complications, and osteoporosis. Glycosylated haemoglobin (HbA1C) can lead to postoperative complications[128].

When antimicrobial cover is deemed necessary, the patients involved should do all they can to reduce oral microbial concentration by improving their oral hygiene routines, using regular antiseptic mouth rinses, and especially quitting smoking.

Diabetic patients with loose complete dentures find themselves in a vicious oral circle where the poor fit of their dentures due to bone loss forces them to eat soft food of poor nutritional value while plaque accumulation on the fit surface encourages widespread mucosal inflammation. Enter denture adhesives, the Magic Carpet.

Denture adhesives can improve denture retention, bite force and masticatory performance of complete denture wearers [129]. Denture adhesives can initially improve denture stability and retention; however, relying on them excessively to compensate for poorly fitting dentures may lead to bone resorption over time due to pressure points or uneven force distribution on the bone. Also, it may irritate soft tissue, which indirectly affects bone resorption. Denture adhesive should not replace a well-fit denture. However, the regular application of denture adhesive paste containing zinc can bring hyperzincemia and, consequently, copper deficiency, myelopathy, pancytopenia (reduction of white and red blood cells and platelets), and neurological complications. Also, it will encourage more bone loss.

Dento-alveolar surgery is not contra-indicated in immunocompromised and HIV-positive patients, especially when CD4 rates are high and the patient is on antiretroviral therapy [130].

CD4 T lymphocytes (CD4 cells) stimulate other immune cells, such as macrophages, B lymphocytes (B cells), and CD8 T lymphocytes (CD8 cells), to fight infection. HIV weakens the immune system by destroying CD4 cells.

Congenital neutrophil deficiency renders the patient prone to infection. This can include severe periodontitis. The patient can still benefit from dental implant treatment if this is coordinated with the patient's doctor and carried out using strict anti-infective measures.

Patients suffering from neuro-psychiatric disorders can benefit from dental implant treatment, but poor oral hygiene and bruxism are common, so this needs to be factored into the treatment plan.

Surgery on smokers is not necessarily contraindicated, but increased bone loss can be expected [131].

Proper use of antibiotics only where absolutely necessary

There is a worldwide concern about what is considered to be the overuse of antibiotics. The consequence has been an increase in the resistance of bacteria to antibiotics. Thirty years ago, one inquiry by the authorities found that dentists in the UK were responsible for 7% of antibiotic prescriptions, with doctors and farmers responsible for the remaining 97%. A more recent figure claimed dentists wrote 10% of antibiotic prescriptions.

Increased bacterial resistance to antibiotics is not the only concern. Dentists need to be aware of potential allergic or toxic reactions. Dental procedures carry a high risk of producing bacteraemia [132].

Failing implants are associated with microbial periodontitis in which the predominant organisms are gram-negative, motile and anaerobic bacteria [133].

It needs to be noted that staphylococci, coliforms and Candida spp, which are not generally associated with periodontitis or dental abscesses, have been isolated in peri-implantitis. Also present on infected metallic biomaterials are staphylococcus aureus, which attaches to titanium surfaces, and coagu-

lase-negative staphylococci [134].

The balance risks of antibiotic resistance, adverse drug reaction, increased cost, and the benefit of decreasing infection have been studied in patients with cardiovascular and prosthetic joints. However, it has been shown that antibiotics reduce the frequency of alveolar osteitis in healthy patients and decrease the rate of dental implant failure [135].

A number of protocols exist for administering a single pre-operative dose or multidose antibiotic, and the decision to administer these is usually left to the dentist's discretion.

The pre-operative use of mouth rinses like chlorhexidine and topical iodine has been advocated in order to minimise postoperative infection in cases where bone graft, bone substitute, or membrane have been placed [136,137]. Other factors which need to be considered are history of smoking, systemic disease, as in the immunocompromised, or a history of endocarditis, recent radiotherapy, or the presence of non-dental implant prostheses. Invasive dental procedures which last more than 45 minutes are associated with an increased likelihood of infection [138].

There is disagreement over the timing and dose of antibiotic prescriptions. It has been suggested that a single pre-operative dose of antibiotics increases the implant survival rate, but the postoperative multidose does not. Against this, the advocates of the multidose claim that 2 gr Amoxicillin or 2 gr Ampicillin post-operatively and 500 mg 4 times a day for two days are necessary [139].

The systemic use of antibiotics in dental implant surgeries does not reduce the infection rate of dental implant surgeries in immunocompromised patients [140].

While the dentist needs to minimise prescribing antibiotics for healthy patients, it is the dentist's responsibility and judgement of how to prevent infection and failure.

The author recommends Amoxicillin 500 mg and Metronidazole 250 mg, three times per day, starting the day of the operation and continuing for five days.

In grafted cases or with compromised patients' antibiotics should be taken for seven days.

Antibiotics are not needed for the second stage of surgery or flapless surgery.

Oral infection of bacterial origin should be treated for 4-7 days. The antibiotics do the hard work, allowing the patient's immune system to take over. There is no doubt that multicentre studies are needed to clarify this critical issue.

Prevention:

Possible sources of direct bacterial contamination during surgery (implant and bone) should be minimised. Surgical instruments, gloves, the air in the operating room, the air exhaled by the patient, saliva, and peri-oral skin are bacterially potent.

Reduction of the salivary flow will be observed by atropine, the supine position of the patient, and the appropriate surgical plan for the oral flap (atraumatic reflection). A Chlorhexidine mouth rinse pre-operatively reduces the level of intra-oral bacteria.

Use separate trolleys for separate procedures, where each trolley has the surgical instruments appropriate to the relevant procedure. A separate surgical trolley for extraction and curettage, bone preparation and implant placement, and bone substitutes/membranes/bone grafts are needed [141].

While a chlorhexidine-alcohol solution is generally used to clean and disinfect the patient's skin, available evidence indicates that it has a limited effect. An alcohol-based povidone iodine paint may be a better disinfectant, but it can be transferred from the patient's skin to the surgical area by a surgical glove or instrument. The potential allergic reaction to this transfer can range from a simple rash to severe respiratory impairment.

It is recommended that a perforated cap be placed to cover the patient's nose.

CTX Value	Risk of ONJ
300 to 600 pg/ml (normal)	None
150 to 299 pg/ml	None to minimal
101 to 149 pg/ml	Moderate
Less than 100 pg/ml	High

Predicting osteonecrosis in bisphosphonate patients due for implant surgery: the serum CTX test.

This test is called the Collagen Type-1 C-Telopeptide (CTX). The serum CTX (C-Terminal Cross-Linking Telopeptide) measures the rate of bone turnover. This information is of great value in assessing the risk of bisphosphonate-induced osteonecrosis of the jaw (ONJ) [142].

The measurement 'pg' in the table stands for 'picogram.'

Neurological disorders, including headache, migraine, migraine neuralgia, raised intracranial pressure and headache due to misuse of medication, need to be diagnosed. Tension in occipitofrontalis that feels like a band-like and gets worse during the day is a tension headache that needs reassurance.

Migraine experiences visual aura, unilateral headache and photophobia, nausea and vomiting, which Oral contraceptive stimulates.

Pain around the eye and nasal stiffness, which onset is in the morning and recurs for several weeks, are signs of the migrainous neuralgia alcohol stimulates.

Headaches, which are worse in the morning, reduced levels of consciousness, vomiting, the absence of pupillary reflexes, and increased blood pressure with a slow pulse rate are signs of raised intracranial pressure.

Epilepsy or fit is characterised by an aura and loss of consciousness with tonic and clonic phases and incontinence. The fit lasts less than 5 minutes. Recent guidelines are not to do anything except take away anything that may harm the patient, loosen any tight clothing around the neck and put him/her in the recovery position after the fit stops.

Psychiatry in dentistry has not been taught enough during undergraduate and postgraduate studies. It will burden the dentist to tackle the case; on the other hand, referring a patient to a specialist for hypertension is more manageable than referring it to a psychologist. Organic brain syndromes range from acute organic reactions and mood swings to clouding of consciousness and disorientation in time and place. Alcohol withdrawal, drugs, and infection can exacerbate the condition. Dementia is the reduction of short-term memory, but depression has the same signs and symptoms. Psychosis, which is the loss of reality, consists of schizophrenia with delusions and Mania, which is euphoria, hyperactivity and bipolar disorder.

Depression, which has been diagnosed, has increased, or has become more important in society, needs to be emphasised. Early morning wakening, tearfulness, inability to concentrate, or worthlessness.

Neuroses are symptoms without organic or psychotic symptoms. Anxiety neurosis is the physical symptoms without physical explanation and coexists with depression—obsessional neurosis, in which intrusive thoughts are repeated purposeless activity.

Personality disorders are not diseases but need to be considered. Obsessional, borderline (seeing everything in black and white) and sociopath in which there is no concept of affection or guilt and irresponsible.

Patients with narcissistic personality disorder are contra-indicated in complicated cases of dental implant treatment and oral rehabilitation.

This mental condition has inflated a sense of their own importance, need for excessive attention and lack of empathy for others. They show extreme confidence, but under this mask, they have a fragile self-esteem, which cannot tolerate the slightest criticism. The narcissistic personality disorder causes problems in relationships, including the dental team. Generally, they are unwilling to play the part they play and do not accept responsibility for their action. They are disappointed when they are not given special favours. The treatment is usually talk therapy (psychotherapy).

Modifying the patient's behaviour could help the patient and the dentist during treatment. Relaxation techniques can help mild phobias but not mental disorders. Modelling imitates positive behaviour with short-term benefits, but rewards can reinforce it. Encouragement helps. Jordan Peterson has wept in his lecture that people need so little encouragement, and that affects not only the child but any patient. It is unbelievable that you cannot overstate that power in the individuals. Praise, reassurance, and encouragement are potent motivators for encouraging behaviour change for oral hygiene and respecting post-operative and post-treatment instructions.

The six stages of the behaviour change are as follows [143]:
1. They do not intend to change
2. They intend to change
3. They have an action plan to change
4. The action plan is made
5. Prevent old behaviour
6. New behaviour established

Self-efficacy is the term for how confident a person is at a task. That could reflect on oral hygiene and respecting the post-operative treatment instructions.

Finally, it is the dentist himself who will need dental or medical treatment. The psychological trauma of the dentist needs to be studied during oral rehabilitation and dental implant treatment. These dentists need the willpower to continue the best treatment for their patients, even though psychological stress, the experience of the lack of appreciation from the patient and other issues would be traumatic for the dentist. The guidelines of each country differ, and the dentist should comply with its regulations. For further information on systemic disease management, detailed guidance is provided in Section 8.4 on "Communication with Other Specialists".

1.6. Blood biochemistry

A general medical examination of the patient is the responsibility of the GMP, and it is essential that the dentist is in touch with the patient's GMP to consult on this.

Since not all countries have an NHS (or equivalent) system to which the attending dentist can refer, it becomes the dentist's responsibility to determine the patient's medical status. This will be discovered either through questions of the patient, referrals to relevant parties for relevant tests, or to an appropriate physician.

Routine blood testing is not recommended, but it might be if the patient is to be treated under sedation or if the history and/or clinical examination indicate a need.

This section will provide concise information, and average values will be quoted with the laboratory reports to enable comparisons to be made.

Blood chemistry

A complete blood count (CBC) is a standard blood test that measures the types and numbers of blood cells in the sample. This test can also reveal the presence of infection, dehydration, and/or anaemia.

The HbA1c test measures the quantity of haemoglobin in the blood that has become glycated (chemically bonded with glucose). Haemoglobin molecules stay in the blood for around three months, so the HbA1c test can measure how glucose has interacted within the blood for up to 3 months. Thus, HbA1c provides a longer-term trend, similar to an average, of how high your blood sugar levels have been over some time.

The blood glucose level is the concentration of glucose in your blood at a single point in time, i.e. the very moment of the test. This is measured using a fasting plasma glucose test, which can be carried out using blood taken from a finger or a blood sample taken from the arm. Thus, fasting glucose tests provide an indication of your current glucose levels only, whereas the HbA1c test serves as an overall marker of what your average levelsare over a period of 2-3 months.

HbA1c can be expressed as a percentage (DCCT unit) or as a value in mmol/mol (IFCC unit). Since 2009, mmol/mol has been the default unit used in the UK.

Since June 2011, the way HbA1c values are reported has switched from a percentage to a measurement in mmol/mol. To make sense of the new units and compare these with old ones and vice versa, use the HbA1c units converter.

The table below summarises the routine blood tests and when they are high or low.

Test	Function	Low	High
Haemoglobin	a protein on red blood cells that carries oxygen	blood loss or anaemia.	When the body requires an increased oxygen-carrying capacity, usually because of smoking or living at a high altitude. The red blood cell production naturally increases to compensate for the lower oxygen.
Platelet Count (thrombocytes):	Part of the blood that makes the blood clot.	the person is receiving chemotherapy, haemolytic anaemia, leukaemia, or recent blood transfusion	anaemia, polycythaemia vera, a recent surgery to remove the spleen, thrombocytosis due to cancer
Blood Urea Nitrogen (BUN)	a measure of kidney function	low in protein diet, malnutrition, severe liver damage, overhydration	kidney disease by diabetes or high blood pressure, dehydration or heart failure and subsequently less blood flow to the kidney.
Carbon Dioxide (CO2)	Is present in the form of bicarbonate, which is regulated by the lungs and kidneys	Metabolic acidosis or the blood is too acidic. Addison disease, an adrenal gland problem. Ketoacidosis. This is a complication of type 1 and type 2 diabetes.	Hypercapnia is caused by hypoventilation or disordered breathing, where not enough oxygen enters the lungs and not enough carbon dioxide is emitted.
Creatinine	produced by the body during the process of normal muscle breakdown	Muscle disease (muscular dystrophy), liver disease, pregnancy, excess water intake and certain medications.	Kidney disease, intense exercise, Dehydration, Increased consumption of protein, medications
Glucose	A blood glucose test measures the glucose levels in your blood. Glucose is a type of sugar and is the body's primary energy source. A hormone called insulin helps move glucose from the blood into the cells.	Hypothyroidism, Too much insulin or diabetes medicine, Liver disease	Diabetes type 1, low insulin Type 2, insulin is not adequate. Eat more than planned or do less exercise. Cold or flu, stress and dawn phenomenon (a surge of hormones that the body produces daily around 4:00 a.m. to 5:00 a.m.). Kidney disease, Hyperthyroidism, Pancreatitis, Pancreatic cancer.
Serum Chloride	Maintains the pH of the blood	congestive heart failure, diabetic ketoacidosis, aldosterone deficiency, prolonged vomiting or gastric suction, Addison disease, chronic lung diseases (causing respiratory acidosis)	Dehydration, Cushing syndrome, kidney disease
Serum Potassium	Role in muscle contraction and cell function	Diuretic drugs (for hypertension)	Kidney disease, Addison disease (low cortisol)

Sodium	Control blood pressure and volume	dehydration, Cushing syndrome or kidney disease, Addison disease, hypothyroidism, severe vomiting or diarrhoea, and drinking too much water. Drugs (diuretic, anti-depressant), Ecstasy.	Diarrhoea, kidney disease, diabetes insipidus, Cushing syndrome
INR	measures of the extrinsic pathway of coagulation to determine the clotting tendency of blood, in the measure of warfarin dosage, liver damage, and vitamin K status.	Hypothyroidism. High vitamin K intake. Nephrotic syndrome.	Liver disease (vitamin K-dependent coagulation factors have been impaired). Prolong use of antibiotics, fat malabsorption syndrome and Anticoagulants.
Creatinine	produced by the body during the process of normal muscle breakdown	Muscle disease (muscular dystrophy), liver disease, pregnancy, excess water intake and certain medications.	Kidney disease, intense exercise, Dehydration, Increased consumption of protein, medications
White Blood Cell Count (WBCs)	the infection-fighting portion of the blood and play a role in inflammation	bone marrow problems, chemical exposure, autoimmune disease, and problems with the liver or spleen	presences of tissue damage (burns), leukaemia and infectious disease.
Red Blood Cell Count (RBCs)	The cells that carry oxygen to the body.	iron deficiency anaemia, blood loss, problems with the bone marrow, leukaemia and malnutrition	indicate heart problems, kidney disease, over-transfusion and dehydration.
Haematocrit	percentage of the blood that is composed of red blood cells.	anaemia, blood loss, bone marrow problems, malnutrition	dehydration, polycythemia vera, smoking, living at a high altitude and congenital heart disease.
Mean corpuscular volume (MCV)	the average volume of the red cells, measured in femtolitres	Microcytic Anaemia	Macrocytic anaemia
Mean corpuscular haemoglobin concentration (MCHC)	the average amount of haemoglobin per red blood cell in picograms	Microcytic Anaemia	Macrocytic anaemia
Red blood cell distribution width (RDW)	the variation in cellular volume of the RBC population.	No concern; RBCs are about the same size.	Nutrient deficiency (iron, folate, vit B12) Macrocytic deficiency
Neutrophil granulocytes	Resolve infection and heal damaged tissue	Infection, cancer treatment	Infection, high stress, RBC cancer, rheumatoid arthritis, trauma, burn, smoking, pregnancy, thyroiditis
Lymphocytes	A type of white blood cell, it is a part of the immune system.	HIV infection	after an infection. Viral infections such as glandular fever and. Leukaemia, cytomegalovirus, Hepatitis (A, B, C), HIV/AIDS, hypothyroidism, syphilis, TB,
Lymphocytes	A type of white blood cell, it is a part of the immune system.	HIV infection	after an infection. Viral infections such as glandular fever and. Leukaemia, cytomegalovirus, Hepatitis (A, B, C), HIV/AIDS, hypothyroidism, syphilis, TB,
Monocytes	A type of white blood cell that can differentiate to macrophage	Chemotherapy, radiation therapy.	Bacterial infection, tuberculosis, malaria, Rocky Mountain spotted fever, monocytic leukaemia, chronic ulcerative colitis, and regional enteritis

Eosinophil granulocytes	the movement to inflamed areas and regulating inflammatory response, trapping foreign bodies, killing cells, anti-parasitic and bactericidal activity, contributing to immediate allergic reactions,	Intoxication from alcohol or excess cortisol, like in Cushing's disease.	In parasitic infections, asthma, or allergic reaction
Basophile granulocytes	Type of white blood cell. Fighting fungal or bacterial infections and viruses. They release granules of enzymes to fight against harmful bacteria and germs.	Granulocytopenia (agranulocytosis), anaemia or leukaemia stop the body from producing new blood cells or damage existing blood cells.	Granulocytosis, Infections, autoimmune diseases, and blood cell cancers.
erythrocyte sedimentation rate (ESR), also called a sedimentation rate	is a non-specific measure of inflammation	polycythaemia, sickle cell, anaemia, hereditary spherocytosis, and congestive heart failure	pregnancy, inflammation, anaemia or rheumatoid arthritis

1.7. Biomechanics and macro design of bone

The internal stress distribution in the mandible is affected not only by forces on the teeth but also by the forces applied to the mandible by the muscles of the masticatory system, like lateral pterygoid that pulls them medially, due to various opening and closing actions required by chewing, speech, and involuntary jaw motions, and by the changes in inter-condylar distance. The inter-condylar distance may be increased from micrometres to more than 1 mm, with the mandibular flexure around symphysis during the opening/closing cycle and induce high tensile stress in the articular disc [144].

To gain insight into the primary stability of dental implants in bone, one must delve into the biomechanical behaviour of bone (e.g., strain), examine how implant design impacts bone, and consider the effects of surgical trauma on bone during implant placement (Fig. 1.14).

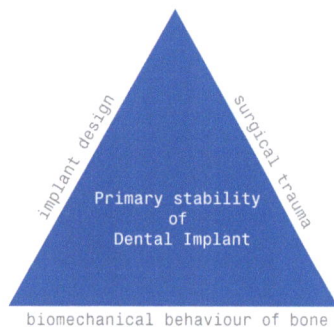

Figure 1.14 three main factors in the primary stability of dental implants in the alveolar bone.

It deforms when a force is applied to any material, such as bone. The amount of deformation in the material, relative to its original length, is called strain.

Strain is a dimensionless unit defined as the change in length divided by its original length ($\varepsilon = \Delta L/L$). The tensile strain occurs when a material is pulled so that it gets longer. Absolute magnitudes of peak tensile strain in bone can rise to 1200 microstrain in tension.

The compressive strain occurs when a material is pushed together to become shorter. During vigorous activity, absolute magnitudes of peak compressive strains in the bone can rise to 3500 microstrains (0.35%).

Shear strain is the angle, measured in radians, through which a material has been deformed by forces acting parallel with, rather than opposed to, the material. A radian is equal to 57.3

degrees. Shear strain arises when layers within a material slide against one another, as might occur with torsion or bending; peak values for the shear strain can rise to 1500 microstrain (figure 1.15,1.16).

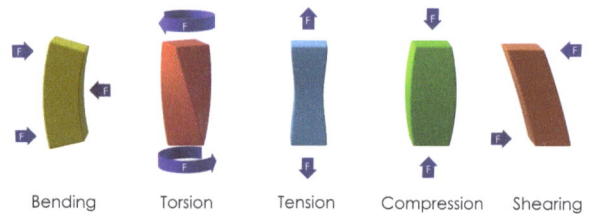

Figure 1.15 Types of stresses in engineering.

It is preferable to report the magnitude of the force in terms of the cross-sectional area of the material on which it is acting. The force per unit area is the stress (σ = Force/Area) and is reported in newtons per square meter (N/m2) or pascals (Pa).

One study applied the re-modelling algorithm for non-homogeneous density/elastic modulus distribution to conical and cylindrical cross-sections of dental implants. It was predicted that bone density increased on the tips of the threads and decreased inside the grooves, but softer bone around the periphery of the threadless implants was observed [145].

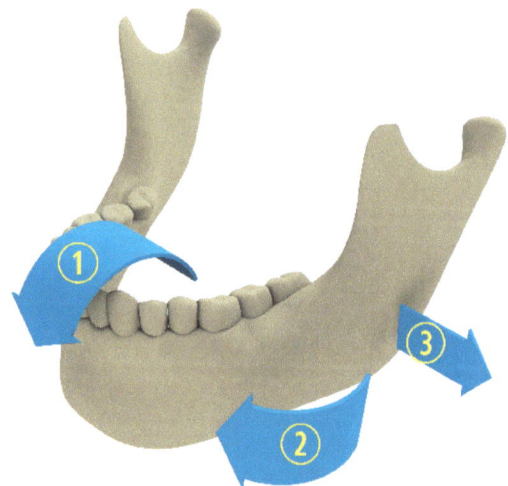

Figure 1.16 types of strain in the mandible during mastication. 1) Sagittal bending, 2) Torsion, 3) Lateral bending.

The bone crest around a newly placed implant comprises dense cortical bone with a minimal blood supply. The bone strain resulting from the procedure is essential in encouraging bone modelling and remodelling. High insertion torque produces transient ischemia, provoking periosteal hyperplasia and, by apposition, bone formation rather than necrosis.

Static bone strain has an effect on implant stability and bone remodelling. Bone adapts its mass and structure in response to load-induced strain, and the resultant remodelling depends on the magnitude of the strain, its frequency, and the rate of stimulus.

The mechanobiology of bone healing is affected by strain. Low stress and strain promote intra-membranous ossification; medium may promote intra-membranous ossification, but high tensile strength promotes fibrous tissue formation [146].

Static strain occurs when a weight is attached to a static material, and the material is allowed to stretch through the attached weight alone. The distortion is permanent. After removing a loading strain, residual strains still exist within the material (bone). These will also have an effect, and the magnitude of damage and strain accumulation will lead to stress distribution.

Differing bone qualities will show different levels of reaction to strain. The cortex has minimal elasticity and varying thicknesses, while cancellous bone has different levels of densities and different levels of elasticity; despite these structural and physical differences, the jawbone functions as a cohesive unit.

Implants with multiple threads seem to dissipate strain more effectively, thereby reducing maximum stress levels. However, threads introduce sharp edges at the implant-bone interface, leading to stress concentrations at the circumference of these edges.

In quantifying the potential strain engendered during and after implant placement, research has not adequately addressed the influence of drill design, implant design, and the size of the resulting space between bone and implant.

In rabbit tibia, where the cortical plate is thin and the cancellous bone is replaced by fatty tissue, an increase in the diameter of the implant by as little as 0.15 mm in the cortical region increases the static strain. This improved both the primary and subsequent biologic stability (osseointegration) of the implant [147].

The terms 'press-fit phenomenon' and 'interference fit' have sometimes been used in relation to screw and cylinder implants. The press-fit dental implant's primary stability will be governed by the design of the dental implant, the interference fit, the quality of the bone, and its frictional properties.

'Press-fit' indicates a mechanical connection between two structures related to the implant design based on contact pressure, and the term 'interference fit' is used when two parts are fastened by frictional push. A typical example is the press fitting of shafts into bearings—the two parts are shaped with slight differences in size (Figure 1.17).

This is also called 'interference fit' because one part slightly interferes with, or imposes upon, the space of the other.

Interference press fit could be used to generate the deformation since each component mutually interferes. The actual viscoelastic behaviour of the bone tissue implies that the elastic recoil or rebound of the bone decreases over time. When a hole smaller than an implant is prepared, 'pre-load' is applied to the implant and primary stability is achieved. The displacement field over the hole's surface depends on the elastoplastic behaviour of both the bone and the implant material, and the strain in the peri-implant bone evolves. The inelastic effects in bone secure the implant in the bone, called 'the press fit phenomenon'.

Implants are usually made cylindrical, although they can be slightly tapered to reduce excessive abrasion during insertion. Remember, the dentist needs friction on the soft bone.

Bone is viscoelastic and exhibits creep and stress relaxation, which means it has fluid and solid properties. The bone's deformation and its elastic recoil depend on the density of the bone tissue.

A viscoelastic material under a time-dependent increase of constant strain is called viscoelastic creep. Stress relaxation is the decrease in tensile stress over time when the body is held at a fixed length.

There is a difference between cortical and cancellous bone, which is less viscoelastic.

When cortical bone is stressed, it can deform significantly even by moderate levels of interference-fit. Nevertheless, its elasticity is not as important as its thickness. When the thickness of the cortex is 1mm or less, it can fracture and collapse into the cancellous bone.

Bone's visco-elastic performance also depends on the level of the initial elastic deformation to which it is subjected when the press-fit is achieved. The assembly strain (i.e., the deformation of the bone tissue upon the introduction of the implant) has an

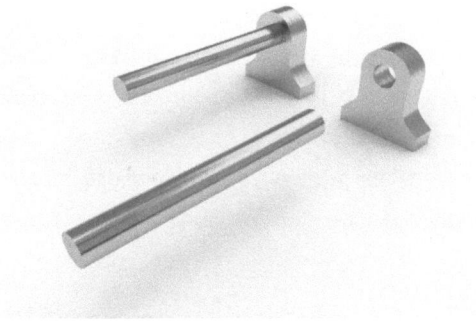

Figure 1.17 shaft to bearing interaction to provide stability.

effect on both the contact pressure between bone and implants (e.g., the initial press-fit) and the rate at which the press-fit-engendered stress is dissipated through deformation and elastic relaxation.

The relationship between bone quality and stress distribution has not been thoroughly researched and, therefore, understood. In poor bone quality (type D), a cylindrical screw implant produces maximum stress level at the neck and in the middle of the body, but in other types of bone, concentrated only at the crest. The interaction between the macro design (of the implant) and the prosthetic connection should not be underestimated.

A cylindrical implant with a Morse taper connection induces lower shear stress and strain in the peri-implant region compared with an external connection and conical implant [148] (figure 1.13). Press-fitting implants rely in part on implants' frictional resistance to the elastic opposition of the bone. The bone is compacted into the rough surfaces during the push of the implant inside the bone cavity, with its interference fits [149].

For implant placement to be successful, it is essential that the bone be protected during all three stages - osteotomy, implant placement, and following implant placement. The best scenario following surgical trauma was a 0.5 mm border zone of bone became necrotic, and 28 days after placement of a press-fit cylindrical implant, the formation of bone lacunae was observed.

If the difference between the diameter of the prepared hole by drill and the width of the screw implant is high, the torque will be higher than the elastic limit of the bone, new bone formation is delayed, and bone resorption will be observed, but this does not apply when the cortex is thin, and the cancellous bone quality is poor.

Greater roughness increases the interference fit and implanta-

tion force, but the relation between stability, implantation force, and bone damage has not been thoroughly researched and addressed.

NB, In the dental implant literature, cylinder and screw implants have been used in disarray. The dental implants can be placed like a screw in a wood by spinning a few turns in the hole using a screwdriver which sits firmly on the head of the screw. The body of these screws can be horizontal or conic. Sometimes the screw with the horizontal body is called cylindric. However, a surgical mallet inserts dental implants like a nail in the wood. In this book, cylindrical implants are the ones placed by a surgical mallet. The blade dental implants are also inserted using a surgical mallet.

Placement of cylinder implants has demonstrated that compaction of bone increases the fixation of implants inserted with exact fit and press fit between the implant and bone. In soft bone, cylinders are inherently more stable on insertion than screws.

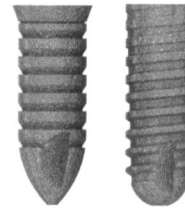

Figure 1.18 the left implant is a cylinder implant which is placed like a nail using a surgical mallet, and the right implant is placed by screwing in the bone.

The spring-back effect of compact bone reduces the initial gap between implant and bone. This gap reduction enables bony bridging to develop more quickly. Over-compaction of bone can affect its viability such that gap healing may be impaired.

Compaction increases peri-implant bone density, bone-implant contact, and primary stability. The inherent elasticity of compacted bone will lead to a degree of spring-back (by about 9%), enhancing the primary stability level. In other words, the cavity into which the implant has been forced will automatically be reduced by 9% [150,151].

There is a concern regarding the negative effect of time after dental implant placement, as the osseointegration has not been finalised, and the cell death can increase the prepared hole's size and reduce its stability.

The peri-implant density can be enhanced by bone compaction during the first two weeks in dogs (which is equivalent to 6 weeks in humans); also, it increases the bone implant contact (BIC) over the four weeks in dogs (which is equivalent to 12 weeks in humans) and non-vital bone observed around dental implants [152]. In dogs, femora with a funnel-shaped medullary canal are best suited for a press-fit implant as they permit a concentric conical interlock between the implant and bone. This has been demonstrated using a conical bone drill preparation followed by placing a press-fit implant into the low-density bone [153].

1.8. Factors Influencing Primary Dental Implant Stability (Remain Unclear)

Primary implant stability is the mechanical stability established between bone and dental implants and refers to the stability of an implant immediately after implantation.

That initial (primary) stability matures, and that maturity develops in three stages.

The first stage starts immediately after implant placement and depends on implant design, bone preparation, bone-condensing techniques, and both the cortical bone's thickness and the trabecular bone's strength.

The second stage comes with mature bone healing in direct apposition to the implant surface, where the bone quality and implant surface preparation can have an effect. The third stage arrives when the bone succeeds in adapting functionally around the implant under loading [154].

Insertion torque

The need to obtain primary stability and force distribution is not a problem when dealing with a normal cortex and good-quality bone. However, dealing with a thin cortex and poor-quality bone presents a challenge. The approach most often adopted is to place an oversized implant in the prepared cavity. In the dense bone, it becomes unpredictable; when it fails, one of two complications may follow. In the first, the implant screws in satisfactorily up to the last millimetres or so and then will not go further. In the second, the implant screws in quickly until it cannot go further, but now turns fruitlessly without tightening; the screw just spins in bone.

The dental implants are placed in the prepared cavity with two approaches, screwing and hammering. A screw is able to fasten by to draw two pieces (e.g., wood) together. There is a major grip strength when force is applied vertically to the screw. The screws do not have much shear force but much tensile strength; the screw keeps parts (e.g., wood blocks) together when faced with vertical force. The nails use the shear strength that the force can handle from the sides. Nails can bend under pressure and have much shear strength but not much tensile strength. In carpentry, when it is going to bear weight/gravity, like a table, the screw is the best option, but if it bears side-to-side movement, the nail is preferred (Figure 1.19).

It is essential to understand the difference between tensile strength and shear strength. Putting it in succinctly, if tensile strength (grip) is needed, use a screw, and if shear strength is needed, use a nail. In the real world of mechanics, it is recommended to use phronesis and choose the best option when it does not matter.

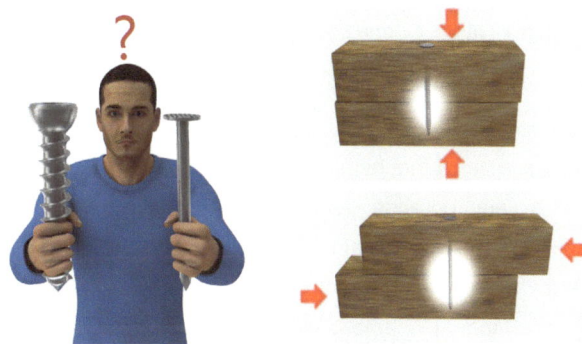

Figure 1.19 Should I use a nail or a screw?
In summary, screws exhibit grip strength (upper right), and nails exhibit shear strength (lower right).

Both types of dental implants, which were placed by a surgical mallet (the author calls it cylindrical implant) and the implants fastened by screwing (the author calls it screw implant), have had comparable long-term success rates [155].

The author has had 25 years of experience, and the cylindrical implants are still functioning.

The author's experience regarding cylindrical dental implants (Bicon, IMZ, Frialit-2, S&S Biomat) was unpredictable implant placement in the hard bone during the surgery.

Regarding screw implants, it is necessary to emphasise that despite advertisements of the companies, the thread designs V-shaped, trapezoid, buttress and reverse buttress do not affect the quality of the primary stability [156].

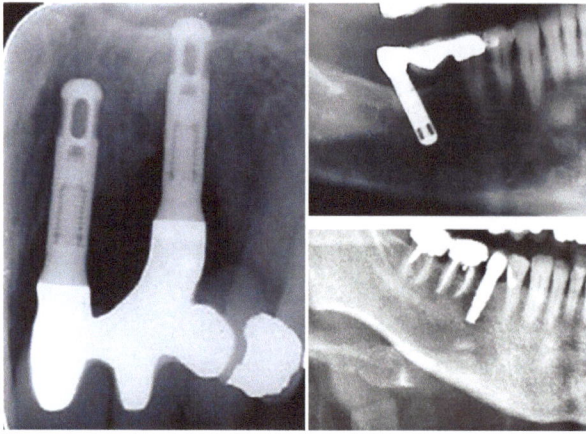

Figure 1.20 Left: periapical x-ray of the IMZ cylindrical implants after 24 years. The patient had a car accident, and the bone was grafted with a chin block to increase the width. 4-5 mm bone loss after 24 years. Upper right: DPT of the cylindrical IMZ replacing 47 attached to the 45 natural teeth; after 18 years, the implant was placed mesial-apically to avoid an Inferior Dental Canal. Lower right: DPT of the replaced 45 with Frialit-2 cylindrical implant; after 18 years, there is no bone resorption.

There is a belief that high resistance torque is mandatory in implant osseointegration, but two implant preparation techniques were compared in a study. Both implants were buried under the gum. The first technique used conventional serial drilling with customary placement and the second employed oversized socket preparation. It was shown that the conventional implant technique, using serial drilling, does not require high torque primary stability. It was also shown that osseointegration will still occur when oversized socket drilling is adopted and excludes high mechanical engagement, as long as the implant is undisturbed during the healing process and that rotational and vertical mobility of the implant is prevented. This will be confirmed by feedback from the implant adaptor (the instrument which is mounted to the implant to screw it into the implant site).

In the customary scenario, for the first few weeks of mechanical engagement between the implant and the bone, the bone/implant contact (BIC) was high compared to the oversized scenario. However, after a few weeks, it was matched by that in the oversized cavity scenario, where it seems that new bone formed from the bone adjacent to the sandblasted acid-etched implant surfaces [157,158].

NB: during function, the level of BIC is a prerequisite for implant stability.

Implants in the anterior mandible have a lower risk of primary stability failure compared with those in the maxillae. Females have a higher risk of primary implant stability failure than men, and implants less than 15 mm in length have a higher risk of primary stability failure than longer implants, which are better able to withstand immediate loading [159].

The quantity and location of cortical bone and trabecular bone surrounding the implant are important factors for stability, as they contribute to bone-implant contact [160].

Higher primary stability was found in the mandible than in the maxillae, and the results were statistically significant [160,161]. This may be one of the reasons for the higher failure rate in the maxillae [162].

Bone quality and implant stability are lower in the posterior area. For this reason, the posterior implant success rate is lower than in the anterior [163]. The thick cortical and dense trabecular bone will increase primary stability in the anterior area.

There is a controversy in the literature [164-166] over the use of longer and/or broader implants in order to increase primary stability. Proponents argue for the increased support from the expanded bone-implant contact surface, and there is no doubt that by increasing the length or diameter of the implant with the expanded inner cortical engagement along the maximum length of the implant, primary stability will be increased.

It is generally agreed that when the loading of the implant reaches between 500-3000 u strain (physiological loading), this leads to mature bone formation and reduces the bone healing period of osseointegration. The tension exerted by the attainment of physiological loading has a direct effect on cell behaviour. It does this by activating signalling pathways and regulating gene expression. The clinical relevance is that this may enhance osseointegration at the immediately loaded bone-implant interface [167,168].

The value of primary implant stabilisation decreases gradually with the reconstruction of bone tissue around the implant. This takes place in the first weeks after surgery and gives way to establishing secondary stability, the ongoing process of osseointegration. When the healing process is complete, the initial mechanical stability will have been entirely replaced by biological stability. The most dangerous moment for implantation success is the moment of the lowest initial stabilisation, which occurs during the 3–4 weeks after implantation when the primary stability is minimal and the biological stability has not been completed. Stability is found to increase up to the 10th week [169-172].

If insufficient primary stability occurs after implantation, leading to increased implant mobility, it can contribute to implant failure. The attainment of primary stability immediately after dental implant placement and before osseointegration is an important factor for dental implant success; it is essential with one-piece dental implants with immediate loading.

The highest interfacial stresses are faced in the implant collar, which engages the cortical bone near the apex of the implant in the trabecular bone. The interfacial shear stress is high in the buccal side of the body. Positive collar slop, larger implant diameter, and longer implant collar reduce the magnitudes of the interfacial stresses. Nevertheless, bear in mind that the dentist does not have the luxury of an acceptable alveolar ridge width [173].

Also, the amount of the occlusal load should need to be considered, besides the prominent biophysical properties of the cortical bone and marrow [174,175].

The cortex has an essential role in increasing primary stability. Bone quality has more influence on primary stability than implant design, but the research did not demonstrate poor bone quality.

There are many factors influencing the primary stability, and there is chaos implementing in the relationships between the prepared bone cavity (drill design), implant body (cylindric or conic) and types of threads, the differences between the dimensions of the drill and the implant. The differences arise in tolerances of dimensions of the drills, the implant body and the threads and the effect of the quality of the bone (the cortical thickness and the trabeculae's density).

How to increase the primary stability of dental implants

When the bone is soft, primary stability is an issue and has to be achieved using different techniques,

Surface roughness can affect interfacial shear stress, resulting in increased resistance to loading. The roughness is made up of a mass of tiny pits of different sizes and shapes. Each pit on the rough surface is an element that is resistant to shear. The density of the pit has been studied, and a direct significant effect of the increased roughness and the primary stability has not been observed.

However, the implants with treated surfaces showed greater roughness and a higher friction coefficient and demanded a more significant insertion torque than machined implants during placement [176-178].

Screw implants with a cylinder or tapered body do not affect the primary stability, but it has been shown that in type IV bone, tapered-screw implants significantly provide higher primary stability. The bone preparation shape cylinder and tapered body implant increased the primary stability in poor bone quality, and in straight-screw type implants, lateral compression force seems to have had only a tiny effect on primary stability [179].

Different options exist for the relationship between the implant body design and the bone cavity. The prepared bone cavity and the implant may have different types of relationships (figure 1.21).

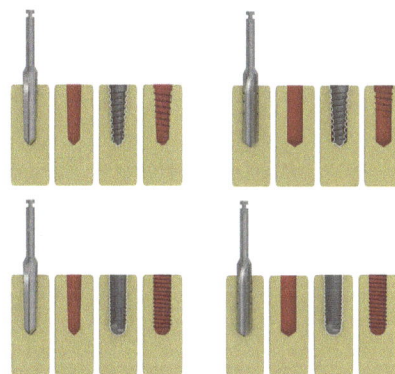

Figure 1.21 Besides the tolerance between the prepared cavity, the difference between the prepared cavity's geometry and the threads' surface affects the primary stability.

The drills are conic or cylindrical, as are the implant's body and the threads' outer surface. The threads are perpendicular to the long axis of the implant and are inserted like a nail, or threads are angulated, which is screwed into the bone cavity.

There are not many studies to compare them, with different types of bone quality and inner cortical engagement and the tolerances between the bone cavity and implant diameter [180].

Different techniques have been recommended to increase bone quality when bone quality is poor.

One surgical technique used to increase initial implant stability in low-density bone is to prepare an implant receptor site that is smaller in diameter than the implant to be placed. In this way, an osteocompressive fit is achieved between the implant surface and the bone bed. By drilling 0.6mm less than the company's protocol and enhancing primary implant stability, the undersized drilling technique might also achieve a translocation of bone particles from the cortex to cancellous bone. This biological phenomenon, comparable to the autologous bone graft, positively influences the osteogenic response [181]. However, the bone tissue is sacrificed by drilling, and this shortcoming is exacerbated in situations where limited bone or bone of lesser density is available.

Reducing the depth of final bone preparation also increases the primary stability in tapered screw implants. This may have been caused by the morphological characteristics of the tapered-screw type implant, in which the diameter of the cavity formed in the bone preparation site reduces when bone preparation decreases.

Osteotomes are wedge-shaped instruments with varied steepness of taper, designed to compress, cut and deform the soft bone to provide space in the bone for future dental implants. The osteotome gives the surgeon a tactile sense of the bone quality.

The osteotome was introduced to increase the primary stability of dental implants. This technique consists of first preparing a small-sized pilot hole, then compressing the bone tissue laterally and apically with a series of spreaders or drill-shaped instruments pressed in by a surgical mallet. A high degree of stability can be achieved without removing additional bone. There are contradictory results of the effect of the osteotome technique.

Simultaneous undersized and osteotome techniques result in bone compression around the implant, but in the osteotome technique, the compression is clearly higher because of force-fitting stresses that arise when an implant is placed into an implant bed of a smaller diameter.

The bone density of the implant recipient site and the shape and height of the implant surface should determine the amount of required misfit between the implant diameter and drill hole.

Research: Dr Nik

Two in vitro and other in vivo studies were performed in 2004.

A. In-vitro

The soft part of cow ribs was used, the cortex was reduced to a maximum of 1 mm, and the implants were placed after bone preparation.

In this research, a new design conical drill was used, which, when used counterclockwise, the tip could penetrate the bone but could not remove bone and compress the bone trabecula laterally without increasing the vibration of the drill.

In the first research, cylindrical implants were used with parallel reverse buttress threads perpendicular to the axis of the dental implant, which was inserted like a nail; the preparation was different in each case. In each group, ten dental implants were used and compared.

1. With drill 2mm clockwise and immediate placement (tapped in like a nail – 3.4mm implant)
2. With drill 2mm clockwise, 3mm and 3.4 anticlockwise, and implant placement – 3.4mm implant
3. Drill 2mm clockwise, and then serial surgical mallet and osteotomes 3mm, 3.4, were used, and a 3.4mm implant was placed
4. Conventional drilling sequences 2, 3, 3.4mm clockwise and implant placement

Using a pull-out test machine, researchers observed a decrease in the primary stability of the implants from the top to the bottom one hour after placement.

The results and more details are in Chapter 4.3, Hard Tissue Management.

B. In-vivo

In the In-vivo research, the rabbit tibia was used as a poor-quality bone model; it has a thin cortex, and the cancellous bone is poor and mainly fatty tissue (figure 1.22).

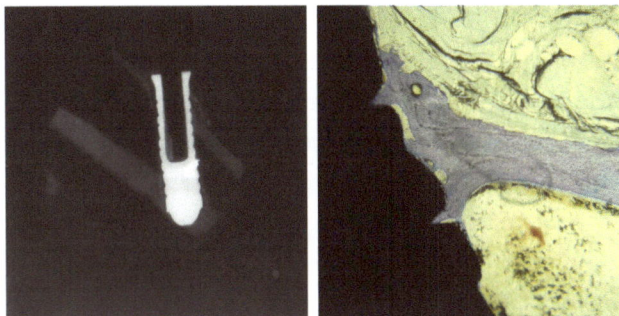

Figure 1.22 Right, light microscopy, undecalcified resin section, toluidine blue staining, a dental implant placed in the rabbit's tibia, the cortex is thin with the fatty medullary bone. Left, the microradiograph of the Osseointegrated implant in the rabbit's tibia and the lack of cancellous bone is evident.

The 2 mm diameter drill was used in one rabbit tibia, and cylindrical implants with a 3.4mm diameter were immediately placed. Furthermore, conventional serial drilling was applied on the other tibia, diameters 2,3 and 3.4 mm, and the implant was placed. Twenty dental implants were placed in ten rabbits. After two months of using a torque meter (CDI torque products, USA), the implants were removed, and the osseointegration quality was compared. A significant difference was observed between the quality of the two groups, and the quality of using only the 2 mm drill was higher than the other group, with an average of 54 Ncm compared to 31 Ncm in the control group. In the application of undersize drilling, during dental implant placement, the cortex may push inside the cancellous region like batwing doors and increase the BIC (figure 4.19).

The dentist needs to use every trick in the book to deliver short- and long-term success when dealing with poor-quality bone with a thin cortex.

Other surgical techniques for improving the primary stability of implants, such as obtaining bicortical anchorage, tuberosity and pterygo-maxillary implantation, have been introduced [182-184].

Fibrin tissue glue was introduced as a hemostatic agent and adhesive material composed of purified fibrinogen and thrombin, bonding with the coagulation's physiological cascade. The glue is successful as a sealant in conjunction with sutures or clips and is used in posterolateral spinal infusions. However, studies need to be implemented in dental implant cases [185].

There is a demand from the patient that immediately after implant placement, enjoy having a fixed prosthesis during the healing period. The need for immediate load dental implant techniques has been more pronounced.

High insertion torque is a prerequisite for immediate single-tooth implants for successful early loading procedures [186-188].

The primary mechanical stability of a dental implant is a critical factor in the success of immediate loading.

There may be a misconception as to what represents adequate primary stability. A minimum of 30N/cm has been the default treatment for one-piece dental implants or immediate load implants. Some studies have also preferred insertion torque as a determinant of implant stability, and torque values of 32, 35, 40 Ncm and higher have been chosen as thresholds for Immediate Load [189,190].

Even though it was recommended that it is preferable in single implant placement with a high insertion torque [191], the immediate load has been placed with a high survival rate with low insertion torques. Extraction and immediate implant placement and provisionalisation using a low-insertion-torque protocol of ≤25Ncm have been stated. Low rotational stability was not a contraindication to treatment unless there was a lack of axial stability [192,193].

Measurement of the primary stability

Some dentists prefer to measure the primary stability of the dental implants. The initial stability at the time of implant placement is influenced by both the cortical bone thickness and the strength of trabecular bone [194].

These factors are mostly nonlinearly correlated (the behaviour is random) with ITV (insertion torque value), PTV (Periotest value), and ISQ. ITV and PTV seem more suitable for identifying the primary implant stability in osteoporotic bone with a thin cortex.

The ITV can be measured during screw dental implant placement by manual or electric ratchets. Manual ratchets are in two families: spring (toggle-type) and frictional (beam-type). The spring type is more reliable than the frictional, but some believe the frictional type is more reliable in lower torques which are used on some of the abutments' screws only [195].

Different torques can be adjusted for the spring type and do not have a mechanical stop, so the torque applied is not limited, but only a single torque set by the manufacturer delivered for the friction type. The friction type may become corroded, and the autoclave hardens the lubricants and affects its precession [196].

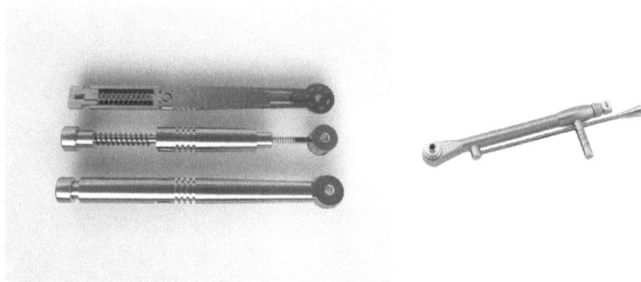

Figure 1.23 The original author designed a spring-type torque meter (left) compared to a friction-type (right).

Also, papers have published that age, the amount of sterilisation, and the torque applied do not significantly affect the precision of the manual ratchets [197].

Using an electric device, resonance frequency analysis (RFA) determines the implant stability quotient (ISQ). RFA involve sending magnetic pulses to a small metal rod attached to the dental implant. The rod vibrates, and the probe reads its resonance frequency and translates it into an ISQ value with a standard range of 55-80. This device was developed for research, but some clinicians like to use it in the clinic. The device has been manufactured with wire (Ostell) and wireless (Penguin).

Any measurable device needs to be calibrated, and manufacturers have no guidelines on how many times of use it needs to be calibrated. Some authors recommend annually, which is arbitrary and undermines the application of these types of devices in everyday life.

The author believes in the clinic, the best way to measure the primary stability of the screw implant is the ITV using a manual spring ratchet which is used during implant placement. However, for cylindrical implants, which are indicated in soft bones, the rod inside the implant, and with manual dexterity, the dentist will feel the stability as all the dentists do have experience with other types of treatment. When we are dealing with soft bone after dental implant placement, it is not a good idea to disturb the stability by any means, including PTV and ISQ.

Assessment of primary stability of dental implant

It is recommended that the radiographic assessment subchapter be studied first in the patient assessment and treatment plan chapter.

The three main dangers of implant success are lack of primary stability, overheating, and overloading. Assessing and predicting the primary stability of the implant during the treatment plan is an important issue which needs to be addressed.

The assessment of quality bone is classified as before the surgery, immediately after implant placement and after dental implant placement.

• Before the surgery, the only option was different types of radiographs.

The main aim is for the dentist to realise when the bone quality is poor, to warn the patient, and to protect himself from high expectations of the patient. He cannot do magic to improve patients' bone quality even though there are techniques to increase bone quality. Also, one must understand what poor bone quality means, the need for maximum dimensions of the dental implant and the increase in the number of dental implants, which reflects the position of the implants, and to purchase the dental implants, which reflects the cost of the treatment. The dentist cannot tell the patient that because during bone preparation, I realized the quality of bone is poor, and I must increase the number of dental implants, and the cost of treatment will increase. On the other hand, if the dentist continues as planned and ignores the problem, it will affect the success of the treatment after a few years.

Periapical, panoramic, CT, CBCT and DXA (DEXA) have been proposed.

Digital image analysis computed tomography (CT) using the Hounsfield Unit has limitations. Plain digital radiographs can be used to study cortical and cancellous bone texture [198].

CBCT is used to study the dimensions of the alveolar bone, but no CBCT models are the same. Finding a specific CBCT model does not apply to other models, and thus, the Gray Values (GVs) cannot be considered truth [198,199] (figure 1.24).

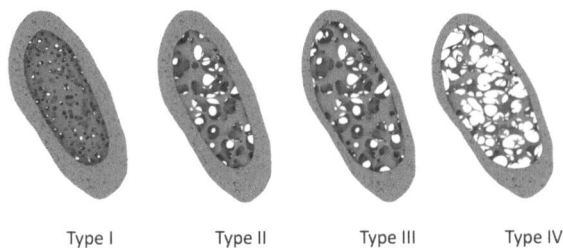

Type I   Type II   Type III   Type IV

Figure 1.24 cross-section of different types of alveolar bone quality.

The quality of the bone, as indicated by the CT scan, has been classified into four categories: types I, II, III, and IV. However, it is not easy to distinguish radiographically between types II and III.

Regardless of the relative usefulness of CT scans, the clinician must be reminded of the attendant risk with computed tomography, which delivers a higher radiation dosage than conventional radiographs.

DXA separated the bone mineral, fat tissue and fat-free soft tissue. The elements attenuate photons' high and low energy levels, hydrogen as low and calcium as high. The X-ray scan is pixel-by-pixel; the summed estimate is the molecular component.

Each manufacturer uses different attenuations for the X-ray beam. Usually, the spine, hip, and forearm are studied. The effective dose is small, and it is safe to use. The precision is less for obese and osteoporotic cases. There are major differences in the results between each manufacturer.

DXA dose is small, but the precision cannot distinguish the cortical and trabecular bone mass. This device cannot be a gold standard for body composition [200,201].

There is not enough evidence that there is a correlation between skeletal and jawbone mineral density, which makes it more questionable to use in the assessment of bone quality in dental implantology [202].

Using a film holder and referencing an aluminium step-wedge with each exposure is recommended to standardise the bone quality assessment using periapical X-rays. The equal thickness of mineralized tissue and Aluminium produces similar densities [203].

Panoramic (OPG, DPT) is usually used; the Klemetti index may be the closest we can get to diagnosing poor bone quality bone,

but it could never be accurate for an individual site.

Calibrating the panoramic radiographs using a step wedge phantom (using DXA) is recommended. Five steps of copper ranging from 0.1-0.5 mm thick which, each step is measured using DXA. During the exposure, the copper wedge is placed on the bottom of the radiographic film cassette to provide a reference image on the radiograph [204].

• DURING THE SURGERY

The perception can be noticed by reflecting a flap. The dentist may observe the cortical bone cracking while reflecting the flap when the bone quality is very poor. Also, major bleeding points from the cortex can be observed.

Perception of bone quality by bone classification is the most reliable and objective scale of bone density using the bone entrapment method. This subjective classification has also been used to characterize the perception of bone quality during the drilling procedure by providing comparative materials of differing resistance to drilling to aid classification. Indeed, the concept of intra-operative drilling resistance is being used as an objective quantitative assessment of bone quality. The implant's design and the drill's wear can bias the perception.

Other methods for assessing bone quality are impractical for the practising implant surgeon.

Evaluation is always a problem because prior diagnosis and assessment can never compete with actual discovery, either at the time of osteotomy preparation or even subsequent to implant placement. It may provide accurate data, but it is retrospective unless the dentist has pre-assembled stock with different types of implants designed for different types of bone. Provided the patient has been adequately advised of any uncertainties, the availability of pre-assembled stock allows the surgeon to adapt readily to any operational requirement.

The Bone Debris Entrapment (BDE) method is more predictable and safer. Based on the hand-felt perception of the drilling resistance, only class 1, with a mean histomorphometric density of 76.5% and class 4 (28.8%) can be distinguished, and anything in the middle can be distinguished by class 2. It is not possible to predict the subtle differences between classes 2 (66.8%) and 3 (59.6%), which have been recommended and used as default. Thus, bone density can be classified into three groups [205]. The 'Bone Debris Entrapment' system used by the Nik dental implant drills provides a quantitative bone-quality classification and offers a predictable osteotomy technique. Using the pilot 2mm drill of the Nik system, prepare the implant site to the required depth. The BDE System is based on the amount of debris entrapped within the drill's flutes. When the amount of debris fills 0-1/3 of the flutes, it indicates soft bone and is type III; between 1/3-2/3 indicates medium quality bone (type II), and more than 2/3 indicates hard bone (type I). Knowledge of the relevant bone quality will allow the surgeon to choose the appropriate osteotomy technique to ensure predictable implant stability.

• IMMEDIATELY AFTER IMPLANT PLACEMENT

There is controversy regarding the ideal insertion torque. Many clinicians and implant manufacturers assume that high insertion torque is a prerequisite for successful osseointegration, especially when an implant is to be placed under immediate functional load. This has been supported in no small part by evidence from the literature that insertion torque is correlated with an Implant Stability Quotient (ISQ) [206-209].

A Cochrane systematic review on the effectiveness of immediate single-tooth implants stated that high insertion torque was a prerequisite for successful early loading procedures. However, immediate-load implants with insertion torques of 20-50 Ncm in a single implant/crown were equally successful when compared with the conventional method [210].

Cases have been reported where immediate loads have been placed, with low insertion torques and high survival rates [211]. Bone density thresholds for different levels of insertion torques vary [206-208]. Torques up to 100 Ncm reduce axial micromotions [212] but will produce more significant marginal bone loss, as has been shown in vivo for implants subjected to a torque of > 40 Nc [213].

The average insertion torque values for both female and male and younger and older patients differ significantly. Higher insertion torque values have been recorded for men and older patients. Differing bone qualities at implant sites may explain this. It appears that the age and gender of patients have an influence on insertion torque values [206].

The author believes alternative placement strategies may be needed for poor bone quality. These may include placing different bone compression techniques and longer implants to engage the implant's apical part in the cortex's inner layer. Another method is to engage the body of the implant in the inner layer of the buccal and lingual of the cortex.

CT examinations can help dentists predict primary stability before surgery, but authentic assessments can only be made at the moment of surgery.

The most practical ways to assess the level of primary stability likely to be achieved and the level of stability achieved is by the use of four indicators: first, the bone quality as predicted by the radiographs, then the quality discovered at the moment of cavity preparation (more of this later), then the maximum insertion torque measured at the final placement of the implant, and finally the degree of stability as measured by the OssTell machine immediately after the placement [206].

• AFTER DENTAL IMPLANT PLACEMENT

Primary stability immediately after dental implant and prior osseointegration is a crucial factor of dental implant success; it is essential with a one-piece dental implant and needs to be assessed by the dentist.

There are different types of devices to measure the stability of dental implants, which may be used to determine the primary stability, like Periotest values (PTV), Resonance Frequency Measurements (RFM) and ISQ (Implant Stability Quotient). RFM and the ISQ are invasive in calculating primary stability and can reduce the primary stability. Torque measures are the best method of measurement of screw-type dental implants. The measurement of the primary stability of cylindrical dental implants using torque measure is unattainable.

Applying PTV, RFM, or ISQ causes of concerns are abutment length and its stability [213], which is only in one piece implant has resolved; also, the prosthetic stability could bring a bias. Age, gender, anatomic location, and bone quality may produce variable results [214-216].

An objective, quantitative classification of bone density that can be applied and is not operator experience-dependent is needed.

1.9. Splinting Dental Implants

When an implant is placed in poor-quality bone and lacks acceptable primary stability, the condition can improve by splinting to other stable implants or placing a conventional 3-piece implant in a 2-stage procedure.

The need for splinting the abutments of dental implants should be addressed and discussed in two separate stages, before and after osseointegration.

The main reason for considering the need for splints pre-osseointegration is to improve the chances for acceptable primary stability of immediate-load dental implants, especially when such primary stability is not certain. This might be due to poor bone quality or inadequate surgical dexterity, which has not achieved acceptable primary stability. In immediate loading cases, published papers indicate a potential lack of patient co-operation, bone split fractures, and implant loss, in which splinting may prevent failure [207-220].

Splinting a single-tooth immediate load implant to the neighbouring teeth is not advised. A natural tooth moves 50 - 200 um, but a dental implant only moves 10. The consequence of splinting the implant to its neighbouring tooth is that the dental implant becomes mobile and will not osseointegrate [221].

The author recommends that in the single tooth and up to three implant cases, the provisional prosthesis, which may act as a splint, should be out of occlusion by at least 1 mm.

Generally, immediately after placing multiple immediate load implants, they should be splinted to increase the chances of success, especially effective in cross-arch stabilisation.

Our research shows that splinting can:

- Increase resistance to overloading,

- Provide improved aesthetics,

- Protect the soft tissue like cheeks or tongue.

Indications for the need for splinting or provisional prosthesis:

- In the mandible, when there is major vertical bone resorption, the floor of the mouth is level with alveolar bone or even above it.

- When there is macroglossia

- When the buccal space between the cheek and abutment is limited in the posterior maxillae, the latter can erode the buccal soft tissue.

A splint can act as a provisional prosthesis to allow the dentist to evaluate aesthetics, the patient's phonetics, or tolerance of the new tongue space. After a long period of edentulism, while tolerating mobile or labialised teeth or a mobile denture, a fixed and stable bridge is new and unfamiliar and can make the patient uncomfortable. A provisional prosthesis can allow for some prosthetic adjustment and help the patient adjust to the new environment.

Timing the Provision of Splinting:

Splints can be provided, either.

- On the day of surgery, prior to suturing, or

- On the day of surgery, immediately after suturing the mucosa or

- One to two weeks after implant placement.

If one-piece dental implants are used, the titanium one-piece dental implant is divided into three parts: the first part has a rough surface which attaches to the bone, the second part is flared with a polished surface which attaches to the gingival tissue, the third part which is also polished attaches to the crown. The finishing margin of the abutment needs to be shielded from the overgrowth of gingival tissue. Some companies provide rigid plastic rings; if not, they can be made in the dental laboratory.

Methods and Procedures for Splinting

Two delivery approaches can be taken immediately after implant placement or one to two weeks after implant placement.

• ON THE DAY OF SURGERY, PRIOR SUTURING

Prior to implant placement, take a silicone impression of the surgical region, an alginate impression of the opposite jaw, and a rigid bite. The laboratory fabricates a provisional bridge, but the lingual/palatal surface should be 1-2 mm thicker. This reduces the chances of its fracturing. A wire or metallic mesh can also be added to the lingual surface.

If the patient has an acrylic removable denture, this can also be transferred to a provisional fixed bridge used as a splint.

After adjusting the bridge/splint at the chairside, ensure the soft tissue supports the bridge/splint in the edentulous region, controlling its buccal-lingual position and is about 1 mm off occlusion. Then, a gutter is prepared inside the bridge, leaving 2mm of the buccal and palatal surface intact. After implant placement, a rubber dam may now be prepared to prevent the ingress of resin into the marginal undercuts under the ring and protect the gum and any exposed bone from the acrylic. Use a sterile rubber dam to cover the bridge area, punch holes over the abutments, and then position the dam.

The rigid plastic ring is placed over each abutment, confirming the fit. If, for whatever reason, the rigid plastic ring is not stable - the abutment may have been modified - stabilise the ring with red wax or silicone wash used like cement. Confirm the fit of the provisional bridge and adjust as necessary, ensuring that the gutter is large enough to allow a passive fit. Prepare a length of sterile aluminium foil (0.1-0.5mm thick). The occlusal clearance will increase before the bridge cements when the patient bites down on this. Now, place a couple of drops of cold cure resin liquid on the surfaces of the gutter, and then cold cure resin of a putty texture inside the gutter is placed. Holding the aluminium foil onto the occlusal surface, place the bridge on the abutments with the rigid plastic ring and ask the patient to close it.

Before the final stage of polymerisation, the bridge is removed to allow the undercuts to be released and put back again; this can be repeated a couple of times. After final polymerisation, the bridge is removed, trimmed of excess, and adjusted from inside the Rigid Plastic Ring if necessary.

Place the provisional bridge over the abutments with the zinc phosphate cement in the rigid plastic ring. Sterile coconut oil can be wiped over the dam to act as a separator between the dam and the acrylic. If this is unavailable, the patient's saliva can be used. When the cement reaches a putty consistency, trim the surplus, wait for it to set, then wash around the abutment margin, remove the rubber dam, vigorously wash under the flap, and use the suction tip to remove the last remnants of cement.

If the inclinations of the abutments are too great to be fully adjusted at this stage, section the bridge and cement the sectioned bridge, splint the parts with polymethylacrylate resin in the mouth, and polish them.

Alternatively, the rigid plastic rings can be cemented onto the unparalleled abutments and then prepared and paralleled. The gutter in the provisional bridge can be filled by cold cure acrylic, and the hybrid bridge can be cemented onto the rigid plastic rings. The advantages of this approach are that prefabricated finishing margins are more accurate and that adjusting acrylic is much easier than adjusting metal. The disadvantage is that the preprepared gutter now needs to be more significant.

If the prefabricated rigid plastic rings do not allow the bridge to be placed in position, do not place the rigid plastic ring and then attempt to reline close to the finishing line of the abutments. Because acrylic shrinks, the internal layers of the bridge need to be removed, but a minimum of 1 mm of the finishing margin of the bridge or the provisional crown should be left intact.

The dentist should accept that perfect finishing margins of the abutments will not be achieved at this stage, and the clinical problems encountered should be documented in the patient's file. How these problems can be overcome will be discussed later. Due to the time limitation (e.g., patient's run-down), the polymethacrylic resin can be used inside the gutter or the prepared cavity, and when the consistency becomes putty-like, it is inserted in the mouth and just left as it is. Immediately remove the excess and leave it to be polymerised. Usually, due to contraction, it cannot be removed and is stable; leave it and review it every two weeks. Because it has not been isolated, the saliva will act as a cooling agent and, if any doubt, cool it with irrigation during the polymerisation. Occlusion should be off by 1mm unless more than three abutments are splinted. The patient should be reminded not to chew hard food in all circumstances. It is important to note that the bridge may need to be cut out to remove it.

• ON THE DAY OF SURGERY, IMMEDIATELY AFTER SUTURING THE MUCOSA

When there is uncertainty over the primary stability of one of the one-piece or immediate load implants, the dentist prefers to minimise physical interference. The dentist sutures the mucosa before splinting the abutments by placing the rigid plastic rings over the abutments and adding zinc phosphate cement. Remove the excess from the finishing margin with a dental probe and irrigate. After suturing, splint the rigid plastic rings with composite or acrylic, shape them, and polish them. If composite is used, it is preferred to use flow composite first to splint the abutments immediately with minimum manipulation and then use composite; macro fill composite is preferred. If controlling moisture is difficult due to saliva or bleeding, splinting with cold-cure acrylic resin is preferred as the contraction of the resin helps adhere to rigid plastic rings or abutments.

• ONE TO TWO WEEKS AFTER IMPLANT PLACEMENT

If, for any reason, splinting is not convenient at the surgery visit, wait for two weeks for the removal of sutures, take an impression for a provisional bridge to be made, and then cement. A flow composite can be used between the sessions to splint the implants. It is important to remember that the newly inserted implant must be protected from external forces as much as

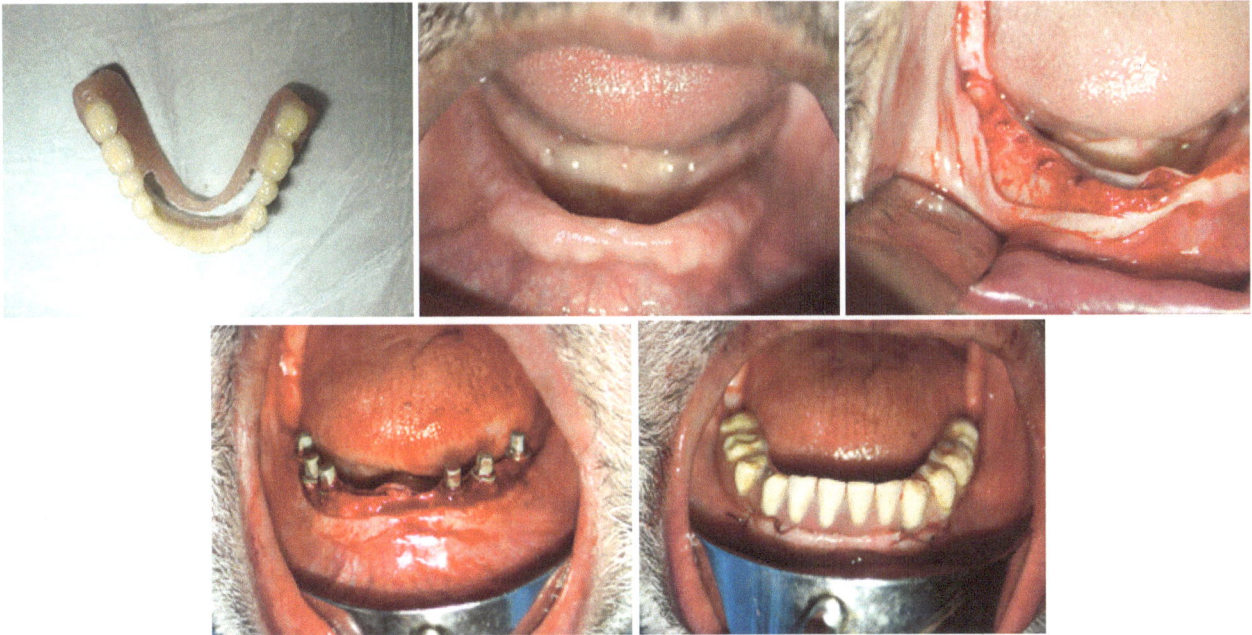

Figure 1.25 Prior to the surgery, the denture is adjusted, and after implant placement, the denture is relined with autopoly-mersing acrylic resin (PMMA) and cemented with zinc phosphate cement. Before suturing, the cement remnant is removed using a sharp excavator, and the mucosa is sutured after rinsing under the flap.

Any physical interference is unwelcome. It follows that if abutment undercuts deny an acceptable path of insertion, they need to be dealt with by the laboratory rather than the surgeon. Thus, laboratory personnel must handle significant or moderate undercuts. If undercuts are too large, the laboratory reshapes the cast, making a jig for the surgeon to use – unwelcome though it may be.

Remember, the provisional bridge's finishing margin is essential, so the laboratory must use a spacer of 0.3mm from the finishing margin for a maximum distance of 1mm. From that point on, the acrylic can be happily removed. The dentist controls the bridge, and if more retention is needed, the dentist can add acrylic resin inside the provisional prosthesis, even though a thick zinc phosphate cement usually provides the retention.

Intra-oral welding:

Intra-oral welding is another option for splinting. The abutments can be splinted directly, or prefabricated titanium abutments or telescopic attachments can be welded to a 1-2 mm titanium bar. If it is welded to titanium abutments or telescopic attachment, take a pickup impression after welding. Before the pickup impression, ensure the titanium frame comes off the abutments. If needed, the abutments should be prepared.

After the pickup impression, the laboratory adds acrylic or composite for aesthetics where necessary. The provisional bridge can be cemented. Use Vaseline on the abutments and inside the titanium frames prior to cementation. Some dentists prefer to add Vaseline to the cement. If removing the provisional metal-based bridge with a crown remover is complex, the dentist may have to cut the bridge into sections for the final impression. That said, it is a rigid and reliable splint.

This method is time-consuming and expensive, but it is recommended for patients with heavily-attritted natural teeth and masticatory solid muscles when the dentist is unsure if they will respect the post-operative instruction regarding not chewing hard food.

The author has experience using it as an inter-maxillary fixation after orthognathic surgery.

• AFTER OSSEOINTEGRATION

Splinting of multiple unit implant-retained components must be considered, especially when implants are flared because of bone configuration, aesthetic needs or the poor quality bone on of the regions (e.g. upper molars); this is more frequent in the maxillary arch.

42

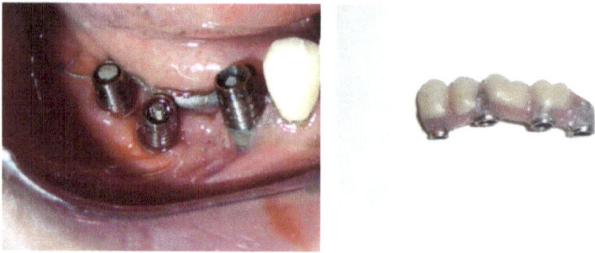

Figure 1.26 Left: the titanium wire is welded to the titanium abutment; right: acrylic or composite can be added. However, that means the splint will be cemented to the abutment instead of being delivered on the same day and splinted to the vulnerable implants.

ing an abnormality is crucial, as the dentist can get a second opinion from a dental radiologist regarding the diagnosis. In this chapter, we will review the necessary anatomic landmarks. Practice makes perfect, as there are normal variations.

This section provides a very brief overview of CBCT reading. In the UK, dentists must complete a specialised CBCT course to take and interpret CBCT scans. The course ensures that dentists are proficient in understanding the complex anatomical details and nuances captured by CBCT imaging. Proper training is essential to diagnose and plan treatments accurately, ensuring patient safety and optimal outcomes.

1.10. Dental X-ray landmarks

Dental X-rays are like a road map in dental implant treatment, used during planning, treatment and after the dental prosthesis delivery. Identifying the anatomical landmarks and recognis

Periapical:

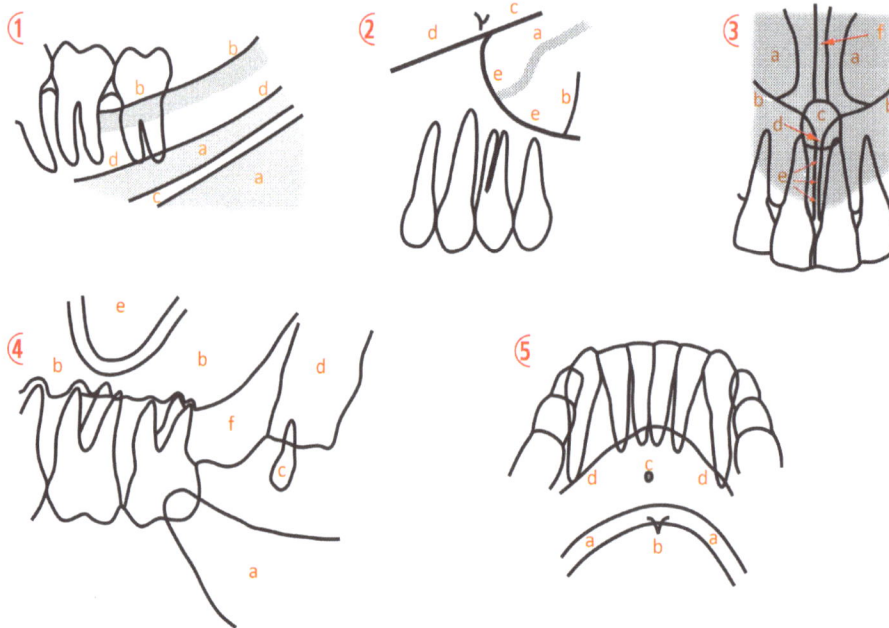

Figure 1.27a Periapical landmarks of the periapical x-rays are upper anterior, upper mid posterior, upper posterior, lower anterior, and lower posterior, respectively.

View 1, Posterior Mandible: a) Mandibular fossae, b) External oblique ridge, c) Cortical margins of inferior Dental Canal, d) Mylohyoid line.

View 2, Maxillary Canine: a) Nutrient canal, b) a septum in the floor of the maxillary sinus, c) medial wall of the maxillary sinus, d) floor of the nose, e) floor of the maxillary sinus.

View 3, Anterior Maxillae: a) inferior concha, b) floor of the nose, c) incisive foramen, d) anterior nasal spine, e) mid-palatal suture, shade) shadow of the nose).

View 4, Posterior Maxillae: a) Coronoid process, b) Floor of the antrum, c) Pterygoid hamulus, d) Lateral Pterygoid plate, e) Zygomatic buttress, f) Tuberosity.

View 5, Anterior Mandible: a) Cortex of lower of the mandible, b) Genial Tubercle, c) Lingual foramen, d) Mental ridge.

DPT:

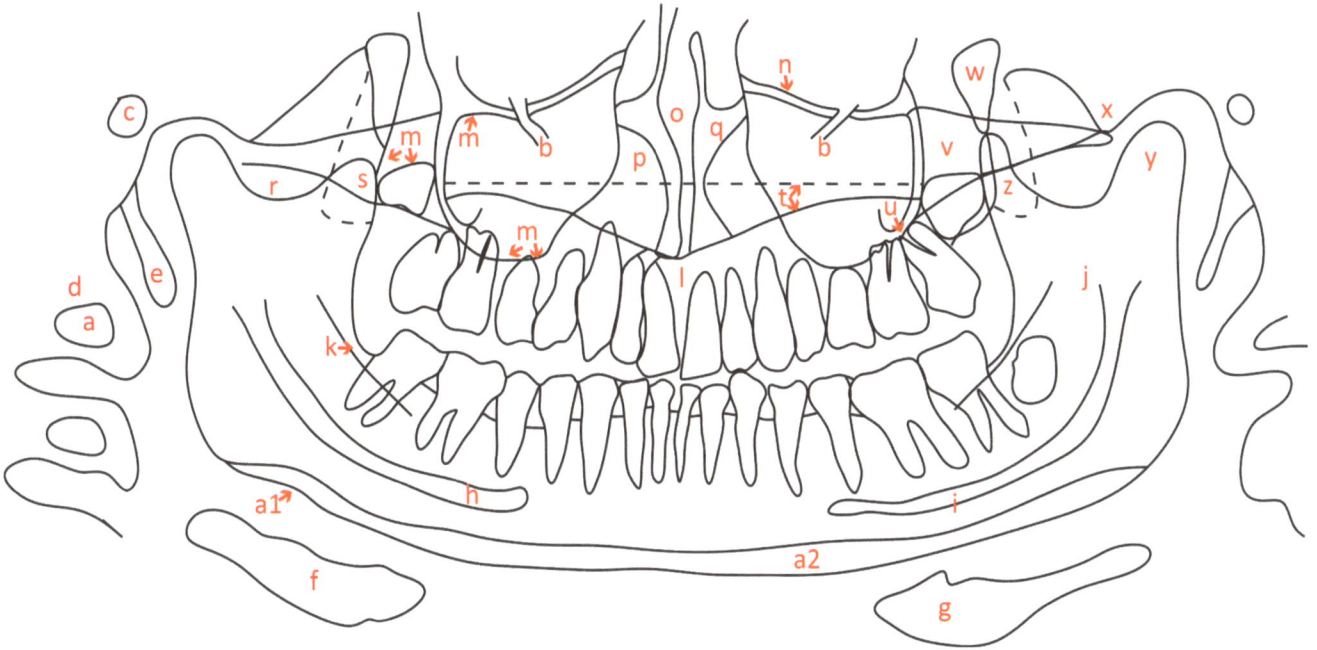

Figure 1.27b DPT radiopacities landmarks.

a) Foramen transversarium, a1) Antegonial notch, a2) Lateral border of the mandible (cortex), b)Infra-orbital canal, c) External auditory meatus), d) Cervical vertebra Infra-orbital rim, e) Styloid process, f&g) Hyoid bone, h) Mental foramen i) Inferior dental canal, j) Mandibular foramen, k) External oblique line, l) Anterior nasal spine m) maxillary sinus walls, n) infraorbital rim, o) Nasal septum p) Inferior concha q) Nasal cavity, r) Sigmoid notch, u) Zygomatic buttress, v) Zygomatic arch, x) Articular eminence, w) Pterygo-maxillary fissure, y) Mandibular condyle, z) Lateral pterygoid plate.

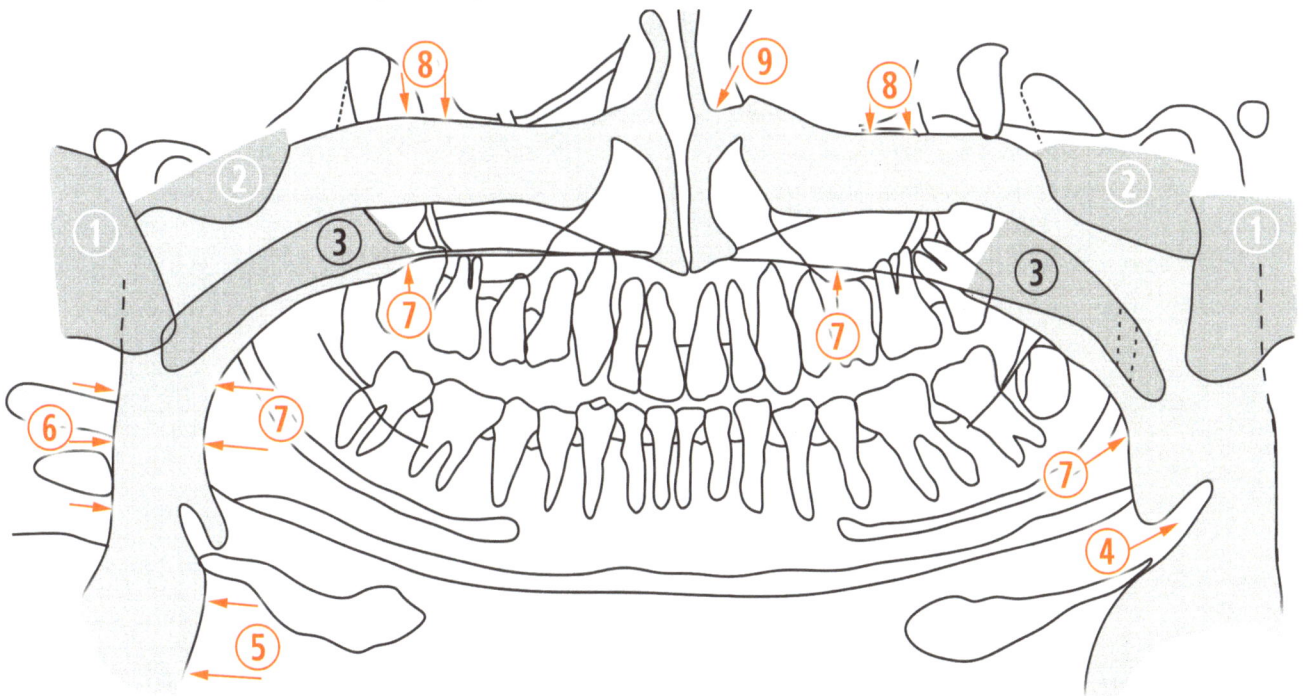

Figure 1.27c DPT radiolucency landmarks.

1) ear lobe, 2) adenoid, 3) soft palate, 4) epiglottis, 5) anterior wall of the oropharynx, 6) posterior wall of the oropharynx, 7) dorsum of the tongue, 8) Air in the nasopharynx, 9) Air in the nasal cavity.

44

CBCT:

Outside showing the ridge morphology, the landmarks need to be familiarised.

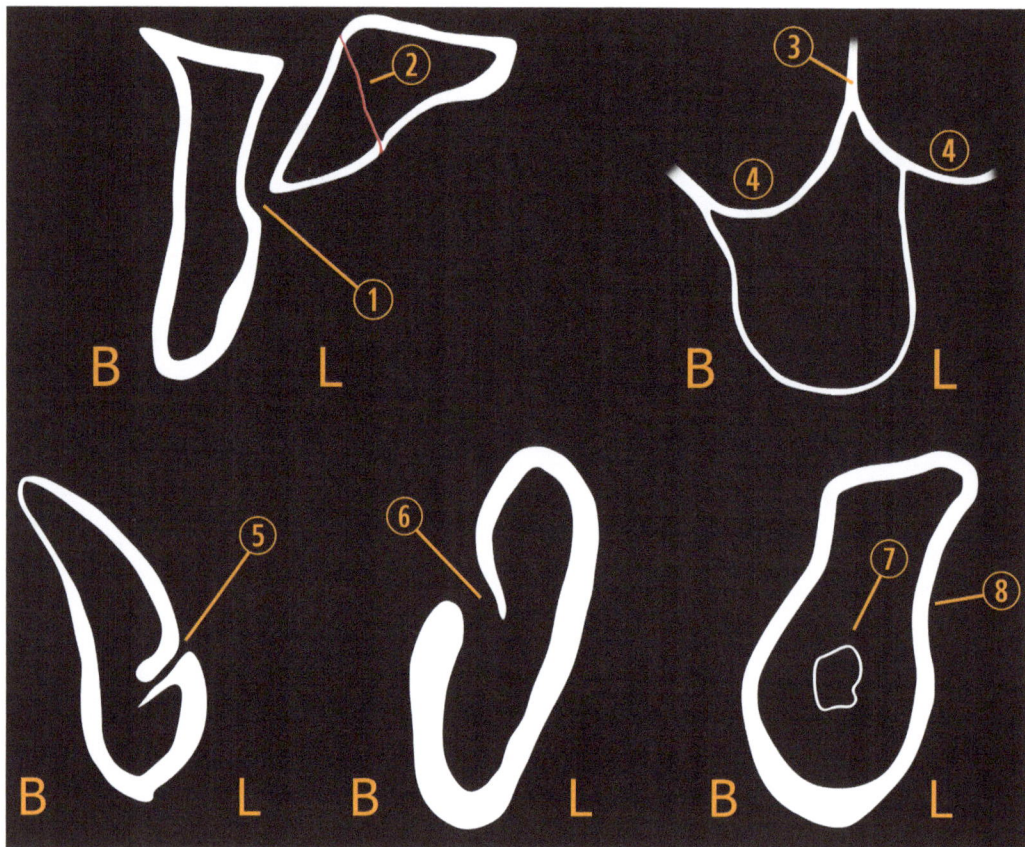

Figure 1.27d CBCT radioopacity landmarks.

Upper left, anterior maxillae: The floor of the nasal fossa, Nasopalatine canal (1), labial concavity, sinus septa in the floor of the sinus, accessory bone channels within the anterior maxillae (2)

Upper right, posterior maxillae: The sinus (4) and sinus floor, sinus septa (3), anterior recess, and sinus health, such as the absence of sinus membrane thickening.

Lower left, anterior mandible: Bone structure, labial and lingual cortical plates, Mandibular lingual canal (5)

Lower middle, premolar region: Mental foramen (6)

Lower right, posterior mandible: Inferior Dental canal (7), submandibular gland fossae (8).

References:

1. Nowjack-Raymer RE, Sheiham A. Number of natural teeth, diet, and nutritional status in US adults. J Dent Res 2007;86:1171-5.

2. Ikebe K: Significance of oral function for dietary intakes in old people. jNutr Sci Vitaminol 2015;61:S74-5.

3. Jacobs R, Wu C-H, Goosen K, van Loven K, van Steenberghe D: Perceptual changes in the anterior maxillae after placement of endosseous implants - Clin.Implant Dent. Relat. Res. 2001:3:148-155.

4. Jacobs R, van Steenberghe D: Role of periodontal ligament receptors in the tactile function of teeth: a review - J Periodontal Res 1994: 29: 153-167).

5. Jacobs R, Wu C-H, Goosen K, van Loven K, van Steenberghe D: Perceptual changes in the anterior maxillae after placement of endosseous implants - Clin.Implant Dent. Relat. Res. 2001:3:148-155.

6. Proske U, Schaible HG, Schmidt RF. Joint receptors and kinaesthesia. 9] Exp Brain Res. 1988;72;219-24.

7. Jacobs R, Vansteenberghe D. From osseoperception to implant-mediated sensory-motor interactions and related clinical implications. J Oral Rehabil. 2006;33:282–92.

8. Lambrechts K, Creemers J, van Steenberghe D: Morphology of neural endings in human periodontal ligament, an electron microscopy study - J Periodontal Res 1992: 27: 191-196.

9. Linden RW, Scott BJ: The effect of tooth extraction on periodontal ligament mechanoreceptors represented in the mesencephalic nucleus of the cat - Arch. Oral Biol. 1989:34:937-941.

10. dos Santos Corpas L, Lambrichts I, Quirynen M, Collaert B, Politis C, Vrielinck L. Peri-implant bone innervation: Histological findings in humans. Eur J Oral Implantol. 2014;7(3):283–92.

11. Bhatngar VM, Karani JT, Khanna A, Badwaik P, Pai A: Osseoperception: An implant mediated sensory motor control- A review. J Clin and Diagnostic Res 2015,9(9):18-20.

12. El Sheikh AM, Hobkirk JA, Howell PGT, Gilthorp MS; Changes in passive tactile sensibility associated with dental implants:2003:18:266-272.

13. Mason R. Studies on oral perception involving subjects with alterations in anatomy and physiology. In: Bosma JF (ed) Second symposium on oral sensation and perception. Charles C Thomas Publisher, Springfield, III; 1967: pp 295–301.

14. Bou Serhal S, van Steenberghe D, Oral stereognosis: a review of the literature -Clin Oral Investig. 1998:2:3-10.

15. Bouvier M, Hylander: Effect of bone strain on cortical bone structure in macques (Macaca mulatta). J Morphol 1981;167(1):1-12.

16. Eriksson RA, Albrektsson T. The effect of heat on bone regeneration: An experimental study in rabbit using the bone growth chamber. J Oral Maxillofac Surg 1984;42:705–711.

17. Eriksson, R.A., Adell, R., 1986. Temperatures during drilling for the placement of implants using the Osseo integration technique. J. Oral Maxillofac. Surg. 44, 4–7.

18. Albrektsson T, Sennerby L: Direct bone anchorage or oral implants: Clinical and experimental considerations of the concept of osseointegration. Int J Prosthodont 1990; 3:30-41.

19. Eid K, Zelicof S, Perona BP, Sledge CB, Glowacki J: Tissue reaction to particles of bone-substitute materials in intraosseous and heterotopic sites in rats: discrimination of osteoinduction, osteocompatibility, and inflammation. J Orthop Res, 19 (5) (2001), 962-969.

20. Sennerby L, Ericson LE, Thomsen P, Lekhom U and Astrand P. Structure of the bone-titanium interface in retrieved clinical oral implants. Clin Oral Impl 1991;2:103-11.

21. Tehemar SH: Factors affecting heat generation during implant site preparation: A review of biologic observations and future considerations. Int J Oral Maxillofac Implants 1991;14:127-136.

22. Aspenberg P, Goodman S, Toksvig-Larsen S, Ryd L, Albrektsson T: Intermittent micromotion inhibits bone ingrowth. Acta Orthop Scand 1992; 63:141-45.

23. Osborn JF, Willich P, Meenen N: The release of titanium into human bone from a titanium implant coated with plasma-sprayed titanium. In Heimke G, Soltesz V, Lee AJC (eds). Clinical implant materials: Advances in Biomaterials, Amsterdam: Elsevier, 1990;9:75-80.

24. Schliephake H, Reiss G, Urban R, Neukan FW, Guckel S: Metal release from titanium fixtures during placement in the mandible: An experimental study. Int J Oral Maxillofac Implants 1993;8:502-1.

25. Ghalegolab K, Kashani IR, Namjou I, Namjoy Nik S. Evaluation of the effect of adipose tissue-derived stem cells on the quality of bone healing around implants. Connect Tissue Res 2016,57(1);10-19.

26. Namjoynik A, Islam MA, Islam M. Evaluating the efficacy of human dental pulp stem cells and scaffold combination for bone regeneration in animal models: a systematic review and meta-analysis. Stem Cell Res Ther, 2023 May 15;14(1):132.

27. Jaffin RA, Berman CL: The excessive loss of Branemark fixtures in type IV bone: A five year analysis. J Periodontol 1991; 62:2-4.

28. Albrektsson T, Sennerby L: Direct bone anchorage or oral implants: Clinical and experimental considerations of the concept of osseointegration. Int J Prosthodont 1990; 3:30-41.

29. von Wowern N: Bone mineral content of mandibles: Normal reference values-rate of age-related bone loss. Calcif Tissue Int 1988;43:193-8.

30. Baxter KC: Relationship of osteoporosis to excessive residual ridge resorption. J Prosthet Dent 1981;46:123-5.

31. Kribbs PJ, Chesnut CH III, Ott SM, Kilcoyne RF: Relationships between

mandibular and skeletal bone in population of normal women. J Prosthet Dent 1990; 63:86-9.

32. Chen H, Liu N, Xu X, Qu X, Lu E. Smoking, radiotherapy, diabetes and osteoporosis as risk factors for dental implant failure: a meta-analysis. PLoS One. 2013 Aug 5.

33. Moghaddam A, Zimmermann G, Hammer K. Cigarette smoking influences the clinical and occupational outcomes of patients with tibial shaft fractures. Injury 2011;42:1435–1442.

34. Chen F, Smoking and bony union after ulna-shortening osteotomy. Am J Orthop. 2001 Jun;30(6):486-9.

35. Al-Hadithy N, Sewell MD, Bhavikatti M, Gikas PD. The effect of smoking on fracture healing and on various orthopaedic procedures. Acta Orthop Belg 2012;78:285–290.

36. Patel, R A; Wilson, R F; Patel, P A; Palmer, R M. The effect of smoking on bone healing: A systematic review Bone & joint research, 2013, Vol.2(6), pp.102-11

37. Vervaeke S, Collaert B, Cosyn J, Deschepper E, De Bruyn H: A multifactorial analysis to identify predictors of implant failure and peri-implant bone loss. Clin Implant Dent Relat Res 2015 Jan;17 Suppl 1:e298-307.

38. Ralho A, Coelho A, Ribeiro M, Paula A, Amaro I, Sousa J, Marto C, Ferreira M, Carrilho E. Effects of Electronic Cigarettes on Oral Cavity: A Systematic Review. J Evid Based Dent Pract. 2019 Dec;19(4):101318.

39. Rouabhia M, Alanazi H, Park HJ, Gonçalves RB Cigarette Smoke and E-Cigarette Vapor Dysregulate Osteoblast Interaction With Titanium Dental Implant Surface. . J Oral Implantol. 2019 Feb;45(1):2-11.

40. Souza JG, Bianchini M, Ferreira C. Relationship between smoking and bleeding on probing. J Oral Implantol 2010 .

41. Strietzel FP, Reichart PA, Kale A, Kulkarni M, Wegner B, Küchler I.Smoking interferes with the prognosis of dental implant treatment: a systematic review and meta-analysis. J Clin Periodontol. 2007 Jun;34(6):523-44.

42. Alomarni AN, Hermann JS, Jones DA, Buser D , Schoolfiled, J, Cochran ML: The effect of a machined collar on coronal hard tissue around titanium implants: A radiographic study in the canine mandible. Int J Oral Maxillofac Implants 2005; 20(5) 677-686.

43. Ricomini Filho AP, Fernades FS, Straioto FG, da Silva WJ, Del Bel Cury AA. Preload loss and bacterial penetration on different implant-abutment connection system. Braz Dent J 2010, 21(2):123-9.

44. Mangano C, Mangano F, Piatteli A, Lezzi G, Mangano A, Lacolla L: Prospective clinical evaluation of 1920 Morse taper connection implant: results after four years of functional loading. Clin Oral Implants Res 2009;20:254-61.

45. Deborah Meleo, Luigi Baggi, Michele Di Girolamo: Fixture-abutment connection surface and micro-gap measurements by 3D micro-tomographic technique analysis. Ann Ist Super Sanità 2012 | Vol. 48, No. 1: 53-58.

46. Dohan Ehrenfest DM, Coelho PG, Kang BS, Sul YT, Albrektsson T.Classification of osseointegrated implant surfaces: materials, chemistry and topography. Trends Biotechnol. 2010 ;28(4):198-206.

47. Wennerberg A, Albrektsson T, Albrektsson B, Krol JJ. Histomorphometric and removal torque study of screw-shaped titanium implants with three different surface topographies. Clin Oral Implant Res 1996;6:24–30.

48. Becker W, Becker BE, Ricci A, Bahat O, Rosenberg E, Rose LF. A prospective multicenter clinical trial comparing one- and two-stage titanium screw-shaped fixtures with one-stage plasma-sprayed solid-screw fixtures. Clin Implant Dent Relat Res.

49. Hansson S, Norton M. The relation between surface roughness and interfacial shear strength for bone-anchored implants. A mathematical model. JBiomech 1999;32:829–36.

50. Esposito M, Coulthard P, Thomsen P, Worthington HV. Interventions for replacing missing teeth: different types of dental implants. Cochrane Database Syst Rev2005;25:CD003815.

51. Perren SM. Evolution of the internal fixation of long bone fractures. The scientific basis of biological interface fixation: choosing a new balance between stability and biology. Journal of Bone and Joint Surgery (Br) 2002;84:1093–110.

52. Pilliar RM, Lee JM, Maniatopoulos C. Observations on the effect of movement on bone ingrowth into porous-surfaced implants. Clin Orthop Relat Res 1986; (208): 108–113.

53. Brunski JB. Avoid pitfalls of overloading and micromotion of intraosseous implants (interview). Dental Implantology Update 1993;4:77–81.

54. Family R, Solat-Hashjin M, Namjoy Nik S, Nemati A. Surface modification for titanium implants by hydroxyapatite nanocomposite. Caspian J Intern Med 2012,3:460-5.

55. Family R, Solat-Hashjin M, Namjoy Nik S, Nemati A. Protection of titanium metal by nanohydroxyapatite coating with zirconia and alumina second phases. Protection of Metals and Physical Chemistry of Surfaces. 2012, 48:688-91.

56. Shalabi MM, Gortemaker A, Van't Hof MA, Jansen JA, Creugers NH. Implant surface roughness and bone healing: a systematic review.J Dent Res. 2006 Jun;85(6):496-500. Review. Erratum in: J Dent Res. 2006.

57. Shalabi MM, Wolke JG, de Ruijter AJ, Jansen JA. A mechanical evaluation of implants placed with different surgical techniques into the trabecular bone of goats. J Oral Implantol. 2007;33(2):51-8.

58. Pillar RM, Lee JM, Maniatopoulos C. Observations on the effect of movement on bone ingrowth into porous-surfaced implants. Clin Orthop Relat Res 1986; 208:108-113.

59. Perona PG, Lawrence J, Paprosky WG: Acetabular micromotion as a measure of initial implant stability in primary hip arthroplasty. An in vitro com-

parison of different methods of initial acetabular component fixation. J Arthroplasty 1992; 7(4):537-547.

60. Shan-Shan Gao, Ya-Rong Zhang, Zhuo-Li Zhu and Hai-Yang Yu. Micromotions and combined damages at the dental implant/bone interface. International Journal of Oral Science (2012) 4, 182–188.

61. Uhthoff HK, Germain JP. The reversal of tissue differentiation around screws. Clin Orthop Relat Res) 1977; (123): 248–252.

62. Akagawa Y, Hashimoto M, Kondo N. Initial bone-implant interfaces of submergible and submergible endosseous single-crystal sapphire implants. J Prosthet Dent 1986; 55(1): 96–100

63. Sagara M, Akagawa Y, Nikai H. The effects of early occlusal loading on one-stage titanium alloy implants in beagle dogs: a pilot study. J Prosthet Dent 1993; 69(3): 281–288

64. Pilliar RM, Lee JM, Maniatopoulos C. Observations on the effect of movement on bone ingrowth into porous-surfaced implants. Clin Orthop Relat Res 1986; (208): 108–113.

65. Brunski JB. Avoid pitfalls of overloading and micromotion of intraosseous implants. Dent Implant Update 1993; 4(10): 77–81.

66. Huang YM, Chou IC, Jiang CP, Wu YS, Lee SY: Finite element analysis of dental implant neck effects on primary stability and osseointegration in a type IV bone mandible, Bio-Medical materials and engineering. 2013;24(1)1407-15.

67. Berglundh T, Abrahamsson I, Lang NP, Lindhe J. De novo alveolar bone formation adjacent to endosseous implants. Clin Oral Implants Res 2003;14:251-62.

68. Franchi M, Fini M, Martini D, Orsini E, Leonardi L,Ruggeri A, Giavaresi G, Ottani V. Biological fixation of endosseous implants. Micron 2005;36:665-71.

69. Futami T, Fujii N, Ohnishi H, Taguchi N, Kusakari H, Ohshima H, Maeda T. Tissue response to titanium implants in the rat maxilla: ultrastructural and histochemical observations of the bone-titanium interface. J Periodontol 2000;71:287-98.

70. Sandborn PM, Cook SD, Spires WP, Kester MA. Tissue response to porous-coated implants lacking initial bone apposition. J Arthroplasty 1988;3:337-46.

71. Germanier Y, Tosatti S, Broggini N, Textor M, Buser D. Enhanced bone apposition around biofunctionalized sandblasted and acid-etched titanium implant surfaces. A histomorphometric study in miniature pigs. Clin Oral Implants Res 2006;17:251–7.

72. Mendonça G, Mendonça D, . Arago F, Cooper L: Advancing dental implant surface technology – From microntoNanotopography, Biomaterials 29 (2008) 3822–3835.

73. Current issue Forum. Based on what is currently known from scientific investigation and published clinical experience, what should a contemporary definition of osseointegration include? Int J Oral Maxillofac Implants 1992;3:416-9.

74. MG Newman and TF Fleming, period ontal considerations of implant and implant associated microbiota, J Dent Educ 52(1988)pp 737-744.

75. T Bergulundh, J. Lindhe, J. Ericsson ?, C.P. Marinelle, B. Liljenberg and P. Thomsen, The soft tissue barrier at implant and teeth, Clin Oral Implants Res2(1991),pp81-90.

76. D. Buser, HP Weber, K. Donath, JP Fiorellini, D.W. Paquette and R.C. Williams, Soft tissue reactions to non-submerged unloaded titanium implants in beagle dogs, J Periodontol 63(1992), pp.225-235.

77. Abrahmsson I, Berglundh T and Lindhe J: Soft tissue response to plaque formation at different implant systems. A comparative study in the dog, Clin Oral Implants Res 9(1988),pp73-79.

78. Quaranta A, Piattelli A, Scarano A, Quaranta M, Pompa G, Iezzi G. Light-microscopic evaluation of the dimensions of peri-implant mucosa around immediately loaded and submerged titanium implants in monkeys. J Periodontol 2008 Sep;79(9):1697-703.

79. Hermann JS, Buser D, Schenk RK, Higginbottom FL, Cochran DL. Clin Oral Implants Res. 2000 Feb;11(1):1-11.

80. Broggini N, McManus LM, Hermann JS, Medina RS, Oates TO, Schenk RK, Buser D, Mellonig JT, and Cochran DL: Persistent Acute Inflammation at the Implant-Abutment Interface, Dent Res 2003, 82(3): 232-237.

81. F.F. Todescan, F.E. Pustiglioni, A.V. Imbronitio, T. Albrektsson and M. Giuso, Influence of the microgap in the peri-implant hard and soft tissues: a histomorphometric study in dogs, Int J Oral Maxillfac Implants 17(2002). pp.467-472.

82. Bouri A Jr, Bissada N, Al-Zahrani MS, Faddoul F, Nouneh I. Width of keratinized gingiva and the health status of the supporting tissues around dental implants. Int J Oral Maxillofac Implants. 2008 Mar-Apr;23(2):323-6.

83. Linkevicius T, Apse P. Biologic width around implants. An evidence-based review. Stomatologija. 2008;10(1):27-35.

84. Bengazi F, Wennstrom JL and U. Lekhom U: Recession of the soft tissue margin at oral implants. A 2-year longitudinal prospective study, Clin Oral Implants Res 7(1996), 303-310.

85. Oates TW, West J, Jones J, Kaiser D and Cochran DL: long-term changes in soft tissue height on the facial surface of dental implants, Implant Dent 11(2002), pp. 272-279.

86. Small P and Tarnow D: Gingival recession around implants: a 1-year longitudinal prospective study, Int J Oral Maxillofac Implants 15(2000), 527-532.

87. Tarnow D, Elian N, Fletcher P, Froum S, Magner A and Cho SC: Vertical distance from the crest of bone to the height of the interproximal papilla between adjacent implants. J Periodontol 74 (2003),pp. 17895-1788.

88. Cho SS, Wallace SS, The effect of inter-implant distance on the height of

inter-implant bone crest, J Periodontol 71(2000), 546-549.

89. Chaytor DV, Zarb GA, Schmitt AW and Lewis DW: The longitudinal effectiveness of osseointegrated implants The Toronto study: bone level changes, Int J Periodontics Restorative Dent 11 (1991),112-125.

90. 1a. Lauer G, Wiedmann-Al-Ahmad M, Otten JE, Hübner U, Schmelzeisen R, Schilli W. The titanium surface texture effects adherence and growth of human gingival keratinocytes and human maxillar osteoblast-like cells in vitro. Biomaterials. 2001 Oct;22(20):2799-809.

91. Abrahamsson I, Zitzmann NU, Berglundh T, Linder E, Wennerberg A, Lindhe J. The mucosal attachment to titanium implants with different surface characteristics: an experimental study in dogs. J Clin Periodontol. 2002 May;29(5):448-55.

92. .Schierano G, Ramieri G, Cortese M, Aimetti M, Preti G. Organization of the connective tissue barrier around long-term loaded implant abutments in man. Clin Oral Implants Res. 2002 Oct;13(5):460-4.

93. Kim JI, Choi BH, Li J, Xuan F, Jeong SM. Blood vessels of the peri-implant mucosa: a comparison between flap and flapless procedures. Oral Surg Oral Med Oral Pathol Oral Radiol Endod. 2009;107(4):508-12.

94. Hermann JS, Buser D, Schenk RK, Schoolfield JD, Cochran DL: Biologic Width around one- and two-piece titanium implants. Clin Oral Implants Res. 2001 Dec;12(6):559-71.

95. Broggini N, McManus LM, Hermann JS, Medina RS, Oates TO, Schenk RK, Buser D, Mellonig JT, and Cochran DL: Persistent Acute Inflammation at the Implant-Abutment Interface, Dent Res 2003, 82(3): 232-237.

96. Kuppusamy M , Watanabe H,nd Kasugai S, Kuroda S. Implant Dent. 2015 Dec;24(6):730-4. Effects of Abutment Removal and Reconnection on Inflammatory Cytokine Production Around Dental Implants.

97. Quirynen M, Bollen CM, Wyssen H, van Steenberghe D: Microbial penetration along the implant components of the Branemark system. An in vitro study. Clini Oral Implant Res 1994;5:239-244.

98. Subramani K, Jung RE, Molenberg A, Hammerle CHF: Biofilm on dental implants: A review of the literature. Int J Oral Max Fac Impl 2009, 616-626.

99. João Paulo da Silva-Neto; Marcel Santana Prudente; Thiago de Almeida Prado Naves Carneiro; Mauro Antônio de Arruda Nóbilo: Micro-leakage at the implant-abutment interface with different tightening torques in vitro. J Appl Oral Sci 2012;20(5):581-7.

100. Hermann JS, Schoolfield JD, Schenk RK, Buser D, Cochran DL. J Periodontol. 2001 Oct;72(10):1372-83. Influence of the size of the microgap on crestal bone changes around titanium implants. A histometric evaluation of unloaded non-submerged implants in the canine mandible.

101. Mascarell S, Citterio H, Le Roux E, Berdal A, Lescaille G, Friedlander L. Oral prosthetic rehabilitation in patients with Epidermolysis Bullosa Hereditaria: a systematic review. Int J Prosthodont . 2023 Dec 14;0(0):1-38.

102. Enhos S, Duran I, Erden S, Buyukbas S: Relationship Between Iron-Deficiency Anemia and Periodontal Status in Female Patients. Journal of Periodontology 2009. 80(11):1750-5.

103. Koo S, Koning Jr B, Mizusaki CI, Allgrini Jr S, Yoshimoto M, Carbonari MJ: Effect of alcohol consumption on osseointegration of titanium implants in rabbits. Implant Dentistry 2004;13:232-7.

104. Kammerer, P.W., Frerich, B., Liese, J., Schiegnitz, E. & Al-Nawas, B: Oral surgery during therapy with anticoagulants – a systematic review. Clin Oral Invest, 2015 19: 171–180.

105. Johnson-Leong, C. & Rada, R.E: The use of low-molecular-weight heparins in outpatient oral surgery for patients receiving anticoagulation therapy. Journal of the American Dental Association 2002, 133: 1083–1087.

106. Bailey, B.M. & Fordyce, A.M: Warfarin anticoagulant therapy. BDJ 1984, 156: 310.

107. Öztürk K, Kuzu TM, Ayrıkçil S, Gürgan CA, Önder GO, Yay A. Effect of systemic atorvastatin on bone regeneration in critical-sized defects in hyperlipidemia: an experimental study. Int J Implant Dent. 2023 Dec 14;9(1):50.

108. Wahl MJ, Pinto A, Kilham J, Lalla RV: Dental surgery in anticoagulated patients–stop the interruption. Oral Surg. Oral Med. Oral Path.Oral Rad. 2015, 119:136–157.

109. Gomez-Moreno G, Aguilar-Salvatierra A, Fernandez-Cejas E, Delgado-Ruiz RA, Markovic A., Calvo-Guirado JL: Dental implant surgery in patients in treatment with the anticoagulant oral rivaroxaban. Clinical Oral Implants Research 2016, 27(6):730-3

110. Clemm R, Neukam FW, Rusche B, Bauersachs A, Musazada S, Schmitt CM: Management of anticoagulated patients in implant therapy. A clinical comparative study. Clin Oral Impl Res 2016, 27(10), 1274-82.

111. Napenas JJ, Hong CH, Brennan MT, Furney SL, Fox PC, Lockhart PB: The frequency of bleeding complications after invasive dental treatment in patients receiving single and dual antiplatelet therapy. JADA 2009;140:690-5.

112. Scully C. Medical problems in dentistry. 7th ed. London: Churchill Livingstone;2014.

113. Alshami A, Romero C, Avila A, Varon J: Management of hypertensive crises in the elderly. J Geriatr Cardiol. 2018 Jul; 15(7): 504–512.

114. https://www.sdcep.org.uk/media/qvpj2kfb/sdcep-antibiotic-prophylaxis-implementation-advice.pdf

115. Larvin H, Kang J, Aggarwal VR, Pavitt S, Wu J. Risk of incident cardiovascular disease in people with periodontal disease: A systematic review and meta-analysis. Clin Exp Dent Res 2021 Feb;7(1):109-122.

116. Norowski PA Jr, Bumgardner JD Norowski PA Jr, Bumgardner JD . Biomaterial and antibiotic strategies for peri-implantitis: a review. .J Biomed Mater Res B Appl Biomater. 2009 Feb;88(2):530-43.

117. Sanz M, Marco Del Castillo A, Jepsen S, Gonzalez-Juanatey JR, D'Aiuto

F, Bouchard P, Chapple I, Dietrich T, Gotsman I, Graziani F, Herrera D, Loos B, Madianos P, Michel JB, Perel P, Pieske B, Shapira L, Shechter M, Tonetti M, Vlachopoulos C, Wimmer G. Periodontitis and cardiovascular diseases: Consensus report. J Clin Periodontol 2020 Mar;47(3):268-288.

118. Lipnick, Michael S Feiner, John R, Au, Paul BS Bernstein, Michael BS, Bickler, Philip E. The Accuracy of 6 Inexpensive Pulse Oximeters Not Cleared by the Food and Drug Administration: The Possible Global Public Health Implications. Anesthesia & Analgesia: August 2016 - Volume 123 - Issue 2 - p 338-345.

119. Sivakumar I, Arunachalam S, Choudhary S, Mahmoud-Buzayan M, Tawfiq O, Sharan J.: Do Highly Active Antiretroviral Therapy Drugs in the Management of HIV Patients Influence Success of Dental Implants? AIDS Rev. 2020;22(1):3-8.

120. Al-Hadithy N, Sewell MD, Bhavikatti M, Gikas PD. The effect of smoking on fracture healing and on various orthopaedic procedures. Acta Orthop Belg 2012;78:285–290.

121. Patel, RA, Wilson RF, Patel PA, Palmer, R M. The effect of smoking on bone healing: A systematic review Bone & joint research, 2013, Vol.2(6), pp.102-11.

122. Kang MH, Lee DK, Kim CW, Song IS. Clinical characteristics and recurrence-related factors of medication-related osteonecrosis of the jaw. Korean Assoc Oral Maxillofac Surg. 2018 Oct; 44(5): 225–231.

123. Advisory Task Force on Bisphosphonate-related Osteonecrosis of the jaw. American Association of Oral and Maxillofacial Surgeons. American Association of Oral and Maxillofacial Surgeons position paper on bisphosphonate-related osteonecrosis of the jaws. Journal of Oral and Maxillofacial Surgery 2007;65:369-76.

124. Landes CA, Kovas AF. Comparison of early loading of non-submerged ITI implants in irradiated and non-irradiated oral cancer patients. Clinical Oral Implants Research 2006;17:367-74.

125. Diz P, Scully C, Sanz M: Dental implants in the medically compromised patient. J Dentistry 2013 (41), 195-206.

126. https://www.addisonsdisease.org.uk/Handlers/Download.ashx?IDMF=26887766-029d-4728-9163-e4ce24eb34a7.

127. Fujimoto T, Nimi A, Saai T, Ueda M. Effects of steriod induced osteoporosis on osseointegration of titanium implants. Int J Oral Maxillofac Implants 1998;13:183-9.

128. Tawil G, Ypunan R, Azar P, Sleilati G. Conventional and advanced implant treatment in the type II diabetic patient: surgical protocol and long-term clinical results. Int J Oral Maxillofac Implants 2008;23:744-52.

129. Shu X, Fan Y, Lo ECM, Leung KCM. A systematic review and meta-analysis to evaluate the efficacy of denture adhesives. J Dent. 2021 May;108:103638. doi: 10.1016/j.jdent .

130. Oliveria MA, Gallottini M, Pallos D Maluf PS jablonka F Ortega JL. The success of endosseous implants in human immunodeficiency virus-positive patients receiving antiretroviral therapy: a pilot study. JADA 2011;142:1010-6.

131. Galindo-Moreno P, Fauri M, Avila-Ortiz G, Fernandez_barbero JE, Carbero-Leon A, Sanchez-Fernandez E. Influence of alcohol and tobacco habits on perio-implant marginal bone loss: a prospective study. Clinical Oral Implants Research 2005;16:579-86.

132. Pallasch T. Antiobiotic prophylaxis: problems in paradise. The Dental Clinics of North America 2003, 47: 665-79.

133. Leonhardt A, Renvert S, Dahlen G,. Microbial findings at failing implants. Clin Oral Implants Res 1999;10:339-345.

134. Harris LG, Richards PG. Staphylococcus aureus adhesion to different treated titanium surface. J Mat Sci Mat med 2004;15:311-314.

135. Dammling C, Gilmartin EM, Abramowicz S, Kinard B. Indications for Antibiotic Prophylaxis for Dentoalveolar Procedures. Dent Clin North Am 2024 Jan;68(1):99-111.

136. Esposito M, Cannizzaro G, Bozzali P: Efficacy of prophylactic antibiotics for dental implants: A multicenter placebo-controlled randomised clinical trial. Eur J Oral Implantol 1:23, 2008)

137. Binhamed A, Stoykewych A, Peterson L: Single preoperative dose versus long-term prophylactic antibiotic regimens in dental implant surgery. Int J Oral Maxillofac Implants 20:115,2005.

138. LaPorte DM, Waldman BJ, Mont MA, Hungerford DS. Infection associated with dental procedures in total hip arthroplasty. J Bone Joint Surg Br 1999;81:56-9.

139. Esposito M, Coulthard P, Oliver R: Antibiotics to prevent complications following dental treatment. Cochrane Database Rev 3: CD004152, 2003.

140. Matias de Assis G, Queiroz SIML, Germano AR. Systemic Use of Antibiotics in Dental Implant Surgeries in Immunocompetent Patients: A Blind Randomized Controlled Trial. Int J Oral Maxillofac Implants, 2023 Dec 12;38(6):1168-1174.

141. Veksler AE, Kayrouz GA, Newman MG. Reduction of salivary bacteria by pre-procedural rinses with chlorhexidine 0.12%. J Periodontol 1991,62:649-651.

142. Marx RE. Oral and Intravenous Bisphosphonate Induced Osteonecrosis of Jaws. History, Etiology, Prevention and Treatment. Quintessence Publishing Co. Inc. Hanover Park, IL 2007. P 84.

143. Prochaska, JO, Velicer WF. The transtheoretical model of health behavior change. Am J Health Promotion,1997;12:38-48.

144. Sivaraman K, Chopra A, Venkatesh SB. Clinical importance of medial mandibular flexure in oral rehabilitation: a review. J Oral Rehab 2016, 43(3),215-25.

145. Chou HY, Jagodnik JJ, Muftu S: Predictions of bone remodeling around

dental implant systems. J Biomech 2008, 48, 1365–1373.

146. Carter DR, Beaupre GS, Giori NJ, Helms JA. Mechanobiology of skeletal regeneration. Clin Orthop Relat Res 1998;355:S41–S55.

147. Halldin A, Jimbo R, Johansson CB, Wennerberg A, Jacobsson M, Albrektsson T, Hansson S: The effect of static bone strain on implant stability and bone remodeling. Bone 201, 49(4):783-9.

148. Andrade CL, Carvalho MA, Cury AA, Sotto-Maior BS: Biomechanical effect of prosthetic connection and implant body shape in low-quality bone of maxillary posterior single implant-supported restorations. Int J Oral Maxillofac Implants 2016;31:92-7.

149. Bishop NE, Höhn JC, Rothstock S, Damm NB, Morlock MM: The influence of bone damage on press-fit mechanics. J Biomechanics 2014(47):1472-1478.

150. Channer MA, Glisson RR, Seaber AV, Vail TP. Use of bone compaction in total knee arthroplasty. J Arthroplasty 1996;11: 743-9.

151. Chareancholvanich K, Bourgeault C, Schmidt AH. Invitro stability of cemented and cementless femoral stems with compaction. Clin Orthop 2002; 394:290-302.

152. 18: Kold S, Rhabek O, Toft M. Bone compaction enhances fixation of weight-bearing titanium implants. Clin Orthop Res 23(2005):824-30.

153. Noble PC, Alexander JW, Lindahl LJ, Yew DT, Granberry WM, Yullos HS. The anatomical basis of femoral component design. Clin Orthop 1988,235:148-65.

154. Hasan I, Bourauel C, Mundt T, Stark H, Heinemann F. (Biomechanics and load resistance of small-diameter and mini dental implants: a review of literature). Biomed Tech (Berl). 2014 Feb;59(1):1-5. doi: 10.1515/bmt-2013-0092.

155. Mau J, Behneke A, Behneke N, Fritemeier CU, Gomez-Roman G, d'Hoedt B, Spiekermann H, Strunz V, Yong M: Randomized multicenter comparison of 2 IMZ and 4 TPS screw implants supporting bar-retained overdentures in 425 edentulous mandible. Int J Oral Maxillofac Implant 2003, 18(6):835-47.

156. Almutairi AS, Walide MA, Alkhodary MA: The effect of osseodensification and different thread design on the dental implant primary stability, f1000Res 2018, 5:7:1898.

157. Jung U-W, Kim S, Kim Y-H, Cha J-K, Lee I-S, Choi S- H. Osseointegration of dental implants installed without mechanical engagement: a histometric analysis in dogs. Clin. Oral Impl. Res. 23, 2012, 1297–1301

158. Sang-Hyun Moon, Heung-Sik Um, Jae-Kwan Lee, Beom-Seok Chang, Min-Ku Lee. The effect of implant shape and bone preparation on primary stability. J Periodontal Implant Sci 2010 October; 40(5): 239–243.

159. Mesa F, Muñoz R, Noguerol B, Dios Luna J, Galindo P, O'Valle F. Multivariate Study of Factors Influencing Primary Dental Implant Stability. Clin Oral Implants Res. 2008 Feb;19(2):196-200.

160. Barewal RM, Oates TW, Meredith N, Cochran DL. Resonance frequency measurement of implant stability in vivo on implants with a sandblasted and acid-etched surface. Int J Oral Maxillofac Implants. 2003 Sep-Oct;18(5):641-51.

161. Bischof M, Nedir R, Szmukler-Moncler S, Bernard JP, Samson J. Implant stability measurement of delayed and immediately loaded implants during healing. Clin Oral Implants Res. 2004 Oct;15(5):529-39.

162. Penarrocha M, Carrillo C, Boronat A, Martí E. Early loading of 642 Defcon implants: 1-year follow-up. J Oral Maxillofac Surg. 2007 Nov;65(11):2317-20.

163. Lazzara R, Siddiqui AA, Binon P, Feldman SA, Weiner R, Phillips R. Retrospective multicenter analysis of 3i endosseous dental implants placed over a five-year period. Clin Oral Implants Res. 1996; 7(1):73-83.

164. Ostman PO, Hellman M, Wendelhag I, Sennerby L. Resonance frequency analysis measurements of implants at placement surgery. Int J Prosthodont. 2006 Jan-Feb;19(1):77-83.

165. Polizzi G, Rangert B, Lekholm U, Gualini F, Lindström H. Brånemark System Wide Platform implants for single molar replacement: clinical evaluation of prospective and retrospective materials. Clin Implant Dent Relat Res. 2000;2(2):61-9.

18. Calandriello R, Tomatis M, Vallone R, Rangert B, Gottlow J. Immediate occlusal loading of single lower molars using Brånemark System Wide-Platform TiUnite implants: an interim report of a prospective open-ended clinical multicenter study. Clin Implant Dent Relat Res. 2003;5 Suppl 1:74-80.

167. Rubin CT, Pratt GW, Jr, Porter AL, Lanyon LE, Poss R. Ultrasonic measurement of immobilization-induced osteopenia: an experimental study in sheep. Calcif Tissue Int. 1988;42:309–312.

168. Huiskes R, Ruimerman R, van Lenthe GH, Janssen JD. Effects of mechanical forces on maintenance and adaptation of form in trabecular bone. Nature. 2000;405:704–706.

169. Araceli Boronat López, José Balaguer Martínez , Joana Lamas Pelayo , Celia Carrillo García , Miguel Peñarrocha Diago . Resonance frequency analysis of dental implant stability during the healing period. Oral Cir Bucal Med Oral Patol Oral Cir Bucal. 2008 ;13(4),244-7

170. Bischof M, Nedir R, Szmukler-Moncler S, Bernard JP, Samson J. Implant stability measurement of delayed and immediately loaded implants during healing. Clin Oral Implants Res. 2004 Oct;15 (5) : 529-39.

171. Boronat-López A, Peñarrocha-Diago M, Martínez-Cortissoz O, Mínguez-Martínez I. Resonance frequency analysis after the placement of 133 dental implants. Med Oral Patol Oral Cir Bucal. 2006 May 1;11(3):E272-6.

172. Ersanli S, Karabuda C, Beck F, Leblebicioglu B. Resonance frequency analysis of one-stage dental implant stability during the osseointegration period. J Periodontol. 2005 Jul;76(7):1066-71.

173. Faegh S, Müftü S. Load transfer along the bone–dental implant interface. Journal of Biomechanics. Volume 43, Issue 9, 18 June 2010, Pages

1761–1770.

174. Shalabi MM, Wolke JG, de Ruijter AJ, Jansen JA: Histological evaluation of oral implants inserted with different surgical techniques into the trabecular bone of goats. Clin Oral Implants Res 2007, 18(4):489–495.

175. Dhore CR, Snel SJ, Jacques SV, Naert IE, Walboomers XF, Jansen JA: In vitro osteogenic potential of bone debris resulting from placement of titanium screw-type implants. Clin Oral Implants Res 2008, 19(6):606–611.

176. Skelak R, Zhao Y. Similarity of stress distribution in bone for various surface roughness heights of similar form. Clin Implant Dent Related Res 2000:2:225-30.

177. Skelak, Zhao. Interaction of force-fitting and surface roughness of implants. Clin Implant Dent Related Res 2000.2:219-24.

178. Dos Santos MV, Elias CN, Cavalcanti Lima JH. The effects of superficial roughness and design on the primary stability of dental implants. Clin Implant Dent Relat Res. 2011 Sep;13(3):215-23.

179. Oh GY, Park SH, Kim SG. Influence of implant fixture design on implant primary stability. J Korean Acad Prosthodont. 2007;45:98–106.

180. Moon SH, Um HS, Lee JK, Chang BS,1 Min-LeeMK. The effect of implant shape and bone preparation on primary stability. J Periodontal Implant Sci. 2010 Oct;40(5):239-43.

181. Tabassum A, Walboomers XF, Wolke JG, Meijer GJ, Jansen JA: Bone particles and the undersized surgical technique. J Dent Res 2010, 89 (6):581–586.

182. Martinez H, Davarpanah M, Missika P, Celletti R, Lazzara R. Optimal implant stabilization in low density bone. Clin Oral Implants Res. 2001;12:423–432.

183. Olsson M, Friberg B, Nilson H, Kultje C. MkII--a modified self-tapping Branemark implant: 3-year results of a controlled prospective pilot study. Int J Oral Maxillofac Implants. 1995;10:15–21.

184. Turkyilmaz I, Aksoy U, McGlumphy EA. Two alternative surgical techniques for enhancing primary implant stability in the posterior maxilla: a clinical study including bone density, insertion torque, and resonance frequency analysis data. Clin Implant Dent Relat Res. 2008;10:231–237.

185. Zarate-Kalfopulos B, Estrada-Villasenor E. Use of fibrin glue in combination with autologous bone graft as bone enhancer in posterolateral spinal fusion. An experimental study in New Zealand rabbits. Cir. Cir. 75(3), 201–205 (2007).

186. Martinez H, Davarpanah M, Missika P, Celletti R, Lazzara R. Optimal implant stabilization in low density bone. Clin Oral Implants Res. 2001;12:423–432.

187. Olsson M, Friberg B, Nilson H, Kultje C. MkII--a modified self-tapping Branemark implant: 3-year results of a controlled prospective pilot study. Int J Oral Maxillofac Implants. 1995;10:15–21.

188. Turkyilmaz I, Aksoy U, McGlumphy EA. Two alternative surgical techniques for enhancing primary implant stability in the posterior maxilla: a clinical study including bone density, insertion torque, and resonance frequency analysis data. Clin Implant Dent Relat Res. 2008;10:231–237.

189. Degidi M, Piattelli A. 7-Year follow-up of 93 immediately loaded titanium dental implants. Journal of Oral Implantology.2005;25:31

190. Lorenzoni M, Pertl C, Zhang K, Wimmer G, Wegscheider WA. Immediate loading of single-tooth implants in the anterior maxilla. Preliminary results after one year Clinical Oral Implants Research 2003;14:180-7.

191. Cannizzaro G, Leone M, Ferri V, Viola P, Federico G, Esposito M. Immediate loading of single implants inserted flapless with medium or high insertion torque: a 6-month follow-up of a split-mouth randomised controlled trial. Eur J Oral Implantol. 2012;5:333–342.

192. Norton MR. The Influence of Low Insertion Torque on Primary Stability, Implant Survival, and Maintenance of Marginal Bone Levels: A Closed-Cohort Prospective Study. Int J Oral Maxillofac Implants 2017; Jul/Aug;32(4):849-857.

193. Norton MR. The Influence of Insertion Torque on the Survival of Immediately Placed and Restored Single-Tooth Implants, Int J Oral Maxillofac Implants 2011;26:1333–1343.

194. Hsu JT, Fuh LJ, Tu MG, Li YF, Chen KT, Huang HL. The Effects of Cortical Bone Thickness and Trabecular Bone Strength on Noninvasive Measures of the Implant Primary Stability Using Synthetic Bone Models. Clin Implant Dent Relat Res. 2011.

195. M. C. Vallee, H. J. Conrad, S. Basu, and W.-J. Seong, "Accuracy of friction-style and spring-style mechanical torque limiting devices for dental implants," Journal of Prosthetic Dentistry, vol. 100, no. 2, pp. 86–92, 2008.

196. M. Mahshid, A. Saboury, A. Fayaz, S. Jalil Sadr, F. Lampert, and M. Mir, "The effect of steam sterilization on the accuracy of spring-style mechanical torque devices for dental implants," Clinical, Cosmetic and Investigational Dentistry, vol. 4, pp. 29–35, 2012.

197. Gutierrez J, Nicholls JI, Libman WJ, Butson TJ. Accuracy of the implant torque wrench following time in clinical service. Int J Prosthodont 1997; 10: 562-7.

198. Merheb J, Graham J, Coucke W, Roberts M, Quirynen M, Jacobs R, Devlin H. Int J Oral Maxillofac Implants. 2015 Mar-Apr;30(2):372-7. Prediction of implant loss and marginal bone loss by analysis of dental panoramic radiographs.

199. R Pauwels, R Jacobs, S R Singer, and M Mupparapu. CBCT-based bone quality assessment: are Hounsfield units applicable? Dentomaxillofac Radiol. 2015 Jan; 44(1).

200. M A Laskey: Dual-energy X-ray absorptiometry and body composition. Nutrition 1996 Jan;12(1):45-51.

201. Mary B. Leonard MD, MSCE, Craig B. Langman MD, in Bone Disease of Organ Transplantation, Pediatric Transplant Bone Disease, 2005.

202. Calciolari E, Donos N, Jung-Chul P, Petrie A, Nikos Mardas N : A systematic review on the correlation between skeletal and jawbone mineral density in osteoporotic subjects. Clin Oral Implants Res 2016 Apr;27(4):433-42.

203. Gulsahi A, Paksoy C, Yaziciaglu N, Terziaglu H: Assessment of bone density differences between conventional and bone-condensing techniques using dual energy x-ray absorptiometry and radiography. December 2007. Oral Surgery, Oral Medicine, Oral Pathology, Oral Radiology, and Endodontology 104(5):692-8.

204. Sinan Ay, Gursoy UK, Taner Erselcan, Taner Erselcan, İsmail Marakoğlu, İsmail Marakoğlu. Assessment of mandibular bone mineral density in patients with type 2 diabetes mellitus. December 2005 Dentomaxillofacial Radiology 34(6):327-31.

205. Trisi, P, Rao W. (1999) Bone classification: clinical-histomorphometric comparison.Clinical Oral Implants Research10: 1–7.

206. Turkyilmaz I, Tumer C, Ozbek EN, Tözüm TF. T. Relations between the bone density values from computerized tomography, and implant stability parameters: A clinical study of 230 regular platform implants. J Clin Periodontol 2007;34:716–722.

207. Turkyilmaz I, McGlumphy E. Influence of bone density on implant stability parameters and implant success: A retrospective clinical study. BMC Oral Health 2008;24:8–32.

208. Turkyilmaz I, Sennerby L, McGlumphy E, Tozum T. Biomechanical aspects of primary implant stability: A human cadaver study. Clin Implant Dent Relat Res 2009;11:113–119.

209. Kahraman S, Bal BT, Asar NV, Turkyilmaz I, Tozum TF. Clinical study on the insertion torque and wireless resonance frequency analysis in the assessment of torque capacity and stability of self-tapping dental implants. J Oral Rehabil 2009;36:755–761.

210. Benic GI, Mir-Mari J, Hämmerle CH.Loading protocols for single-implant crowns: a systematic review and meta-analysis. Int J Oral Maxillofac Implants. 2014;29 Suppl:222-38.

211. Toljanic JA, Baer RA, Ekstrand K, Thor A. Implant rehabilitation of the atrophic edentulous maxilla including immediate fixed provisional restoration without the use of bone grafting: A review of 1-year outcome data from a long-term prospective clinical trial. Int J Oral Maxillofac Implants 2009;24:518–526.

212. Trisi P, Perfetti G, Baldoni E, Berardi D, Colagiovanni M, Scogna G. Implant micromotion is related to peak insertion torque and bone density. Clin Oral Implants Res 2009;20:467–471.

213. Duyck J, Corpas L, Vermeiren S. Histological, histomorphometrical, and radiological evaluation of an experimental implant design with high insertion torque. Clin Oral Implants Res 2010;21:877–884.

214. Lachmann S, Laval JY, Jager B, Axmann D, Gomez- Roman G,Groten M. Resonance frequency analysis and damping capacity assessment. Part 2: Periimplant bone loss follow-up. An in vitro study with the Periotest and Osstell instruments. Clin Oral Implants Res 2006;17:80-4.

215. Quesada-Garcı´a MP, Prados-Sa´nchez E, Olmedo-Gaya MV, Mun˜oz-Soto E, Gonza´lez-Rodrı´guez MP, Vallecillo-Capilla M. Measurement of dental implant stability by resonance frequency analysis: a review of the literature. Med Oral Patol Oral Cir Bucal 2009;14(10):e538-46.

216. Turkyilmaz I. A comparison between insertion torque and resonance frequency in the assessment of torque capacity and primary stability of Branemark system implants. J Oral Rehabil 2006;33:754-9.

217. Chee W, Jivraj S. Efficiency of immediately loaded mandibular full-arch implant restorations. Clin Implant Dent Relat Res. 2003;5:52–56.

218. Ganeles J, Rosenberg MM, Holt RL, Reichman LH. Immediate loading of implants with fixed restorations in the completely edentulous mandible: report of 27 patients from a private practice. Int J Oral Maxillofac Implants. 2001;16:418–426.

219. Matsuzaka K, Nakajima Y, Soejima Y, Kido H, Matsuura M, Inoue T. Effect on the amount of bone-implant contact when splining immediate-loaded dental implants. Implant Dent. 2007 Sep;16(3):309-16.

220. Glauser R, Lundgren AK, Gottlow J, Sennerby L, Portmann M, Ruhstaller P, Hämmerle CH. Immediate occlusal loading of Branemark TiUnit implants placed predominantly in soft bone: 1-year results of a prospective clinical study. Clin Implant Dent Relat Res. 2003;5 Suppl 1:47-56.

221. Pesun IJ. Intrusion of teeth in the combination implant-to-natural-tooth fixed partial denture: a review of the theories. J Prosthodont 1997 Dec;6(4):268-77.

CHAPTER TWO:

DOCUMENTATION, RECORD KEEPING AND TREATMENT PLANNING

2. DOCUMENTATION, RECORD KEEPING AND TREATMENT PLANNING

Aim:
The chapter on "Documentation and Record Keeping" aims to stress the critical role of accurate and comprehensive documentation in dental practice, focusing on best practices for maintaining detailed patient records to ensure quality care and regulatory compliance.

Necessary Knowledge:
It is assumed that at this stage, you have a general knowledge of the science related to dental implantology.

Learning Outcome:
After completing this chapter, the reader will have gained a basic knowledge of the medicolegal aspects of consent, treatment planning and decision-making.
1.   Informed consent
2.   Consent and medicolegal aspects
3.   Treatment planning

> Patient consent is a process, not a one-off event.
>
> If there is doubts about embarking on a particular course of treatment for a given patient then consult your indemnity organization.
>
> The pros, cons, and risks of each treatment plan should be explained carefully.
>
> Making a checklist for each phase of treatment, starting with the initial examination.

2.1. Informed Consent
Documentation serves as a cornerstone in dentistry, particularly in the context of dental implant treatment. It fulfils several crucial purposes, including legal and ethical accountability, continuity of care, clinical decision-making, and quality assurance. Comprehensive records document the patient's journey and provide a roadmap for dental professionals to navigate treatment complexities and optimize outcomes.

Medicolegal Aspects: Informed Consent
In view of the UK's Brexit policy, the legislation referred to in this segment may be altered, and the legal requirements demanded by it may be similarly altered. Accordingly, should these changes be instituted, the reader will need to consult his/her indemnity organisation to confirm the then-current requirements. However, until any government action is taken towards such an end, the legal requirements referred to here are still current - but be aware and warned.

GDC's standards
GDC guidance on the principles of informed patient consent states that 'Giving and getting consent is a process, not a one-off event. It should be part of an ongoing discussion between the dentist and the patient'.

From a general European perspective, the obligations that medical and dental professionals have towards both their patients and themselves are to ensure that any treatment plan which has been developed for that particular patient has been based upon:

A clear understanding of the reasons for the patient's visit and what the patient sees as their need, a full and holistic assessment of the patient's clinical and relevant psychological needs, and the presentation to the patient of any appropriate alternative treatment plans - ideally developed with the patient, a full explanation of the clinical pros, cons, and risks of each treatment plan, giving the patient a choice and a clear presentation the length of treatment and number of sessions and the cost(s) of any proposed treatment plans is needed.

The conversations between the patient and dentist must be carefully recorded in the patient's notes [1].

The author recommends providing documentary video animation clips to discuss the options, cons and pros of each type of treatment. The patient first watches the clips to gain good background knowledge. After the dentist explains the options, review the abstract of the plan with the patient, print it, and hand it to the patient. Ask the patient politely to explain it back to the dentist. The dentist must understand that the patient's knowledge of dentistry is limited, and the patient's stress and bashfulness would reflect that the patient will be nodding the head up and down but really does not know the treatment plan and why.

Indemnity organisations:

If you have any doubts about embarking on a particular course of treatment for a given patient, then consult your indemnity organisation. They will no doubt emphasise many of the points.

Usually, there are more than one treatment plan and a hierarchy of complexity. The risks of each option, including no treatment, should be explained. There are always compromised plans and not 100 per cent right plans.

The patient's needs:

The patient needs to know that they have been listened to and their concerns understood. The patient should appreciate that the subsequent examination has been careful and has addressed their concerns. The resulting treatment plan(s) should be presented to the patient using radiographs and photos. Each treatment plan's pros, cons, and risks should be explained carefully. The costs will have been clearly explained.

If necessary, the first consultation can be followed by a second consultation, especially if a second opinion or specialist advice needs to be sought.

In any event, the patient must be provided with a printed copy of the highlights of the clinical discussions, copies of the radiographs and photos, a clear exposition of the relevant costs, and a note of each treatment possibility's clinical pros, cons, and risks. The patient will also need an idea of the time frame for the course of treatment and the likely completion date of each treatment plan.

The above should provide the patient with all the information necessary for informed consent to be given.

The author recommends that a member of the family or friend be on the day of delivering the treatment plan with the patient's consent, especially in complicated cases.

It is a good idea to provide the treatment plan in a relaxed consultation room; if the patient consents, record a video of your discussion with the patient. Each country's regulations and culture differ.

The dentist's needs:

The dentist must ensure that the patient's concerns have been fully understood, that the clinical assessment has been thorough and has taken account of the patient's concerns, that the treatment plans which have been developed are realistic and achievable, that the pros cons and risks of each treatment plan have been carefully explained, that the costs have been adequately communicated, even though they will be noted in the printed copy of the conversation and proposals which will be sent to the patient. Above all, be sure that what you are proposing to accomplish for the patient is achievable and that your skills match your promise to the patient. Failure to do so could be costly.

The dentist must ensure careful contemporaneous notes are made and entered on the patient's record card. Written notes are delicate as long as they are comprehensive and legible. Computerised notes are usually more reliable.

The notes must include the patient's current, full medical history. The notes must include the patient's presenting complaints and expressed wishes. There must be clear evidence of a systematic clinical assessment and a note of the clinical implications derived from any radiographs and photographs. Make clear, full notes of any conversations you have with the patient.

Always be prepared to offer assistance in seeking a second opinion if requested or if you detect uncertainty in the patient. Never be offended by the prospect. A second opinion may produce useful suggestions besides demonstrating open-mindedness and engendering trust.

If any complaint is made, it may be referred to the General Dental Council. The GDC has published guidelines on implant dentistry and approved training, and you are urged to read these. Any realisation on your part that you might be overreaching yourself should trigger a reassessment. If necessary, seek a second opinion from a specialist.

Planning and checklists:

Making a checklist for each phase of treatment, starting with the initial examination, can be invaluable. Note everything you need to examine, along with the resulting assessment.

Note every aspect of the anatomy and consider its implications for successful implantation.

Prior to the operative phase, a checklist for the instrumentation is needed. A discreetly placed checklist for each stage of the operation may prove to be a useful aide-memoire.

As noted above, the above principles are echoed in published European and international ethics standards.

Have too many goals? Too many goals are not plans; they are only wish lists. You have to prioritise, but each goal has its own constituents; if you don't prioritise, you can not make and implement a plan.

European Law:

From a European perspective, the Charter of Fundamental Rights of the European Union and the Council of Europe's Convention on Human Rights and Biomedicine establish the general rule on free and informed consent in the health field.

The Dental Ethics Manual by the FDI World emphasises that ' a necessary condition [requirement] for informed consent is good communication between dentist and patient '.

It identifies three major obstacles to good dentist-patient communication:

1. Language barrier
2. Culture barrier
3. Inadequate explanation of the possible short-term and long-term impediments for the patient

Language Barrier

Differences in language can present an insurmountable barrier. If you cannot communicate, that means you cannot treat. Even a designated interpreter (maybe family) may have excellent English for use in the street but still not understand the nuances of language, which can lay a future minefield that may blow up in your face a little further down the line.

Therefore, treatment plans, carefully laid out in precise English,

need to be accompanied by an accurately translated version which, whatever complaints may arise, can be shown unequivocally to have been mistranslated by the patient's interpreter and, therefore, cannot be blamed on your very precise English, or your interpreter's translation, which the patient's interpreter has read and acknowledged.

Having a list of recommended interpreters most relevant to your patient pool may be useful.

Clear notes must also be made to show that the minutiae were discussed, understood, and confirmed before treatment commenced.

If sedation is necessary, then an anaesthetist who speaks the patient's language fluently is essential. One writes from experience.

Culture Barrier

Because of different cultural understandings of the nature and causes of illness, the patient may not understand the diagnosis and treatment options provided by the dentist. Moreover, what is considered a disfigurement in one culture may be a sign of beauty in another. These matters should be discussed carefully, settled, and signed off on before treatment begins.

The patient may suffer various impairments during treatment, which needs to be anticipated and communicated. These will include temporary speech impairment, temporary aesthetic impairment, and temporary functional impairment. Where any one or all of these are anticipated, the patient must be informed in advance, along with the dentist's assurances that they will be temporary – as long as these can be honestly given.

Dentists should take steps to ensure that two-way communication between patient and dentist is maintained throughout the treatment period and beyond.

'Beyond' is fundamentally important. The patient must be shown that you care.

The process of obtaining informed consent does not consist simply of the presentation of information. It should reflect the dentist's effort to educate and discuss the findings with the patient [2].

2.2. Consent and medico-legal aspects

Even though there are common grounds in dental law and ethics, they differ between countries, and it is emphasised that before even examining a patient, the dentist must have full knowledge and be indemnified.

However, it is a general legal and ethical principle that dentists must get written, valid, informed consent before starting a treatment or physical investigation. The dentist must repeat the consent (verbally) for every visit. The patient should clearly understand the advantages and disadvantages of each option. The author recommends that before a patient arrives for consultation, he should have preliminary information in a brochure. Animation and models can help the patient understand the information during consultation appointments. At the end of the session, it is recommended to ask the patient to reflect back on what he understood and if there is any doubt. Request another consultation session. Having someone in the session, like a wife or husband, adult sister, brother, or children, would help the patient.

In any session and even in the middle of treatment, the dentist must stop if the patient wants the dentist to stop. During treatment, if verbal communication is not an option, he or she can put his or her hand on the dentist's arm. Acknowledging this fact in official guidelines would further safeguard patients' autonomy and dignity [1].

Elements of Effective Documentation:

a. PATIENT INFORMATION

Adequate documentation starts with gathering comprehensive patient details, such as demographics, medical and dental history, and relevant social factors. This holistic approach helps assess the patient's overall health and identify any potential risks related to dental implant treatment.

b. CLINICAL ASSESSMENT

Thorough clinical assessments are crucial in planning dental implant rehabilitation. Examination findings, diagnostic tests like radiographs, and periodontal evaluations guide decisions on implant placement, bone quality assessment, and prosthetic planning. Documenting these observations supports evidence-based treatment planning and ensures patient safety.

c. TREATMENT PLAN

Documenting a comprehensive treatment plan is essential to align clinical goals with patient expectations. This involves re-cording proposed treatments, considering alternatives, and patient preferences. Clear documentation of treatment rationale, potential risks, and expected outcomes supports informed consent discussions and enhances patient-centred care.

d. INFORMED CONSENT

Comprehensive documentation of informed consent discussions is crucial in dental implant treatment. It ensures that patients are fully informed about implant surgery's risks, benefits, and alternatives. Detailed documentation promotes patient autonomy and mitigates legal risks.

e. DETAILS OF PROCEDURES

Recording procedure details, including materials used, techniques, and any complications, support continuity of care and post-operative monitoring. It aids communication among dental professionals and allows for retrospective analysis of treatment outcomes.

f. POSTTREATMENT (SHORT AND LONG-TERM) INSTRUCTIONS

Clear and concise post-treatment instructions are essential for promoting successful outcomes and patient compliance. Documenting these instructions ensures that patients understand how to care for their implants, supporting optimal healing and recovery.

Best Practices in Record Keeping:

a. ACCURACY

Accurate and timely record-keeping is essential for reliable documentation in dental implant treatment. Records must be clear, detailed, and entered promptly after each patient encounter to ensure continuity of care and easy information retrieval.

b. STANDARDISED FORMAT

Using standardized templates or electronic health record systems ensures consistency and facilitates information retrieval. Standardized formats improve the clarity and completeness of documentation, aiding communication among dental professionals and supporting quality assurance.

c. CONFIDENTIALITY AND SECURITY

Ensuring patient confidentiality and complying with data protection regulations are essential in record-keeping practices. Dental professionals must securely store patient records, limiting access to authorized personnel to protect privacy and meet legal requirements.

d. COMMUNICATION

Using records to communicate among dental professionals supports collaboration and ensures continuity of care. Clear documentation enhances patient safety, reduces errors, and improves treatment outcomes.

Risk Assessment And Nerve Injury

With good planning, the incidence of nerve injuries related to dental implant surgery can be avoided. Iatrogenic implant-related nerve injury may cause persistent neuropathic pain, with significant associated functional problems which seriously affect quality of life. Clinicians, therefore, need to ensure that scrupulous preoperative planning, along with best practice radiographic planning, is always carried out, that associated surgical risks are fully assessed, that surgeons are fully and properly confident of their surgical skills, that patients are fully apprised of anticipated outcomes, and have therefore given properly considered and informed consent.

Post-operative follow-up, which can be inadequate, needs to be assiduously pursued. In the United States, the average payout for implant-related nerve injury is higher than the average payout for IAN injury related to third molar surgery. CBCT can help, but if possible, mental foramina can be identified during surgery, and a visual measurement can provide more precise data.

2.3. Treatment planning and decision making

Evidence-Based Decision-Making

Incorporating evidence from systematic reviews, meta-analyses, and patient-specific factors into treatment planning promotes evidence-based decision-making in dental implant rehabilitation. This approach improves treatment efficacy, success rates, and long-term prognoses by integrating the latest research findings and clinical evidence.

Patient-Centered Care

Incorporating patient preferences, expectations, and values into treatment planning promotes patient-centred care in dental implant rehabilitation. Documenting patient preferences facilitates shared decision-making and fosters a collaborative approach, prioritising patient satisfaction and quality of life.

Risk Assessment

Documenting risk assessments related to treatment options informs planning and supports informed consent discussions. Identifying potential risks enables dental professionals to optimize treatment outcomes.

Follow-Up and Monitoring

Establishing protocols for follow-up visits and monitoring treatment outcomes is essential for documenting progress and adjusting plans as needed. Comprehensive follow-up documentation supports continuity of care and ensures optimal outcomes for patients undergoing dental implant rehabilitation.

In some countries, the initial cost of a single implant crown is getting closer to that of a FPD, and failure rates are similar.

The minimally invasive bridges for single tooth replacement have become a good option as long as the patient knows there is a chance of dislodgement and in strategic positions like canine guidance, need to be cautious, and the rate of bone resorption will be higher than placing a dental implant.

The long-term financial costs could also be similar, depending on the country. However, the utility for the patient of keeping healthy adjacent and neighbouring teeth unprepared makes the implant crown more economical. The economic advantage of preserving bone and gum is an added bonus. This will be more important for the young patient. In sum, the implant can be a better economic choice.

A note on statistics: Important information can be gathered from combined data to estimate event rates related to a specific measure. These rates could be annual or, ideally, projected over 5 or 10 years if sufficient data is accessible. Numerous systematic reviews have been conducted that analyse the risks and outcomes associated with different prosthetic choices for tooth replacement [3,4].

Further systematic reviews conducted meta-analyses to estimate success or survival rates over different observation periods. This was achieved by combining and analysing data from similar clinical studies. The resulting survival or success rates were then used to support recommendations for specific treatment approaches based on the evidence found in the literature [5,6].

Additional aspects that could affect the patient's quality of life must be considered for broader appreciation and evaluation. Patients paying for dental services, insurers allocating resources, or the public funding dental services need to be made aware that implants are much more than a luxury – they can preserve the health of the mouth without damaging other teeth and improve patients' quality of life. Analyses such as cost-benefit, cost-effectiveness, and cost-utility analyses may represent tools for evaluating dental medicine's economic outcomes.

Cost-benefit analyses involve comparing the costs of a certain intervention, like water fluoridation, with the savings in dental treatment costs due to reduced cavities. Cost-effectiveness analyses look at how much improvement in clinical outcomes can be achieved with one therapy (A) compared to another (B), considering the costs involved.

A cost-utility analysis assesses the relationship between monetary investment and quality of life, which encompasses factors such as function and comfort, to determine overall value.

Patients value functionality, aesthetics, and comfort more than the discomfort of the treatment or the consequences of a non-treatment (e.g., a missing tooth). A cost-effective treatment should result in benefits for the patients which exceed the costs [7].

Patient satisfaction is the most critical indicator of success in health care. Patient satisfaction reflects successful clinical outcomes, increases patient retention, and reduces medical malpractice claims. The surgeon should be aware that the high cost of implant treatment can contribute to unrealistic patient expectations, thus leading to lowered satisfaction.

Moderating the patients' expectations and rendering them more realistic may help maintain their ultimate level of satisfaction [8].

The secret to successful treatment planning lies in objectively assessing the patient's expectations, the actual surgical possibilities, the confounding factors rooted in the patient's likely physical response to healing, and the patient's psychological response to the enforced treatment period. It would also be wise to involve the team in contributing to this assessment precisely because other team members will see the patient from a different angle, and their contributions may turn out to be necessary.

Factors we should consider are the patient's functional expectations, psychological expectations and physical condition. Sir William Osler once said that dental treatment's Pankey Philosophy (www.pankey.org) includes the sensible axiom: never treat a stranger.

Does the patient suffer any significant systemic disease, indulge in smoking or other types of chemical abuse? Any of these factors can affect the body's physical response during the healing period, can affect the organs, or the patient's psychological behaviour in a way that may jeopardise the chances of a successful outcome.

The dentist must consider the periodontium scallop, crestal bone level, smile line, morphology of the gingival tissues, inter-implant distance, occlusal contacts, and interproximal bone level.

Treatment planning will be affected by the dentist's training, school of thought, and skill level.

Put simply, dental implant treatment planning is dental prosthetic treatment planning that respects its environment.

However, before we discuss this further, we need to examine possible alternatives that might contraindicate the need for implant placement.

Although several systematic reviews have compared success rates of root canal treatment and survival of implant restorations, they have not been able to conclude which treatment option is likely to have the greater success rate, nor in which circumstances. Attempting retreatment or referring for the same has not been compared. Any difference in opinion would likely be based on the dentist's status (GDP v specialist), access to specialist treatment, the experience of the results (whether by GDP or specialist) and dental school teaching.

When such dilemmas present themselves, it is clearly not easy for the patient to make an informed decision because there are too many variables. This is where the dentist's knowledge of the likely period of implant success when placed by a known implantologist can be weighed against, say, a heavily restored tooth, even when the root treatment is beautiful. Alternatively, are you contemplating placing a bridge that will span an area which currently contains an excellently root-treated tooth but with a proposal for an implant on either side? If the need for implants and bridge is in order to restore function, then the root-filled tooth is a hindrance, regardless of its likely longevity.

This is where the dentist's experience and ability to assess prognosis is called upon - or a second opinion is called for. And remember that visual aids can be particularly useful for showing the patient treatment possibilities. People absorb information through sound (voice), pictures, and reading, often through all three. Never presume to know your patient's preferences. Use brochures, animation, and movie clips to provide the patient with any necessary information. It will be greatly appreciated if the patient realises that you are taking every opportunity to explain possibilities in a way that will enable an informed choice.

Decision-making

In simple clinical cases involving single or multiple procedures, the main question is, 'Should we extract the teeth?'

Do we undertake endodontic treatment or retreatment?

Do we organise periodontal surgery?

Will we need to place a crown or a post-crown?

Should the number of sessions affect the decision or the likely pain and discomfort during or after the treatment?

And what about the cost?

After 25 years of experience and having an endodontic specialist (my father) beside me, I find that it is simple criteria which influence my decisions.

Following successful endodontic treatment, can we provide a crown or post-crown that can function without discomfort or significant periodontal bone loss for at least five years? It becomes more complicated if the tooth has grade 1 mobility without any periodontal pocket, bearing in mind the amount of force which would be on the tooth.

Nevertheless, the most important thing is the patient's expectations.

Say that after multiple sessions of endodontic treatment, with or without periodontal surgery or prosthetic treatment, the patient comes back after a year with the crown having fallen out of the root or with the root now fractured. Did the dentist make the best decision? What might the outcome have been if the dentist extracted that tooth instead of root-treating it and replaced it with an implant? After all, an implant is expensive, treatment takes a few months to complete, and the procedure does have a failure rate, even if it is small.

Which would have been the right decision? Which criteria

should we have adopted in order to do the best for our patient, both morally and in order to avoid litigation?

Maybe we should give the patient plenty of time and let him make the decision, even if it is not a specialist decision. Alternatively, maybe the patient is the specialist.

Navigating Patient Expectations and Informed Consent: A Balanced Approach

In dental practice, obtaining informed consent is a legal obligation and a cornerstone of ethical patient care. As dentists, we must ensure that patients are fully informed about the treatments they will undergo, including potential risks and benefits. However, patient expectations are increasingly high, often viewing dentists as infallible and expecting us to predict and control every possible outcome.

Consider this analogy: Imagine you are a passenger on a flight. Before takeoff, does the airline explain every possible problem that could occur during the flight? This could include human or pilot error, mechanical failures involving the engine, structures, electrical systems, hydraulic controls, lights, or even the unlikely event of being hit by a missile by mistake. Of course not. The airline doesn't seek explicit consent for these potential issues because it would be overwhelming and impractical. Passengers implicitly understand that while flying carries certain risks, they trust in the expertise of the crew and the rigorous safety protocols in place. Individuals make the choice to fly, aware of the general risks, or they might choose alternative modes of transport, none of which offer absolute guarantees of safety.

So why are doctors and dentists subjected to such intense pressure to obtain consent for every conceivable risk? Part of the reason lies in the intimate and personal nature of healthcare. Patients are directly affected by the outcomes of medical and dental procedures, which can have significant impacts on their quality of life. This personal impact drives a need for transparency and reassurance.

However, it is essential to recognise that, like any field, medicine and dentistry cannot guarantee absolute outcomes. Complications can arise despite our best efforts and adherence to the highest standards of care. The legal and ethical framework of informed consent is designed to help patients make educated decisions about their care, but it should also be balanced with realistic expectations.

As practitioners, we must navigate this delicate balance, providing patients with the necessary information without overwhelming them with every possible, albeit unlikely, risk. We must foster trust through clear communication, professional competence, and empathy, acknowledging that while we strive for the best outcomes, some factors remain beyond our control.

By understanding and managing patient expectations, we can reduce undue pressure on ourselves and continue to provide high-quality care. It is crucial for both patients and practitioners to recognise that while we aim to minimise risks, the nature of medical and dental treatment inherently involves uncertainties. Trust and mutual respect are key components of the patient-practitioner relationship, allowing us to work together towards optimal health outcomes.

References:

1. Shaw D: Continuous consent and dignity in dentistry, British Dental Journal, Nov 24, 2007, Vol.203(10), pp.569-71.

2. Adelaide C, Delbon Paola, Laffranchi L, Paganelli C: Consent in dentistry: ethical and deontological issues. Journal Med Ethics, 2013, 39(1), 59-61.

3. Lulic M, Brägger U, Lang NP, Zwahlen M, Salvi GE: Ante's (1926) law revisited: a systematic review on survival rates and complications of fixed dental prostheses (FDPs) on severely reduced periodontal tissue support. Clin Oral Implants Res 2007 Jun;18 Suppl 3:63-72.

4. Aglietta M, Siciliano VL, Zwahlen M, Brägger U, Pjetursson BE, Lang NP, Salvi GE: A systematic review of the survival and complication rates of implant supported fixed dental prostheses with cantilever extensions after an observation period of at least 5 years. Clin Oral Implants Res 2009 May;20(5):441-51.

5. Pjetursson BE, Lang NP: Prosthetic treatment planning on the basis of scientific evidence. J Oral Rehabil2008;35 Suppl 1:72-9.

6. Priest G: Revisiting tooth preservation in prosthodontic therapy. J Prosthodont. 2011 Feb;20(2):144-52.

7. Pennington MW, Vernazza CR, Shackley P, Armstrong NT, Whitworth JM, Steele JG: Evaluation of the cost-effectiveness of root canal treatment using conventional approaches versus replacement with an implant. Int Endod J 2009 Oct; 42 (10) : 874-83.

8. Yao J, Hua Tang H, Gao XL, McGrath C, Mattheos N: Patients' expectations from dental implants: a systemic review of the literature. Health and quality of life outcomes 2014, 12:153, 1-14.

CHAPTER THREE:

PATIENT ASSESSMENT AND TREATMENT

3. PATIENT ASSESSMENT AND TREATMENT

Aim:

Provide a detailed framework for conducting thorough patient assessments and developing comprehensive treatment plans in dental implantology

Necessary Knowledge base:

It is assumed that at this stage, you have a general knowledge of the science related to dental implantology, the medicolegal aspects of consent, treatment planning, and decision-making.

Learning Outcome:

After completing this chapter, the reader will have gained basic knowledge of radiographic and clinical assessments.

DPT, the degree of vertical magnification is, overall, between say 5 to 20% and the horizontal magnification about -26 to 15 %.

The buccal-lingual position of Inferior Dental Canal, influence the vertical position of the canal in the DPT. As the canal is toward buccal, the ID canal in DPT shows toward lower border of the mandible.

The use of Spotchem ST device is not mandatory, however every little information helps.

3.1. Radiographic assessment

Various types of radiographic imaging are recommended for treatment planning for implants. These are panoramic and periapical radiography and conventional and computed tomography (CT).

Panoramic radiography (DPT/OPG) is readily available and is the most commonly used. Panoramic radiographs provide broad coverage and a view of many of the structures of the maxilla and mandible at a low cost, but they have their limitations, and these need to be recognized.

The two main disadvantages are its tendency to magnify the image and its lack of cross-sectional information. The tendency to magnify is observed vertically and horizontally and varies with the studied region.

For instance, the degree of <u>vertical magnification </u>is, overall, between, say, 5 to 20%. In canines and premolars, it is between -2 to 10%, and in molars, it is between -5 to 10%. Always bear in mind that the variables likely in any research (different OPG equipment, radiology centre, head position employed) will often lead to different findings.

The <u>horizontal magnification</u> in the incisor region is about -26 to 6 %; in the canines and premolars, it is -5 to 15%; and in molar regions, -7 to 7%.

The magnification is generally more significant in the mandible than in the maxillae.

The bony roof of the inferior dental canal is more evident in men than in women, and two ID canals have also been reported. The image of the ID canal will depend on its anatomical location within the mandible: the more buccally positioned the canal, the more apical it will appear to be. The reverse is also true: the more lingually positioned the canal, the more occlusal it will appear to be [1].

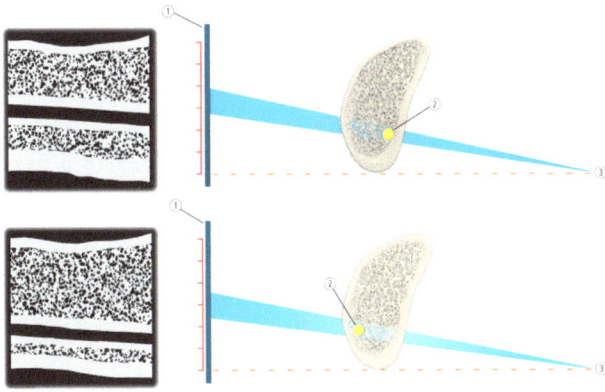

Figure 3.1 The Inferior Dental Canal's buccal-lingual position influences the canal's vertical position in the DPT. As the canal is toward the buccal, the ID canal in DPT shows toward the lower border of the mandible. 1) film plan, 2) Inferior Dental Nerve, 3) x-ray source.

The mental foraminae are not symmetrically placed, and two foramina on each side have been reported. It is crucial to scrutinise the X-ray carefully to verify the number of canals and foramina.

The lower border of the mandible has been used as an indicator of bone quality and classified as C1 - thick and bilaterally uniform, C2 - slightly bowed on one or two sides, C3 - the border has poor quality, with the cortical surface appearing nibbled from the trabecular side (figure 3.2).

The American Academy of Oral and Maxillofacial Radiology recommends cross-sectional imaging for implant site evaluation.

Intra-oral radiography using the paralleling technique is recommended in order to view or identify minute changes; however, the precision is 0.5mm [2].

Identical exposure geometry is complex to repeat when employed for follow-up assessment, reducing its potential accuracy to 0.09 - 0.13 mm. It is even more inaccurate when the inclination of the implant is dictated by the anatomy of the bone remaining after resorption [3].

Digital panoramic images produce adequate image quality, and a mean inaccuracy of 0.21 has been reported thanks to its greater reproducibility. Tomographic images have 0.42 mm inaccuracy, and this represents the least accurate of all techniques.

Current measurement techniques are insufficiently sensitive to enable the measurement of true bone loss until at least 1.0 mm bone loss has occurred [4].

Implants offer advantages in radiological interpretation compared to teeth thanks to the metal's high contrast reference

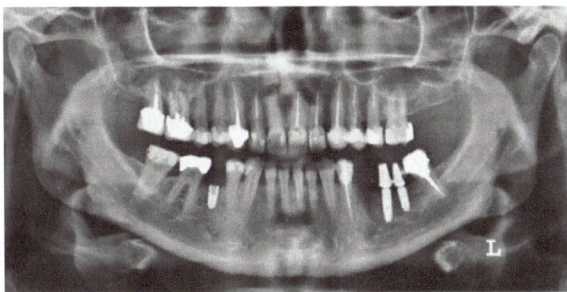

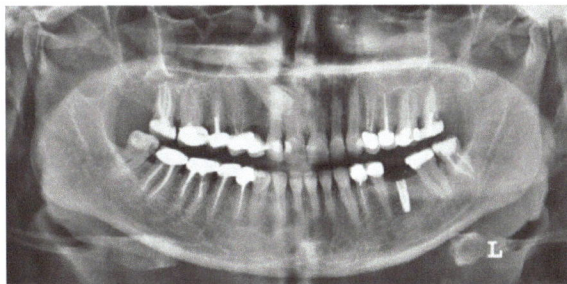

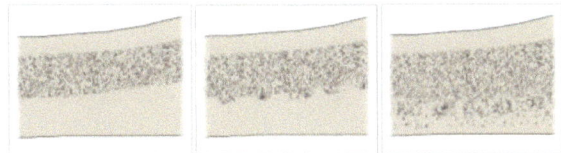

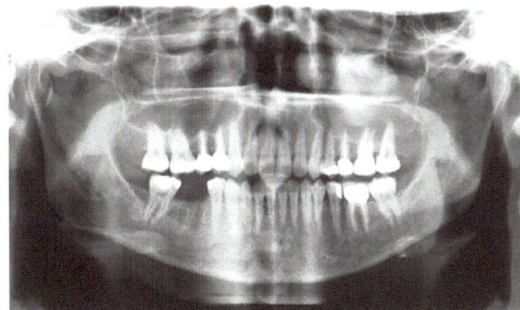

Figure 3.2 The mandible's lower border indicates overall mandible bone quality, upper left: C1 -thick, lower left: C2- slightly bowed, Lower right: C3- nibbled cortex. Upper right: the illustration demonstrates left to right (C1, C2 and C3).

points. The abutment-implant junction is a good reference point. Geometry projection can reduce the error, but accuracy decreases with increasing bone loss [5]. Accuracy below 0.2mm cannot be obtained [6].

In 1987, Schwartz introduced the concept of **computed tomography scans (CT)** for pre-operative assessment of dental implant candidates. The use of CT has continued to grow, although there has been concern regarding the radiation dosage. Such studies have highlighted the higher risk of hypothetical mortality based on absorbed radiation when compared to conventional tomography and quote mortality risks ranging from 8×10^{-6} to 56×10^{-6}, dependent on gender and age. Such risks can be reduced considerably by effectively lowering the dosage output of the scanner without lowering the clarity of the images achieved [7].

Indeed, many clinicians believe that the benefit of this diagnostic tool outweighs the very small risks, which have further decreased with improved scanners and lower dosages [8].

Cone beam tomography has become increasingly critical and allows a precise three-dimensional evaluation of the bone quality and quantity in the maxilla, along with fine details such as the location of the neurovascular bone channels. These become radiographically visible, like the nasopalatine canal, which carries the nasopalatine nerves, arteries, and veins [9].

CBCT can detect anatomical variations. These can include pneumatization, antral septa, hypoplasia, exostoses, and lesions of the sinus such as mucosal thickening, polypoid lesions, discontinuity of the floor of the sinus, air-fluid level, bone thickening, antroliths, discontinuity of the anterolateral wall of the sinus, foreign bodies, and sinus opacification.

Distortion of the Hounsfield Units (CT number) has shown that scanned regions of the same density in the skull can have a different grey-scale value in the reconstructed CBCT dataset. This implies that CBCT should not be used to estimate trabecular bone density. Unfortunately, it presents the best indicator that the implantologist has available at present. It can undoubtedly assess cortical thickness, but its usefulness in the assessment of trabecular bone quality is limited. For this reason, the author does not recommend it but urges implantologists to note the actual quality discovered at bone preparation and compare it with that indicated by CBCT. Some papers suggest that it can be used to assess bone density. It is a powerful tool that can provide a 3D image of the mandible and maxillae for dental implant placement [10,11].

In mandibular and full-head CBCT scans, the C1 and C2 vertebrae can appear, and when they do, They can be used as the mandibular inferior cortex for osteoporosis screening [12].

Cone beam computed tomography (CBCT) has been used to determine the limits of a safe zone within which the surgeon can avoid injury to nerve [13].

CBCT has been recommended for post-operative diagnostic imaging, and it may detect labial bone surrounding the implant, but only when it is more than 0.6mm thick [14].

Based on the systemic review in 2018, CBCT is reliable; however, under and overestimation is expected in the dimensions, and bone quality assessment should be expected [15].

The author recommends that in the vital anatomic areas, like the Inferior Dental Canal and mental foramina, a 2 mm distance or other means is necessary to provide closer drilling, which will be discussed in the other chapters. In the upper canine area, the precision is not reliable, and the dentist may see an overestimation in the CBCT.

A diagnostic (prosthetic) setup or template should be prepared and confirmed in the mouth. The accurate positioning of implants requires careful pre-operative planning. Failure to plan properly can result in implants being unthinkingly placed in embrasures or being so angulated that they would potentially exit through the labial surface of the final crown. That said, there will be times when the only possible implant position will, of necessity, be angled buccally, but knowing this in advance will allow for appropriate post-operative corrections to be planned or inform the patient during treatment planning.

The proper requirements for permanent implant restoration can be assessed by fabricating the provisional restoration in clear or radiopaque acrylic. Vertically, the implant should be placed 3mm apical to the CEJ. The vertical position of the implant should be assessed by applying guidelines described by Block and Chandler.

Using these treatment planning approaches, even with their limitations, allows to explain to the patient the likely outcome of treatment. The proper use of the radiographic stent is essential if accurate information is to be gained. Since the stent is to be fitted in the patient's mouth by a radiological nurse, it must have been adequately adjusted beforehand in the surgery to allow its placement with no interferences. Its proper use is essential [16].

Bone strength plays a significant role in achieving implant success. The trabecular density and microstructure measurements should be combined to improve the prediction of bone strength. This is because those measurements do not always denote each other. For instance, high bone density does not always correspond to high trabecular parameters such as trabecular number and trabecular thickness. Therefore, estimating implant success by assessing trabecular density alone is no longer suggested.

Precise clinical assessment of bone's structural and mechanical properties is essential when planning dental implant treatment and deciding on appropriate implant thread design. PA radiographs with superior resolution and sharpness provide valuable information for evaluating the amount and pattern of trabecular bone structure. Trabecular visibility has been reported to be high on PA radiographs, and the microarchitectural parameters, porosity, connectivity, and anisotropy (homogenetic in all directions) are comparable to those of the 3D method.

However, the panoramic technique applies the rotational principles that structures not centred in the focal trough are not sharply imaged. The formation of geometrical distortions, image magnification, and loss of information are thus commonly observed artefacts on panoramic radiographs. Moreover, the reduced resolution of panoramic images degrades their ability to identify fine trabeculae.

MRI is a non-invasive, non-ionizing system that applies high magnetic fields, transmits radiofrequency waves and detects radiofrequency signals from excited hydrogen protons. The quality of the acquired MRI images is largely influenced by the magnetic field strength, radiofrequency (pulse sequence), pulse-echo time, and the signal-to-noise ratio of the received data. Additionally, the measurements are affected by the selected threshold values, image-processing algorithms, complex analysis, and interpretation of the images. However, the availability and accessibility of MRI machines for dental practitioners remain limited.

Dental magnetic attachments pose no risk from RF heating or magnetically induced displacement at 3.0 T(tesla) MRI [17]. A Tesla is the unit of measurement that quantifies a magnetic field's strength.

The MRI, when compared with CT, has been shown to be reliable with respect to bone measurements for dental implant planning. However, further studies are necessary to determine the technical advantages of resonance at lower fields, com-pared with those of CT and MRI [18].

3.2. Clinical assessment

When the patient arrives at the practice, the staff meets and greets them, offers hospitality, and asks that a medical history form be filled in.

First impression, presenting complaint, dental, social, and medical history asked and noted.

The first intimation of the patient's character may lie in their handwriting on the medical history form. (PubMed has 61 references to graphology. Worth reading and incorporating). Large letters, when used, means 'notice me, understand me'. They want details. Small letters indicate strong focus and concentration on the subject at hand. The patient is reserved but takes everything in.

Consult PubMed on 'Graphology' for more detailed information. Confer with your staff to find out their opinion of the patient's attitude towards them and the prospect of treatment.

This will include details of their oral hygiene routines, which include brushing, flossing, toothpicks, toothpaste type, and use of Waterjet. Smoking and nicotine habits, alcohol, and illicit drugs need to be emphasised. Diet history and occupation, even though some patients may ask themselves why the dentist wants to know my job. It is nice to introduce why you need to know briefly.

The physical examination of the patient starts as they walk into the room. Gait, balance, and bearing can all indicate their current state of health, their attitude to you, and the prospect of treatment. These can change once they get to know you.

The occlusal examination can indicate skeletal factors that may influence their physical success with your treatment. There may be indications for referral to a chiropractor who has appropriate knowledge of the oral connection between posture and occlusion [19].

Other factors to be noted include the condition of the patient's nails, skin, hair and mouth odour. For example, nails - in endocarditis, the nails can be clubbed; in iron-deficiency anaemia, the nails can be spoon-shaped (spoon nails); skin – purpuric papules on the eyelids and extremities indicate amyloidosis; hair – patchy alopecia may indicate sarcoidosis or endocrine diseases: mouth odour (halitosis) can be of oral or non-oral origin. Halitosis of oral origin is dealt with later. Non-oral origins are respiratory tract infection, gastrointestinal reflux disease, diabetic ketosis, and drugs like disulphiram and phenothiazine. At the first visit, the patient should be checked for blood pressure and pulse and undergo a monopolar ECG, spirometer (if the patient suffers from respiratory disease), and blood glucose tests. Should any abnormalities be found, the patient is referred to their GP. If the patient is on any drugs, the amount being taken per day, the reason for their prescription, and for how long they have been prescribed should be recorded. Blood tests including Total Blood Screen: HCT, Red Cell Count, MCV MCH, MCHC, Platelet Count, White Cell Count, Neutrophils, Lymphocytes, Monocytes, Eosinophils, Basophils, ESR, Urea, Creatinine, Calcium, Phosphate, Uric Acid, Blood Glucose, INR, Triglycerides, Cholesterol HDL Cholesterol, HDL, LDL Cholesterol, Iron, Clotting Profile, Prothrombin Time, Vitamin D, Ferritin, ALT, AST, Bilirubin total, HBA1C, TSH (T4 if needed), blood group/type, and urinalysis can eliminate doubts regarding old or medically compromised patients.

The examination continues with screening the patient's face, including skin, eyes, hair, and intra-orally, the mouth's soft tissue. Any abnormalities should be recorded and photographed; for ulcers or bumps, use a ruler to demonstrate the size.

A full dental chart notes teeth present, BPE or six-point chart, existing restorations, types of materials, teeth mobility, missing teeth, and any prosthesis. If the patient knows, the cause of missing teeth should be recorded, such as trauma, genetics, dental disease, tumour, or unknown.

Root-treated teeth are recorded with the details of any shortcomings. Occlusion, malocclusion, tooth wear, and parafunction are noted. Crossbites, especially in the future dental implant site position, are noted. Check the space available for the implant's final crown, especially if the opposing tooth is extruded. Freeway space can be classified as less than 2 mm, 2-6 mm, and more than 6 mm. Attrition and the degree of wear are noted: enamel only, dentin exposed, full surface of dentin exposed.

The Basic Erosive Wear Examination (BEWE) evaluates erosion levels in the mouth by dividing it into six areas and assigning scores ranging from 0 to 3 based on specific criteria:
• 0: No erosion
• 1: Initial loss of surface texture
• 2: Distinct defect with enamel loss less than 50% of the area
• 3: Enamel loss of more than 50% of the area
The total score determines the recommended intervention:

• Total score of 0-2: Routine observation with follow-up every three years
• The total score of 3-8: Oral hygiene and dietary assessment, with follow-up every two years
• Total score of 9-13: Dietary assessment, fluoride measures, and avoidance of restoration, with follow-up every 6-12 months
• Total score exceeding 14: Dietary assessment, fluoride measures, follow-up every 6-12 months, and consideration of restoration if necessary.

The TMJ should be examined, and the maximum opening should be noted. This is critical in dental implant surgery, especially when adequate room is available to place the dental implant handpiece and burs and instruments in the patient's mouth. This is especially so in the lower posterior region.

The author recommends studying the recent clinical guidelines produced by the Faculty's Clinical Standards Committee in March 2024 (https://www.rcseng.ac.uk/dental-faculties/fds/publications-guidelines/clinical-guidelines/).

BPE (Basic Periodontal Examination) needs to be emphasised, and when indicated, six-point full periodontal charting should be carried out. Plaque scores and bleeding scores should be recorded. BPE 4 requires a full-mouth six-point chart.

For the posterior mandible region, the lingual undercut (submandibular gland fossa) can be estimated using the index finger running from the crest toward the apical region, but be careful it may be uncomfortable for the patient as the mylohyoid muscle is pushing down.

Full orthodontic assessment is unnecessary, but significant occlusion abnormalities, such as a large overjet - forward or reverse, traumatic overbite, crossbite, crowding, spaces, and unerupted teeth should be noted. If the canine is missing, check by palpation or study the DPT. The Index of Orthodontic Treatment Therapy Needs (IOTN) can help. Refer for specialist opinion as needed.

A photo and/or intra-oral scan of the edentulous area should show the ridge width, height, and mesiodistal dimensions. This can prove helpful when explaining the treatment plan. It can also be useful for general educational purposes and as evidence if ever needed. Bear in mind that you need to explain to the patient why you need the photos and gain the patient's approval or consent before you take any.

Oral cancer screening must be advocated, using chemiluminescent light Vizitlite Plus with Toluidine blue and Toluidine blue staining but after rinsing the mouth with 1% acetic acid to eliminate mechanically retained stain.

Toluidine blue binds to free anionic groups like sulfate, phosphate, and carboxylate radicals, which stains deoxyribonucleic acid of dysplastic changes and appear as royal blue (dark stain) areas in the mouth.

Autofluorescence can detect abnormal tissue that is not noticed by visual inspection, like VEL scope and Identafi. After using the white light, violet light is used, and then amber light is used, which is absorbed by haemoglobin and highlights the vasculature around the lesions. An abnormal tissue exhibits loss of fluorescence and disorganised vasculature.

Where there is a history of dry mouth, or it is suspected, it should be tested for through sialometry. Testing would be indicated where the patient has undergone head and neck radiotherapy, has been diagnosed with Sjogren's syndrome, lymphoma, sarcoidosis, Graft versus host disease, or is undergoing drug therapy. This last would include anti-hypertensive, anti-cholinergic, anti-depressant, diuretic, or cytotoxic therapy. Sialometry is conducted by having the patient produce a flow of unstimulated resting saliva and deposit this into a funnel attached to a graduated or UltraSal tube. Normal salivary flow will be indicated at 0.25 ml/ minute.

A fuller analysis of the mouth can be conducted with the help of the Spotchem ST device. This uses dual-wavelength reflectometry, and the results can be organised into what is referred to as a radar chart. This displays visually the results of the data obtained. The resulting information is divided into three main categories: tooth health, gum health, and oral cleanliness. Each of these is further subdivided into three indicator categories, which are graded as low, average, or high.

The three main categories are:
Tooth health:
- cariogenic bacteria, where the percentage of cariogenic bacteria is assessed,
- acidity, when a low pH renders the teeth more vulnerable,
- buffering capacity, which indicates the mouth's protective resistance to acid.
Gum Health
- Blood, where the presence of blood in the saliva is detected: high indicates gingival inflammation, ulcer,

- Leukocytes: the number of leukocytes analysed, when high, indicates gingival inflammation.
- Protein: where a high level indicates an increased bacterial population
Oral Cleanliness:
- Ammonia level, when an increased level indicates a high bacterial population, causing bad breath (figure 3.3).

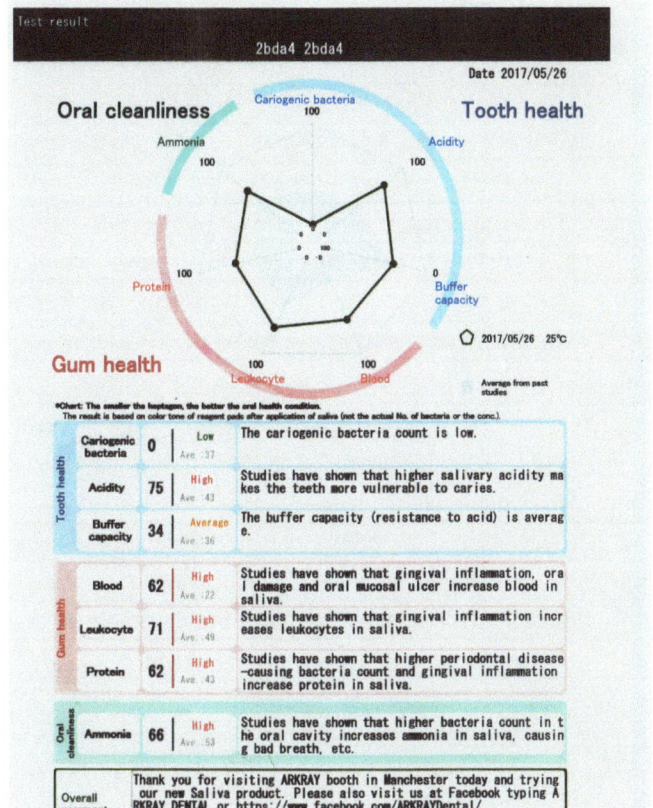

Figure 3.3 A fuller analysis of the mouth bacteria with the help of the Spotchem ST device.

The use of the Spotchem ST device is not mandatory; however, every little piece of information helps.

70

Aesthetic Examination:

Tooth replacement by any means, including dental implants, needs a thorough, systematic, and detailed examination. Regarding dental implants, patient expectations are higher, which may be due to the high cost of treatment. Generally, facial, dental and phonetic analyses are performed. Twenty-four points of what a dentist should observe and note and reflect in the treatment plan as follows:

1	The value of aligning the maxillary dental midline (DM) and facial midline (FM):
	Facial vertical axis (FVA): the nasion (a point between the eyebrows) and the base of the philtrum (also referred to as Cupid's Bow).
	A line connecting these two landmarks should locate the FM and determine the midline's direction.
2	Facial form: square, ovoid, or tapper
3	Lips: thin, normal, or thick and symmetric when relaxing and smiling.
4	Smile line: long or short, normal (only shows papillae) or high
5	Smile zone shape: straight, curved, ellipse, bow, rectangular and inverted.
6	E Plane is a line drawn from the nose's tip to the chin's tip. In Caucasians, the lower lip is 2 mm behind the line, and the upper lip is 4 mm behind the line.
7	Nasio-labial angle: ideally is 90°, and the profile is normal, convex, or concave.
8	Dimension of upper central (width and height) using digital or Castroviejo Calliper
9	Incisal display on rest: upper incisors, average for males is 2.0 mm and females 3.5 mm. With age, the upper display reduces, and lower incisors increase.
10	If the dental vertical axis coincides or is parallel to FVA
11	Dental Horizontal (DH)= Facial Horizontal (FH): The interpupillary line, ophraic line (eyebrows), and commissural line.
	Is FV vertical to the FH? The incisal edge line (incisal plane) and the buccal cusp tips of any posterior teeth on display in a wide smile are to the FH plane.
12	The labial contour of the upper incisors is in three places, and the emergence profile is 15°.
13	Comparing Maxillary Central incisors, position, symmetry, colour/shade, Teeth proportions, and biometrics rules.
14	Does the incisal edge line of the maxillary anterior teeth follow the superior contour edge of the lower lip?
15	Is the incisal edge line, convex, gull-wing, or straight?
16	Speech evaluation: spontaneous clear speck (the F, V, and S) sounds. The patient pronounces Mississippi (for the sibilant sounds) and counts 51-59 for labio-dental sounds.
	S, Z, T, D, N for analysing contact between tongue tip and palate. E.g. if the tooth is thick in the canine area, the patient whistles when pronouncing S.
17	Zenith lines (most apical point).
	The gingival margin of the upper lateral incisor is above, at the level, or below the gum line of the central incisor and canine.
18	The golden proportion of upper anterior teeth: central incisor (1.6), lateral incisor (1), and canine (0.6).
19	Embrasures: The interdental space should be filled with healthy gum at the contact point.
	The papillary contour: is it pointed and fills the interdental space to the contact point?
20	Gingival shape, Zenith point, and longitudinal axis.
21	Axial inclination: Inclination is more toward the midline, more pronounced toward central to the canines, and so on toward premolars, making the mesiodistal size of the crowns less visible toward distal

22	During a smile, the area between the corners of the mouth and the buccal surfaces of the maxillary teeth, the more the space, the less visible concealed. Properly treated upper buccal corridor demonstrated uniformity in colour and alignment of the anterior with the posterior segments in the smile zone. There should not be a shadow on the buccal corridor in the posterior segments.
	The tonicity of the facial muscles, the predominance of the cuspid, and the discrepancy of the value (shade) of the premolars and the anterior teeth influence the appearance of the buccal corridor.
	Buccal corridor: narrow (dark), normal or wide (full)
23	Shade of sclera
24	Tooth colour: use natural light or dental base light LED (of 5500 K and 6500 K with a Colour Rendering Index (CRI) of more than 90.
	Measure respectively:
	1) value (brightness), the grey scale using the middle third of the crown.
	2) Chrome (saturation), using 1/3 of the cervical area of the crown.
	3) hue (red, yellow, blue) using the 1/3 of the incisal of the crown.
	If using the Vita shade guide, sort them as:
	B1-A1-B2-D2-A2-C1-C2-D4-A3-D3-B3-A3.5-B4-C3-A4-C4

Full mouth rehabilitation

When considering full-mouth rehabilitation, it becomes even more complicated.

When there are few teeth plus major vertical bone loss, leaving the teeth in situ reduces aesthetics and leads to food retention. From the surgical point of view, if the patient with systemic disease is accepted for selective oral surgery, then dental implant surgery is applicable. The patient will choose the type of prosthetic treatment based on guidance from the dentist.

Bone quality and quantity should be assessed. The ridge width should be at least 6.5 mm to provide a diameter of 3.5 mm for the implant and 1.5 mm for peri-implant bone.

When the width is between 4-6.5 mm, a ridge expansion, ridge split, or a combined technique can be applied successfully. This cannot be applied when the bone is solely cortex, and the cancellous bone is limited - usually the case in the lower anterior region.

A width of between 3-4mm is problematic. In these circumstances, it is usual to use free bone block grafts or guided bone regeneration techniques. The author prefers to use a ridge split and try to place a stable one-piece or conventional implant, but if this is not possible. Just leave it. Wait three months, go back in, repeat the procedure, and try to place a one-piece implant. Today, a ridge-split and simultaneous one-piece wedge (blade) implant is recommended to replace single root teeth.

When the width is less than 3 mm, split the ridge and wait for 3-4 months for it to heal. Alternatively, we can use a free bone block donated intra-orally by bone harvesting from the mandible's chin, ramus, or external oblique ridge. If this is not possible, it might be harvested extra-orally, usually from the iliac crest, but the success rate is questionable. Different scaffold types with or without membrane, alone or mixed with autogenous bone, have been recommended.

It is very evident that the buccal-lingual position of the implant may not be ideal. The use of different types of prosthetic procedures should resolve the amount of the discrepancy.

Increasing the width is difficult, but increasing the height is much more so.

The soft tissue not only reflects the future aesthetics of the crown but also the survivability of the dental implant.

A few examples may help you make a decision.

Two implants are recommended when replacing a single tooth if the mesiodistal length is more than 11.5mm. Placing three implants to reduce the load in the free-end posterior region is better.

Do not place a minimum number of implants in a full mouth reconstruction, but try to add one implant in each quadrant.

We could discuss cases where everything is in order, but instead, we will concentrate on more realistic cases which present problems that limit the possibilities.

The quality of bone

We need to be able to classify bone quality and quantity because it is important to record this in the patient's notes and provide an algorithm for treatment planning. The author classifies bone based on the cortex's thickness and the cancellous bone's hardness or softness.

The relevant divisions for the cortex are 1) more than 4 mm wide, 2) only 1-4mm wide, 3) less than 1 mm wide. Cancellous bone is classified as hard (like oak), medium (like elm) or soft (like cream cheese), (figure 3.4).

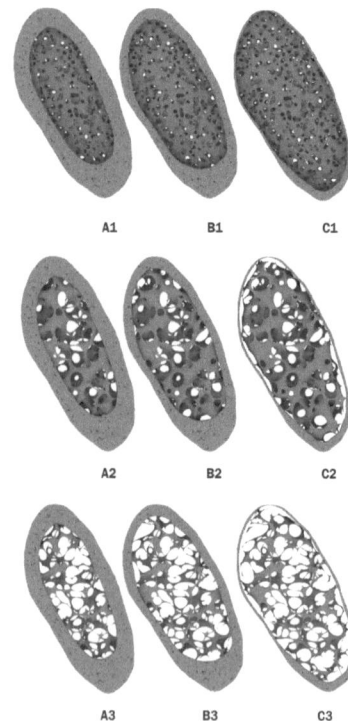

Figure 3.4 The cortex's relevant divisions are 1) more than 4 mm wide, 2) 1-4mm wide, 3) less than 1 mm wide. Cancellous bone is classified as hard (like oak), medium (like elm) or soft (like cream cheese).

The classification of alveolar bone dimensions below provides an algorithm to be used as a guide until the dentist has enough experience to confidently provide a sound treatment plan.

Bone Width	mm	Bone Height	mm	Implant Angle	Crown Height	mm
A	6.5 <	I	8 <	0-15 °	1	Equal
B	3-6.5	II	4-8	15-40 °	2	+ 3
C	3.0 >	III	4>	40 ° <	3	3<

UPPER ANTERIOR

The following factors need to be considered: the length of the final crown, the aesthetics of the soft tissue, and the depth of the undercut of the labial surface of the bone. On the palatal surface, toward the midline, the nasopalatine canal also reduces the alveolar width. We need also to consider the angle between the axis of the implant and the future crown.

If the bone height is type II, there are two options to increase the height,

1. A bone block is used to increase the height toward the coronal and not toward the apex (2.2.a).

2. To increase the height toward the apex (figure 3.5b).

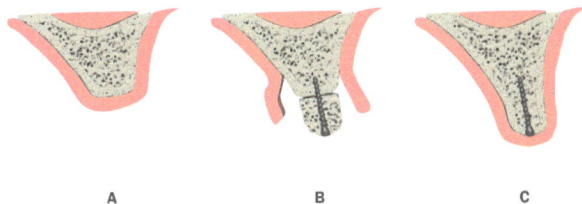

Figure 3.5.a Apical vs coronal bone graft to increase the height of bone.
Increase the height toward the coronal part of the remaining alveolar bone.

There is no doubt the coronal bone graft is more difficult due to the need for soft tissue closure and the increased chance of soft tissue dehiscence, but the length of the implant/crown is reduced, and the lip support is more pleasing.

If the height is about 6-8 mm, pushing up the floor of the cortex using osteotomes invades the cortex at the apical area by up to 0.5 mm, increasing the primary stability and the length.

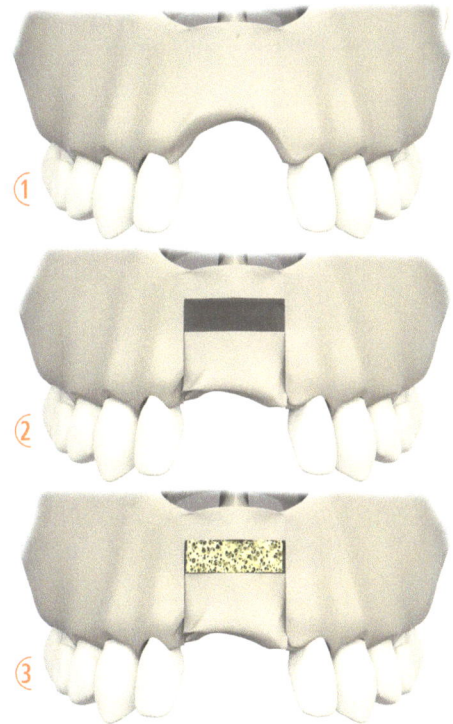

Figure 3.5.b There are two options to compensate for the height: adding to the apical area or adding to the coronal area. Although the first technique has a higher success rate, it is less user-friendly.

We need to use either a drill that does not rag the soft tissue or apply osteotomes to push up the floor of the nose. The cortical at the bone's floor is thick but less invasive with bone block grafting. The technique is not recommended when the cortical thickness of the floor of the nose is more than 3 mm. Make sure that the nasal mucosa has not been perforated. It is also recommended that the nasal floor be elevated through intra-oral access to apply autogenous bone or mixed with bone substitutes to fill the nasal cavity. This technique is more predictable, but the ratio of the length of implant/crown is high and will have mechanical and aesthetic consequences.

The ideal angle is the alpha angle. The beta angle (15-40°) has some limitations which can be circumvented with an angulated abutment. A full ceramic crown is beneficial if there is not enough space buccally.

For delta (> 40°) cases, there are two options: 1) surgery to increase the width with simultaneous placement of the implant, and 2) placing the implant in the available bone and, after the healing period of the dental implant, adjust the angle of the implant by segmental osteotomy, and as you do this, rotate the block with its implant palatal to correct the angle. Simultaneously, the crest of the alveolar bone with the implant will move more coronally. A bone wedge can be harvested from the labial-apical and pushed between the rotated block and the neighbouring bone. The lack of need to use screws, wires/miniplate makes it safer as there is limited space around the rotated block (figure 3.6).

Rotating the bone block and then placing one piece of dental implant may be preferable.

The block rotation technique can avoid the complications of a free graft and the need for a second surgery site to harvest the bone. This procedure is more predictable.

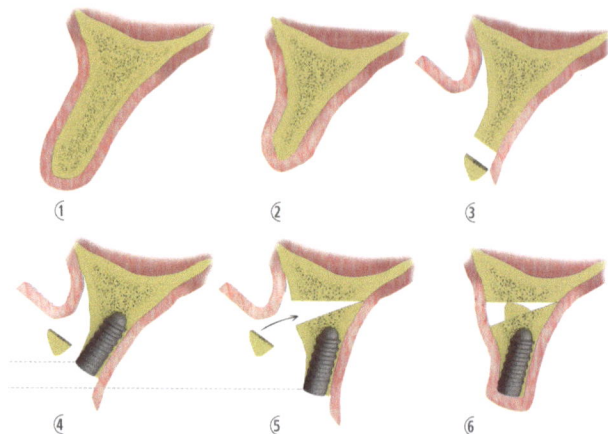

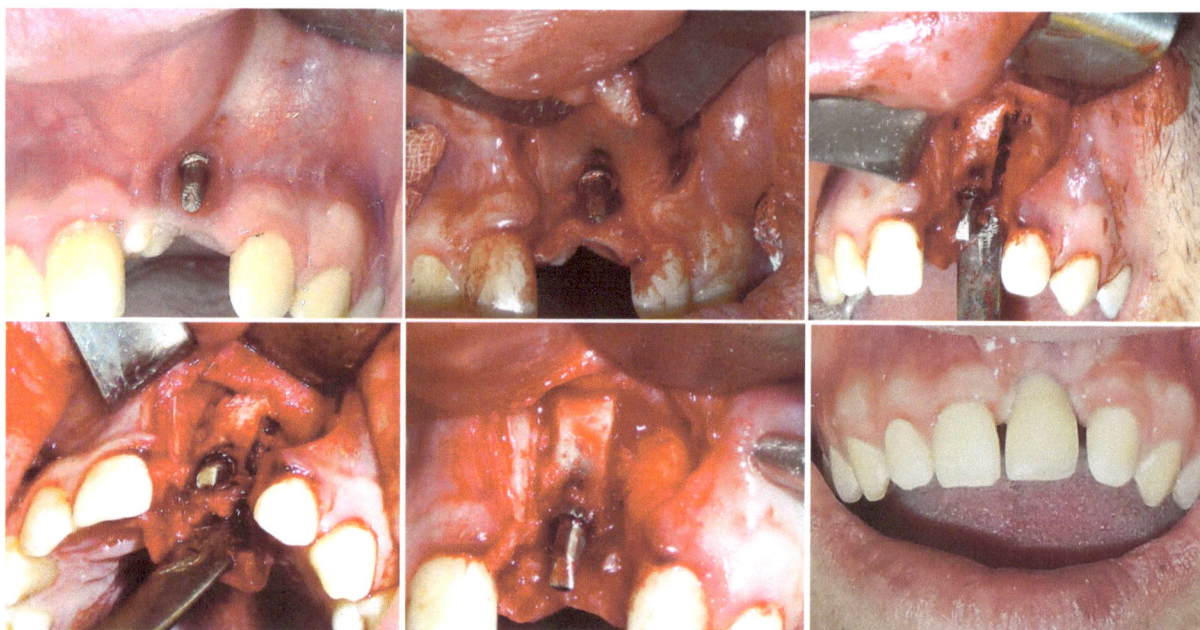

Figure 3.6 a and b. The angle and height can be corrected by placing the implant where the bone is available and then rotating the block by apical osteotomy. Lower right, demonstrate the correction of the angle and height using a provisional acrylic/composite crown till the soft tissue heals.

Predicting/envisaging the final crown: Obviously, the ideal is to provide a natural-looking crown, but there is often a lack of bone and, therefore, gingiva. Short of using bone grafts, what is the best option? The best answer is a one-piece implant or 4 mm gingival height abutment in three-piece implants and waiting three months for healing to occur. This is the easiest and often the best way to produce a few millimetres increase in gingival height by crepitation movement of soft tissue cells on the polish surface towards titanium. It avoids using more complicated techniques, which may produce unpredictable results.

More importantly, with a one-piece implant, the soft tissue healing period overlaps with the bone healing period, saving time. If placing conventional 3-piece implants, during the exposure of the implant at the second surgery, directly place the abutment instead of the temporary healing screw and let the soft tissue run over the titanium surface as much as it can to reduce the clinical height of the crown. The use of pink porcelain helps; it never looks natural; it is just better than nothing.

UPPER POSTERIOR

This is the only segment where bone loss can be observed from the apex and coronal (figure 3.7).

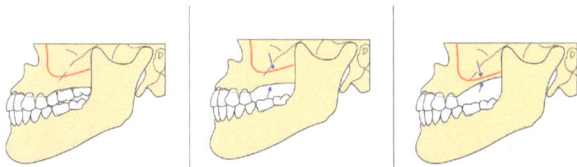

Figure 3.7 Under the maxillary sinus, the upper posterior region is the only area in which bone resorption is by the coronal movement of the sinus floor and apical alveolar crest resorption (left to right).

Usually, dentists prefer to augment the sinus floor rather than increase the height of the alveolar bone or both. However, when coronal bone loss has not been repaired or replaced, high torque will be placed upon the implants, and the poor bone quality will undermine long-term success.

As a blanket rule, if the vertical coronal bone loss is less than 5 mm or the dentist will not calculate the torque, then the options below are recommended.

The quality of the bone dictates the surgical technique to be used. When the bone height is type II (3-6.5 mm), it usually has type A (> 6.5 mm) bone width. Type II bone height can be treated by closed sinus lift (one-stage osteotomy). Type III (< 4 mm) bone height can be treated only by open sinus lift.

The worst scenarios are B III or C III. We cannot expand the ridge and perform a closed sinus lift and implant placement simultaneously because insufficient bone mass can be pushed toward the sinus floor.

When type II and III bone height are observed, If the patient is lucky and a 3mm bone width is found posterior to the maxillary sinus, placing an implant palatal to the sinus is more logical, although an unwelcome angle will be produced. The maximum angle should be type B be due to the prosthesis of type Γ being challenging to manage.

Soft tissue is not a problem. With a more palatal incision, keratinised mucosa can be transferred to the buccal surface using a palatal partial thickness-buccal full-thickness flap. The crown's length is less of a concern, but types II and III exert greater torque on the implants, and if there is poor bone quality in that area, we need to be worried.

There are controversies regarding the placement of short dental implants (6 mm) vs maxillary sinus floor augmentation and 11 mm dental implants [20]. The author's question would be if a 6 mm dental implant suffices in the upper posterior region as the quality of the bone is poor and the force applied to dental implants in the region is maximum. Why don't we use shorter dental implants, like 6 mm or less, in all situations? Companies would not have to make longer implants unless they are for immediate replacement.

LOWER ANTERIOR

We should consider the incisors separately from the canines. 2.5-3mm diameter, one-piece implants provide the best options to enable you to prepare the proximal surfaces of the finishing margins of the abutments and provide space for future crowns. In immediate replacement cases, the cortex may permit a 5mm diameter implant to be placed in the canine area. In any event, the canine replacement must have a minimum diameter of 3.4 mm. Most of the time, ridge expansion, or a ridge split, will be unsuccessful due to limited cancellous bone and thin cortex, which may fracture during extraction, and there is a high potential for bone resorption. The author prefers to use delayed-immediate implant placement in the lower canines.

With single tooth implants, alveolar bone height is always type I, but type II will sometimes occur and may well result in difficulties with aesthetics and problems with food retention.

Due to the anatomical angle of the alveolar bone, Angle alpha is sometimes found. Difficulties will occur, especially if there is consequential occupation of the tongue space.

LOWER POSTERIOR

When the width of the alveolar bone is type B (3-6.5mm), GBR, Bone Block or ridge split are the dentist's options.

Ridge splitting is the least invasive, and the complication and failure are not as severe as bone block grafts, which are the consequence of the soft tissue exposure of the graft. By selecting the ridge split technique, we should bear in mind that in the best scenario, the implants are positioned lingually, and the lingual-buccal cantilever, the offset relative to the centre of the crown, is a biomechanical risk factor, and there is no buccal-lingual space to place the implants in tripod configuration to reduce the workload and need to be applied as much as possible [21] (figure 3.8).

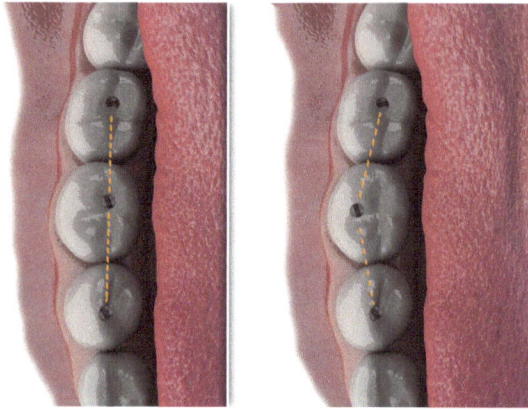

Figure 3.8 The implants are placed offset at the position of the lingual cusp. The occlusal force will be at the caution of danger level. However, if the implants are placed in the tripod configuration, significantly less stress will apply to the implants.

Also, due to the limited space, the metal is exposed on the lingual surface of the crown or bridge, or the surface has an opaque layer only due to lack of space. In these cases, if the patient is concerned, the Zirconia prosthesis does resolve the problem.

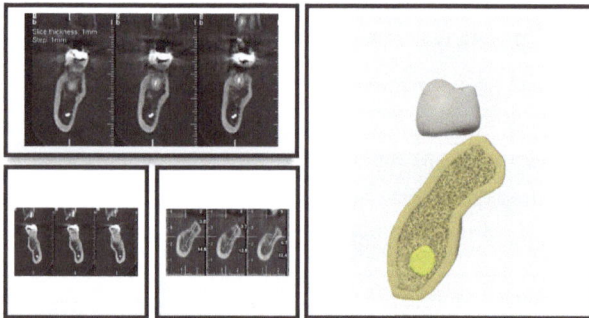

Figure 3.9 A ridge split in the lower posterior region can be limited in the prosthodontic stage as the implant will be inserted lingually compared to the ideal buccal-lingual position. CBCT demonstrates the relationship between alveolar bone, root, and crown in the upper left. The lower left is another scenario. The lower middle and far right demonstrate the relationship between the remaining alveolar bone and the future crown.

The space between the labial/buccal surface and the gingiva of the prosthesis empowers food entrapment under the gingival prosthesis, which needs a skilled laboratory to resolve the problem (figure 3.10, 3.11).

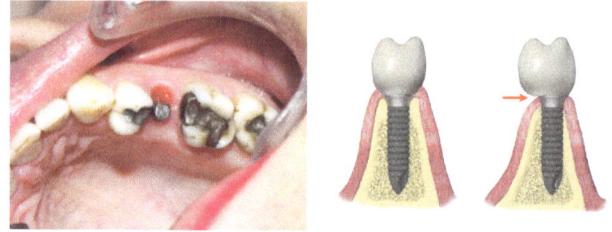

Figure 3.10 Food entrapment could be one of the limitations of ridge splitting in the posterior mandibular region. However, due to mobile soft tissue, it could be limited. However, the patient must be warned. The left photo demonstrates the position of the abutment and the healed soft tissue under a provisional crown. The right photo demonstrates the normal relationship between the implant when there is no bone loss and compares it when the implant is positioned lingual (the red arrow shows the undercut under the crown).

Ridge-splitting is not always successful because the cortex is thick, with a minimum quantity of cancellous bone. Sometimes, though, enough cancellous bone, even if of poor quality, allows ridge-splitting. We should not be surprised to find cases of 3-4mm cortical bone with poor quality cancellous bone, affecting the bone preparation technique.

Planned green-stick fractures: width 3-4 – section as needed, open, leave to heal 3/12 (figure 3.12).

Limitations:

1) when an unplanned green-stick fracture of the lingual cortex occurs (more likely than a fracture of the buccal cortex), especially when the alveolar ridge height has been resorbed to such an extent that the external oblique ridge needs to be displaced.

2) When the patient cannot open the mouth adequately. The procedure is the same - leave to heal for 3/12. Piezosurgery is a marvel in this scenario.

This technique is less invasive and more predictable, with less post-operative pain than guided bone regeneration techniques, which need a more aggressive flap and periosteal reflection.

At least 8.5 mm height of alveolar bone is needed to place a dental implant.

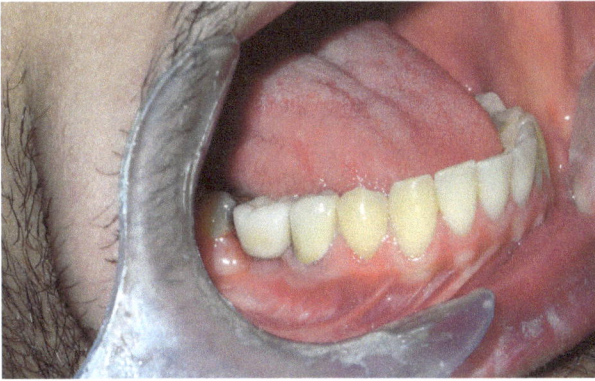

Figure 3.11 The lower right first molar has been replaced by a ridge split in the lingula position; however, the quality of the buccal mucosa is mobile and non-keratinised, and the mobility of the buccal mucosa has permitted to fill the space under the crown, and there is a potential of food entrapment.

The last consequence a dentist wants is to cause an anaesthetised or para-anesthetised lip. There may be an undercut lingually, even though the DPT demonstrates a good height, but the bone preparation can perforate inside the floor of the mouth, which is also hazardous. There are multiple anatomic features which could be damaged.

Sometimes, we have no choice but to respect the undercut and place the implant parallel to the lingual cortex. That means there would be an angulation of alfa- or beta-type. Regarding β type, providing a fixed prosthesis without food retention will require greater attention. Buccal soft tissue is very often mobile and non-keratinised, and this makes it more difficult for the patient to clean. Also, torque may be unwittingly increased. If the implant is placed lingually and sometimes angulated and if the length of the crown is also increased, this will result in increased torque. Bear in mind that cancellous bone is sometimes poor.

The number of implants placed is another controversial issue. The patient and the dentist usually prefer that fewer implants be placed to reduce the cost. However, the factors that need to be considered are high vertical distance and lingula-labial distance, minimum implant length, and maximum occlusal force. On the other hand, due to limited width, the diameter of the dental implant is minimal (3.3-3.5 mm), but the threads of the implant will touch the inner buccal and lingual cortex. The author believes in placing 3 (three pod configuration) dental implants replacing the second and first molar, and if the second premolar is replaced, there is no need to increase the number of dental implants [10].

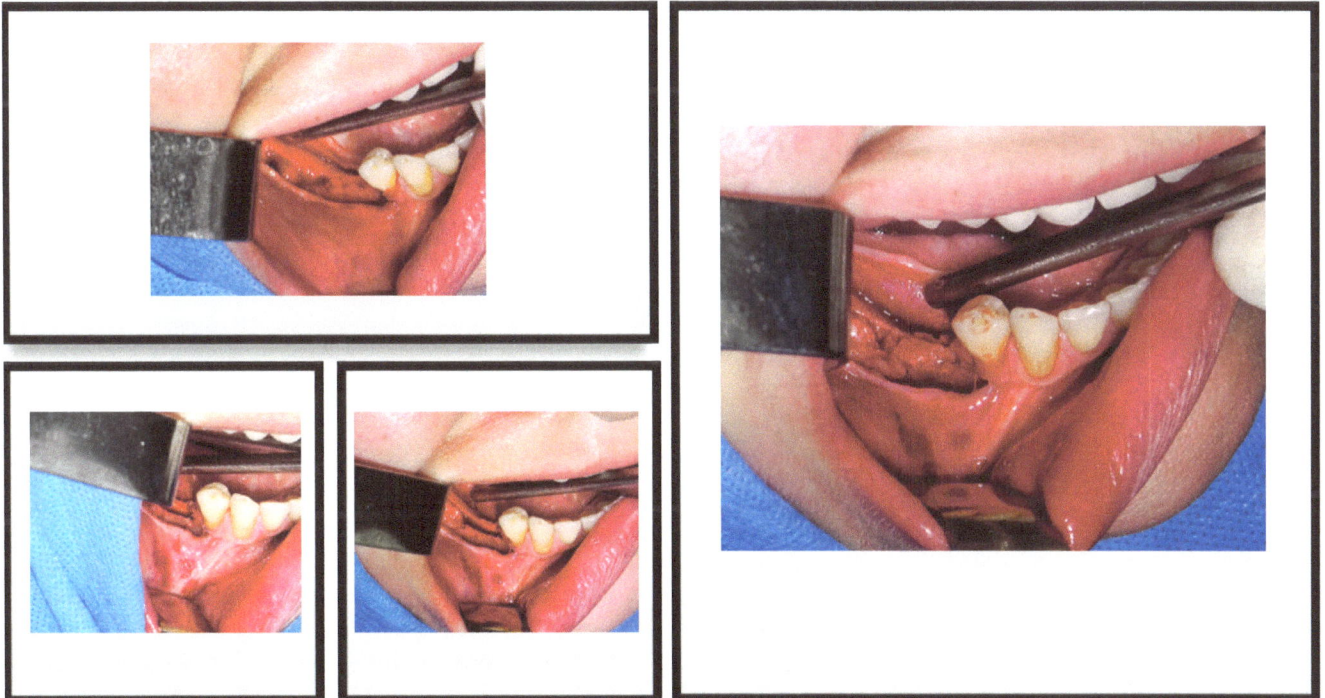

Figure 3.12 Ridge split and placing autogenous bone inside the groove, especially when the buccal and/or lingual cortex is not stable after splitting. Left to right, bone width less than 3 mm with irregular buccal surface; ridge split using disc, pre-elevator and chisel; bone chips were placed on the distal segment, which was the least stable region, and then the top of the groove.

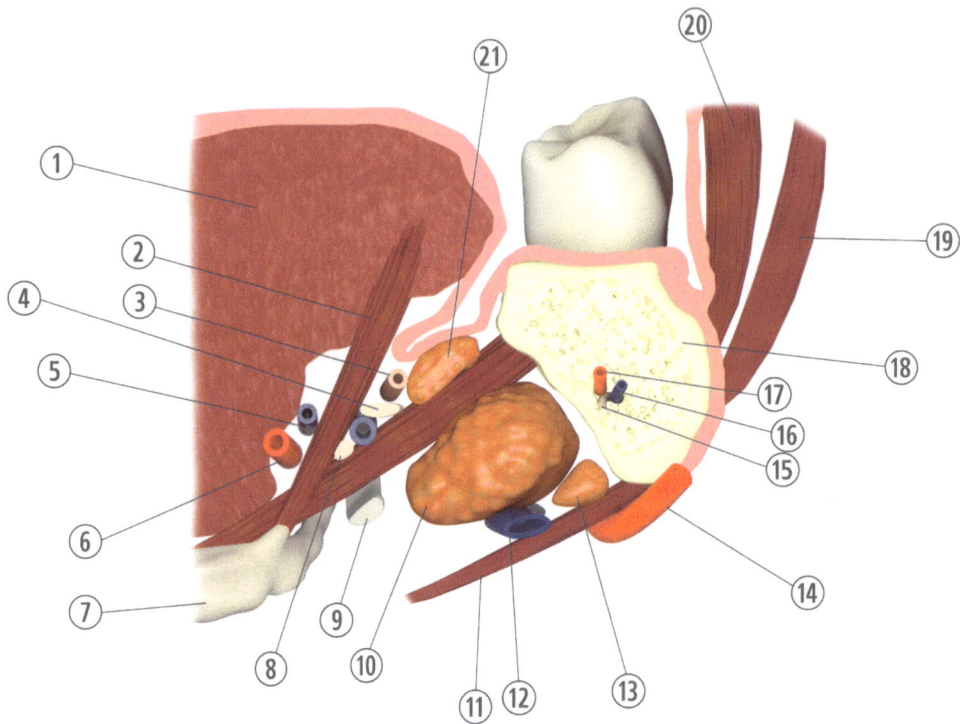

Figure 3.13 Under the Mylohyoid muscle, the facial artery is the first hazardous anatomic feature the dentist needs to worry about; however, the facial vein and submandibular gland are also in access to be invaded. Cross section at the lower first molar: 1) muscles of tongue, 2) Hyoglossus muscle, 3) Submandibular duct, 4) lingual nerve, 5) Lingual vein, 6) lingual artery, 7) Hyoid bone, 8) Mylohyoid muscle, 9) Intermediate digastric tendon, 10) Submandibular salivary gland, 11) Platysma muscle, 12) Facial vein, 13) Submandibular lymph node, 14) Facial artery, 15) Inferior dental nerve, 16) Inferior dental vein, 17) Inferior dental artery, 18) Mandible, 19) Muscles of facial expression, 20) Buccinator muscle, 21) Sublingual salivary gland.

There is a belief that In full arch rehabilitation, the maxillae of the prosthetic unit/implant is recommended to be 1, and for the mandible, two units are sectioned in the midline. Clinical reports show that a 2-unit prosthesis failure is more significant than a 1-unit prosthesis [22].

Why long implants?

The disadvantage of the shorter implant arises from its potential failure to engage sufficient cancellous bone and cortical bone at the apex. The remodelling of the bone at the bone-implant interface is not uniform along its entire length, and this inconsistent osseointegration can result in one region's attaching to the bone and the other not. This is important during the healing period with immediate or early loading. By contrast, the increased length of the longer implant provides primary stability through its more significant contact at the bone-implant interface, whether that is more deeply in cancellous bone or, especially, in contact with the cortical plate.

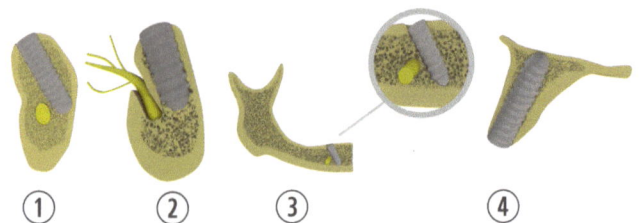

Figure 3.14 Long implants can engage the apex of the implant in the cortical plate, thus increasing the primary and secondary dental implant stability; otherwise, it is unnecessary.

79

The dentist must remember that cortical engagement must be carefully considered. There are two concepts of drill design. The dentist must bear in mind that cortical engagement has to be fully understood as there are two concepts of implant designs regarding drill length/dental implant length.

In one, the implant goes to the tip of the prepared cavity, and in the other, it stops at the base of the tip of the cavity. With such systems, there is a chance that the implant may not seat entirely so that 1-2 mm of the threads remain above the crest. Should the dentist now try to use force in order to seat an implant that has not, and cannot, sit all the way, he will realise that he cannot unscrew the implant to make any corrections.

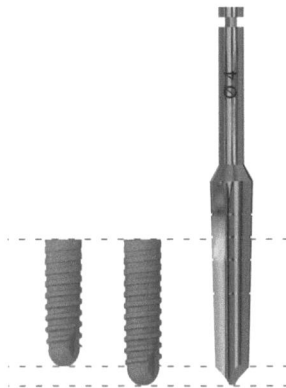

Figure 3.15 The dentist needs to know if the length of the implant coincides with the tip or the base of the tip.

Why short implants?

The short dental implant has been defined as being 6-8mm or under 10 mm.

The highest strain around implants has been observed in the 5mm crestal region. There are reports of short dental implants of 6-8 mm in length being successful in the short term, but there is potential for a compromised implant-crown ratio, and this concern increases in the posterior region with its larger prosthetic table. Even though the author does not recommend these types of dental implants, it has been recommended by others, so if employed, he feels it should be done only in patients with high-quality bone, no history of periodontal disease, and no specific risk factors, whether systemic, such as diabetes, or local, such as bruxism.

Implant diameter and geometry have a pronounced effect on stresses in the cortical plate. Strain values obtained with the short implants were drastically higher (clearly above 10,000 □strain) compared to long implants (5,000 □strain, in general) [23,24].

The main question the author brings forward. Do I want to place a 6mm dental implant where the force of mastication is up to 300N?

Surgical guides:

Surgical guides assist in correctly positioning the dental implant and can predict and prevent some clinical and laboratory complications.

A diagnostic wax-up is prepared, and a surgical guide or template is fabricated after a trial of the teeth arrangement or duplication of the denture.

A guide pinhole is drilled through a clear vacuum-formed matrix. The hole indicates the optimal position of the dental implant. It can also be used as a radiographic template. By adding radiopaque materials (5 mm metal ball bearing), radiographic templates can be used to demonstrate:

- The distance between the alveolar ridge and the labial/buccal surface of the final prosthesis,

- Magnification on the X-ray film,

- Illustrate the relationship between an anatomical landmark (e.g. mental foramina) and the radiopaque material embedded in the template.

The surgical guide is placed in position, the dentist uses the first or pilot drill to initiate the perforation, and the remainder of the cavity preparation is continued freehand.

Drill stops may be used if space has been created in the surgical guide.

A restrictive surgical guide reduces intraoperative decision-making.

It seems promising that prosthetically-directed implant placement uses computer software for precise placement and predictable crown position, but bear in mind that tooth-supported surgical guides are superior to soft tissue-borne guides.

There are two different techniques of computer-aided surgery (CAD/CAM): one is to use the CT data to provide a static virtual implant position which will not allow modification during surgery; the other technique is dynamic in as much as it will allow the surgeon to vary the position for implant placement. This is expensive, time-consuming and not needed by the experienced operator.

Computerised tomography (CT) data are used to plan the implant position. A three-dimensional view of the bone's morphology allows the surgeon to survey the surgical bone site and assess its associated risks more accurately. While the accuracy of CAD/CAM technology in dental implant planning has been documented, it is generally regarded as needing further research. The high cost of introducing implant therapy to one's practice will inevitably restrict its availability to many patients.

The potential errors involved in the CAD/CAM manufacture of surgical guides can occur at any stage – during the scanning process, during software planning thanks to human error, and errors occurring during the rapid prototyping of the stent. Because of its reliability and cost, most dentists prefer the conventional method.

Generally, the author believes that using the surgical guide will only assist in locating the implant's mesiodistal position because it is likely that bone thickness bucco-lingually will be limited, as will be the choice.

There are clinical cases in which the tooth-born surgical guide is not applicable, and the removable surgical guided position is not reproducible after flap reflection.

The other concern is that the touch of the drill inside the tubule (plastic or metal) provides debris that can contaminate the bone cavity and blunt the drill.

With the aim of correct mesiodistal positioning of the implant, the author recommends that at the implant placement area, the surgical guide is to the section in half buccal-lingual; the buccal segment is removed, which can give a direct vision for the dentist (figure 3.16).

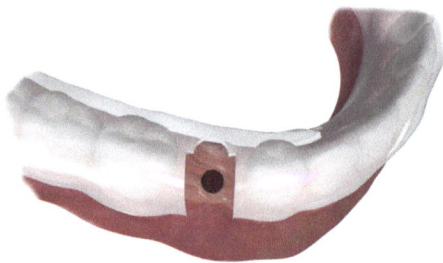

Figure 3.16 For single tooth replacement, a stent is fabricated, and the buccal segment is removed so the dentist can visualise the axis of the drill and the mesiodistal and buccal lingual.

References:

1. Monsour PA, Dudhia R: Implant radiography and radiology. Volume53, Issues1. Special Issue: Oral implant rehabilitation: a state of the art overview of case management. An Australian Dental Journal Special Supplement. June 2008. Pages S11-S25.

2. Schulze RK, d'Hoedt B: Mathematical analysis of projection errors in paralleling technique with respect to implant geometry. Clin Oral Imp Res 2001;12:364-71.

3. Smet E De, jacobs R, Gijbels F, Naert I: The accuracy and reliability of radiographic methpotentialods for the assessment of marginal bone level around oral implants. Dentaomaxillofacial Radiology 2002, 31;176-181.

4. Benn D:. A review of the reliability of radiographic measurements in estimating alveolar bone changes. J Clin Periodontol 1990;17:14-21.

5. Grondahl K, Sunden S, Grondahl H-G: Inter and intra-observer variability in radiographic bone level assessment at Branemark fixtures. Clin Oral Impla Res 1998;9:243-50.

6. Benn DK: Estimating the validity of radiographic measurements of margin bone height changes around osseointegrated implants. Implant Dent 1992;1:79-83.

7. Ekestubbe A, Gröndahl K, Ekholm S, Johansson PE, Gröndahl HG: Low-dose tomographic techniques for dental implant planning. Int J Oral Maxillofac Implants, 1996;11(5):650-9.

8. Norton MR, Gamble C: Bone classification: an objective scale of bone density using the computerized tomography scan. Clin Oral Implants Res 2001 Feb;12(1):79-84.

9. Arx Tv, Lozanoff S, Sendi P, Bornstein MM: Assessment of bone channels other than nasopalatine canal in the anterior maxilla using limited cone beam computed tomography. Surg Radiol Anat 2013;35:783-90.

10. Sukovic P: Cone beam computed tomography in craniofacial imaging. Orthod Craniofac Res. 2003;6(Suppl 1):31-6.

11. Cal ALONSO MBC, VASCONCELOS TV, Luciana Jácome LOPES LJ, WATANABE PCA, FREITAS DQ: Validation of cone-beam computed tomography as a predictor of osteoporosis using the Klemetti classification. Braz Oral Res 2016, 30 (1)1-8.

12. Casselman W, Swenned GRS: Cone-beam computerized tomography (CBCT) imaging of the oral and maxillofacial regon: A systemic review of the literature. Int J Oral Maxillofac Surg 2009;38:609-25.

13. Al-Ani O, Nambia P, Ha KP, Ngeow WC: Safe zone for bone harvesting from the interforaminal region of the mandible. Clin Oral Implants Res 2013, Aug 24 Supple A100:115-21.

14. Naitoh M, Hayashi H, Tsukamoto N, Ariji E. Labial bone assessment surrounding dental implant using cone-beam computed tomography: An in vitro study. Clin. Oral Impl. Res. 23, 2012, 970–974.

15. Fokas G, Vaughn VM, Scarfe WC, Bornstein MM: Accuracy of linear measurements on CBCT images related to presurgical implant treatment planning: A systematic review. Clin Oral Implants Res 2018 Oct;29 Suppl 16:393-415

16. Block MS and Chandler C: Computed tomography-guided surgery: complications associated with scanning, processing, surgery, and prosthetics, J Oral Maxillofac Surg 2009 suppl 3, 67:13-22.

17. Miyata K, Hasegawa M, Abe Y, Tabuchi T, Namiki T, Ishigami T: Radiofrequency heating and magnetically induced displacement of dental magnetic attachments during MRI. Dentomaxillofac Radiol. 2012;41(8):668-74.

18. Pompa V, Galasso S, Cassetta M, Pompa G, De Angelis F, Di Carlo S: A comparative study of Magnetic Resonance (MR) and Computed Tomography (CT) in the pre-implant evaluation. Ann Stomatol (Roma). 2010 Jul;1(3-4):33-8.

19. Westersund CD, Scholten J, Turner RJ: Relationship between craniocervical orientation and center of force of occlusion in adults. Cranio 2017 Sep;35(5):283-289.

20. Guljé FL, Raghoebar GM, Gareb B, Vissink A, Meijer HJA. Single crowns in the posterior maxilla supported by either 11-mm long implants with sinus floor augmentation or by 6-mm long implants: A 10-year randomised controlled trial. Clin Oral Implants Res. 2023 Nov 8. doi: 10.1111/clr.14200. Online ahead of print.

21. Renaurd F, Rangert BO: Risk Factors in Implant Dentistry. Simplified Clinical Analysis for Predictable Treatment, 2008.

22. Degigi M, Piattelli A: . A 7 year follow-up of 93 of immediate loaded titanium dental implants. J Oral Implantology. 31(1):2005, 25-31.

23. I Hasan, F. Heinemann, M. Aitlahrach, and C. Bourauel: Biomechanical finite element analysis of small diameter and short dental implant," Biomedizinische Technik, vol. 55,no. 6, pp. 341–350, 2010.

24. Bourauel, M. Aitlahrach, F. Heinemann, and I. Hasan, Biomechanical finite element analysis of small diameter and short dental implants: extensional study of commercial implants," Biomediziniche Technik, vol. 57, no. 1, pp. 21–32, 2012.

CHAPTER FOUR:

SURGERY

4. SURGERY

Aim:
It explores the surgical techniques and procedures of dental implant placement, including pre-operative preparations, implant placement techniques, and post-operative care protocols.

Necessary Knowledge:
It is assumed that at this stage, you have a general knowledge of the science related to dental implantology, treatment planning, and decision-making—basic knowledge of the radiographic and clinical assessments.

Learning Outcome:
After completing this chapter, the reader will have gained a basic knowledge of the techniques of dental anaesthesia, soft tissue, and hard tissue surgery related to dental implantology. Factors affecting heat generation during bone preparation. How to reduce the heat during bone preparation? What type of irrigation is necessary for bone preparation?

> Mepivacaine and infiltration local anaesthesia is the ideal material and technique.
>
> There are three reasons for the importance of the knowledge of the mandible anatomy:
>
> 1. The potential lingual concavity or angle in the lower region of the mandible,
>
> 2. The presence of the submental space close to the operative site,
>
> 3. the direct access that the submental space has to the submandibular space.
>
> The confluence of these four anatomical features in this region means that any surgical intervention needs to be very carefully prepared for.

4.1. Local Anaesthesia
The success of dental implant therapy is directly related to soft and hard tissue management. Soft tissue management from the incision to peri-restorative component tissue modelling is as important as hard tissue management. Handling the soft and hard tissue is a prerequisite for successful treatment and discomfort. Trust and confidence are the key elements of the dentist-patient relationship, which starts with painless and successful local anaesthesia. Anxiety about dental implant surgery is more prevalent than periodontal surgery, which is more prominent in females. The pain perception is affected by the level of presurgical anxiety. The most uncomfortable experience associated with dental implant surgery is excessive fluid in the mouth, but a trained nurse can eradicate it [1].

There are various local anaesthetics on the market, of which the most commonly used are Lidocaine 2% and Adrenaline 1:80.000, Citanest (Prilocaine 3% with Felypressin 0.03 Unit/ml), Mepivacaine 3%, or Articaine 4% with epinephrine 1:200.000. There are wide varieties of concentrations of the local anaesthetics, plain or different types of vasoconstrictors. Lidocaine and epinephrine were used due to their efficacy and price [2].

During dental implant surgery, systolic blood pressure increases significantly, and pulse rate increases for a short period of time. However, with age, diastolic blood pressure increases, too. During the long period of surgery for multiple implant placement, the systolic, diastolic, and pulse rates increase significantly, even in healthy patients [3].

Epinephrine and norepinephrine are natural hormones and neurotransmitters released during stress and affect the heart and blood pressure. To eradicate the epinephrine reaction of the patients in surgery, the author prefers the use of Mepivacaine without epinephrine and only uses Lidocaine+ epinephrine sparingly - just a few drops subperiosteally - and topically on the sinus mucosa but only if it is not contraindicated. Epinephrine reduces bleeding in the sinus mucosa by contracting the capillaries. Bear in mind the extensive vascular network that is present and the danger of inducing hypertension and tachycardia in a susceptible patient.

Warming the anaesthetic cartridges at about 42°C reduces the pain during injection compared to room temperature, and rubbing the cartridge between the palms of the hand may benefit the patient during the injection [4].

Both local anaesthesia and haemostasis are improved by injecting directly into the gingival margin and interdental papillae until blanching. The author recommends that soft tissue anaesthesia suffices during dental implant surgery, which infiltration can achieve. In the mandible, this is critical when the ID nerve has not been anaesthetised, and the dentist may be warned during the osteotomy.

The infiltration anaesthesia is efficient for dental implant placement in the posterior mandible region where the cortical bone is thick [5].

To reduce pain perception during local anaesthesia injection, comfort the patient by saying that you understand the patient and will do your best. Always have some local anaesthesia in the front of the needle, placing topical anaesthesia before the needle insertion, retract the soft tissue to minimise the thickness of the submucosa and the needle can pierce the mucosa, the bevel of the needle to be parallel to the cortex so it does not pierce the periosteum, every 5 mm penetration inject a small quantity of the local and penetrate the needle more and again a small amount of local is released and between each step wait about 5 seconds. The needle does not need to touch the cortical bone; the local release should be slow and take about 60 seconds. During the injection, asking the patient if he/she is all right is recommended.

Usually, the patients feel uncomfortable when they feel a push, heavy vibration, or tapping. It is essential to warn the patient prior to the stages as they do not like surprises.

The patient feels uncomfortable with mucosa perforation by the needle, raising the flap, especially maxillae, in which the mucoperiosteum is thick, application of a round drill in which the vibration is more than expected, tapping the bone and using osteotomes.

4.2. Soft tissue management

Flapless surgery is the first method of surgery that crosses a young dentist's mind. Generally speaking, the relative effectiveness of flapless surgery is less considered in preference to its low level of post-operative pain [6].

There are controversies about the efficacy of dental implants' long-term success rate and the need for a keratinized gingival zone around them. However, there is no doubt that frequent plaque accumulation provokes soft tissue inflammation and that a keratinized gingival band greater than 2 mm promotes better gingival health [7].

There is insufficient evidence to recommend the best incision technique, suture technique, or material. Well-designed and conducted Randomized Clinical Trials are needed to provide reliable answers to these questions. Many complicated methods have been mentioned in the literature. We shall now discuss the most common ones.

Incision techniques can influence the result. In a two-stage dental implant placement, crestal incisions produce a greater premature exposure rate than palatal incisions.

It is essential to consider carefully the site's geography, where soft tissue reconstruction may be needed. If there are multiple limitations, the dentist's experience and judgment will be relied upon to decide where to use the soft tissue and how.

The author recommends that a 'step-by-step' surgical flap is the method of choice. The lack of papillae should be the dentist's first concern. After making the minimum incision and flap reflection, the bone of the alveolar crest is examined. The incision should allow a buccal repositioning of the peri-implant mucosa. The flap is extended only for the purposes of guided bone regeneration.

On the saddle, the buccal-lingual space is partitioned into three segments. The paracrestal incision is usually made between the second and third segments and extended to the neighbouring sulcus. Then, the buccal surfaces of the neighbouring teeth are also 'divided' into three segments. The incision stops between the first and second segments (figure 4.1).

A triangular or trapezoidal flap is only recommended when a larger exposure of bone is necessary, such as placing or removing the non-resorbable membrane; however, post-operative bleeding, swelling, and pain are expected (figure 4.2).

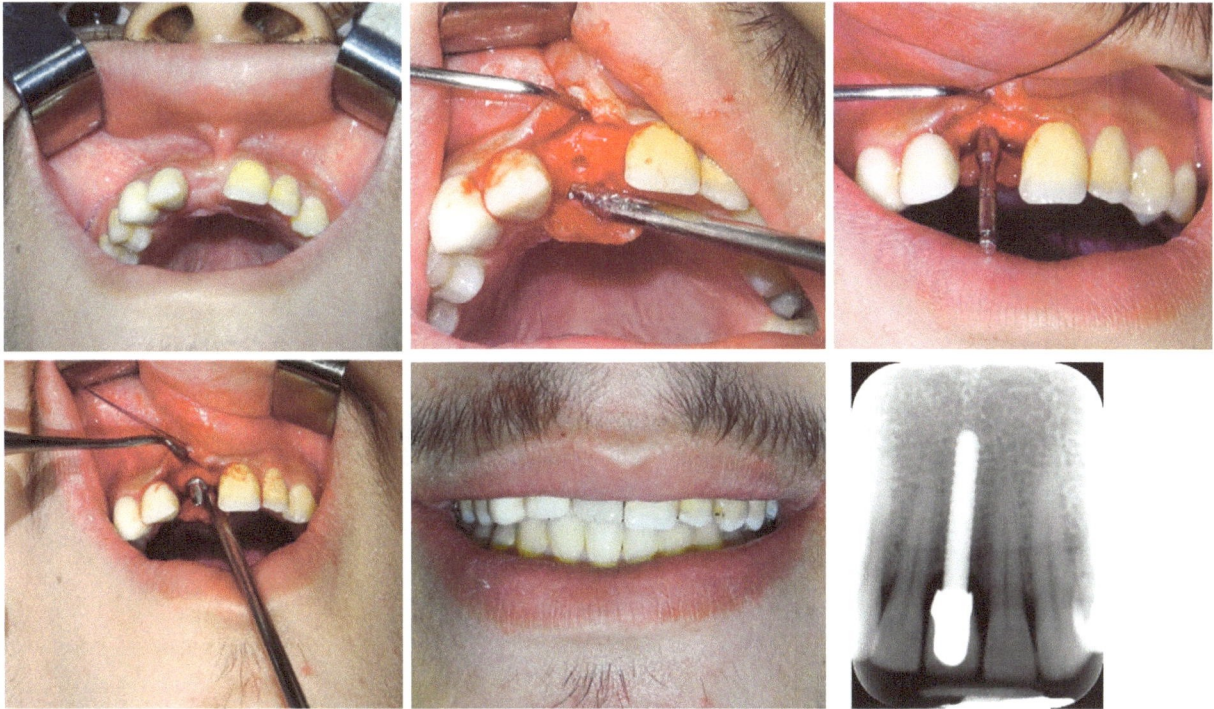

Figure 4.1 Incision- step by step technique:
1. If only needed, relieving incisions: distal and, if necessary, mesial
2. Reflectiong the envelop flap (using Mitche Trimmer and Flat plastic
3. Suturing the flap to labial/buccal mucosa or using a light need holder to pull the suture.

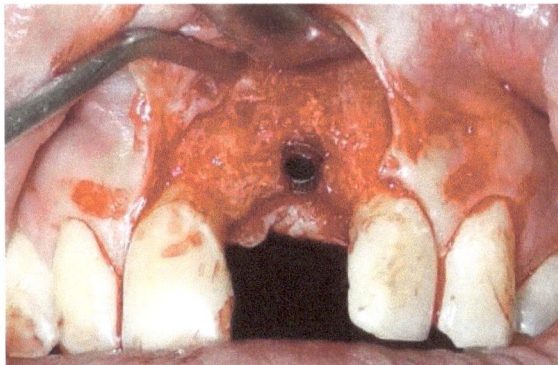

Figure 4.2. A triangular flap or trapezoidal flap is needed to remove the non-resorbable membrane.

Suppose a one-piece implant has been placed, or we are at the second surgical stage of two-stage implant placement. In that case, a T-shaped mucoperiosteal incision should be made to provide soft-tissue closure and interdental papillae reconstruction. Usually, there is not that much bleeding at this stage, but the T-shape incision will bring bleeding, which can be controlled by a sterile cotton roll between the lip/buccal mucosa and labial/buccal gingivae (figure 4.3). The pedicles are rotated to fill the gap between the abutments or abutments and tooth and reconstruct the papillae.

Also, the author has recommended a complicated technique as a full-thickness palatal flap can be provided. The keratinized or connective tissue layer is rotated to fill the papillary space and then stabilised by fine sutures.

An incision not involving the neighbouring papillae is safe, but limited access to the alveolar bone is its disadvantage. If the surgeon needs to extend the flap, the distance of the membrane or grafted area to the vertical incision lines will be reduced, and there will be an increased risk of post-operative infection.

In the upper central region, the nasopalatine neurovascular bundle needs to be incised to free the palatal flap, especially if, due to atrophy, the nasopalatine papillae are on the crest of the alveolar bone.

If the bone width has been increased and bone coverage is not possible, one releasing incision should be performed at the distal aspect of the para-crestal incision. Due to better access, a releasing incision is often/usually recommended on the mesial side, but the distal releasing incision avoids the occurrence of gingival scarring in the aesthetic region. In rare cases, bilateral incisions are needed, and a relieving incision is made parallel to

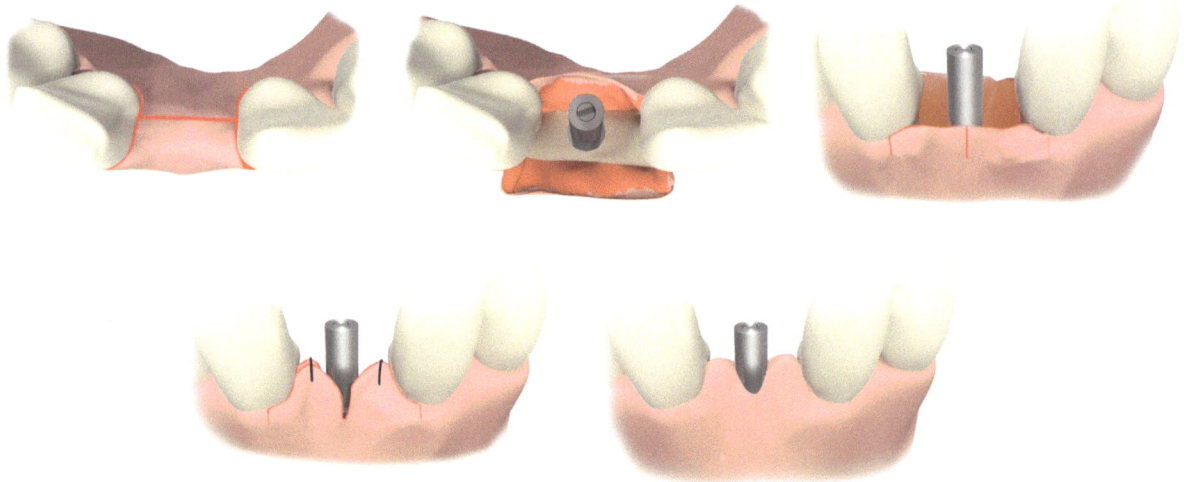

Figure 4.3 Crestal and T vertical incision and retract the mesial and distal triangles towards the papillae.

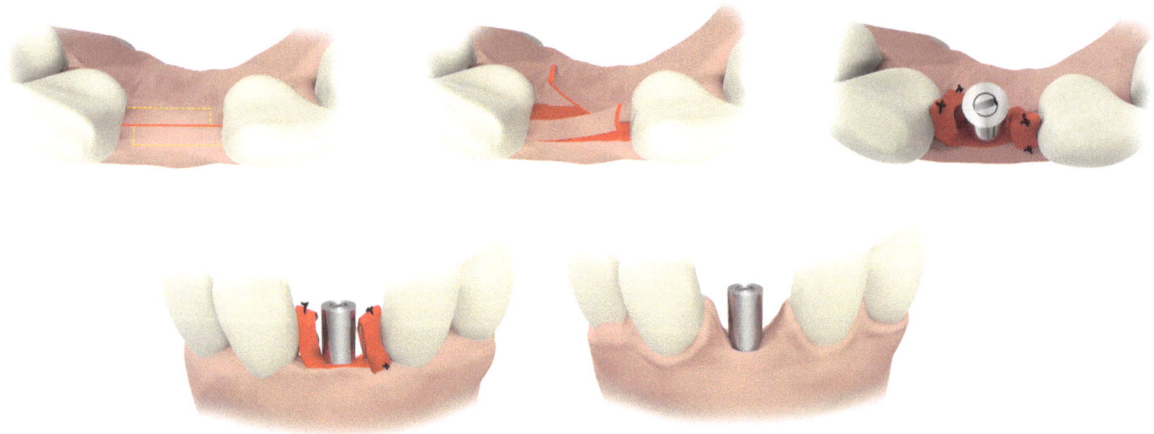

Figure 4.4 Buccal and lingual full-thickness flap and rotation to provide more soft tissue for papillae reconstruction

the alveolar crest to release the flap without perforating it.

Changing the blade used to a new one is recommended to relieve incisions. The dentist may feel the need to push the blade deeper than 1 mm with a blunt blade. It may cut more efficiently if the dentist uses that part of the blade that was not used before, so it is still sharp. However, the consequence could be bleeding and paraesthesia, especially in the mental region.

Whatever technique is used, the dentist must avoid jeopardizing the circulation of the flap margins.

For dental implant placement or bone graft, after the first paracrestal incision, a palatal flap is reflected by Mitchell's trimmer.

The Mitchel trimmer cut pushed the lingual flap and separated the two flaps simultaneously.

Then, the buccal flap reflection is continued with a rigid flat plastic to expose and study the buccal cortex. The lingual flap elevation is completed using a rigid plastic ring.

To protect the periosteum from being crushed by retractors, the author recommends suturing the flap to the vestibule's depth or holding it with a light need holder. This method not only protects the periosteum but also frees up your hand. The periosteum is highly vascularised, especially in the edentulous mandible, and it is the primary blood irrigation source that needs to be protected.

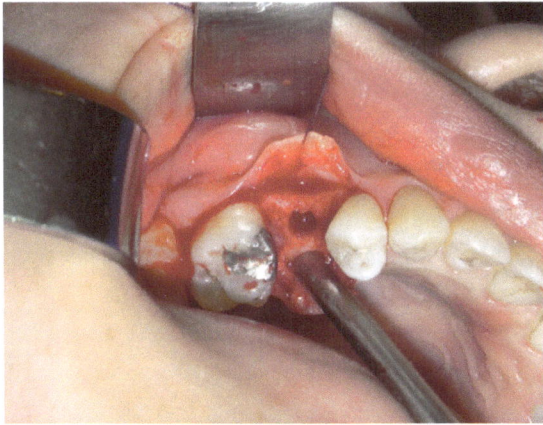

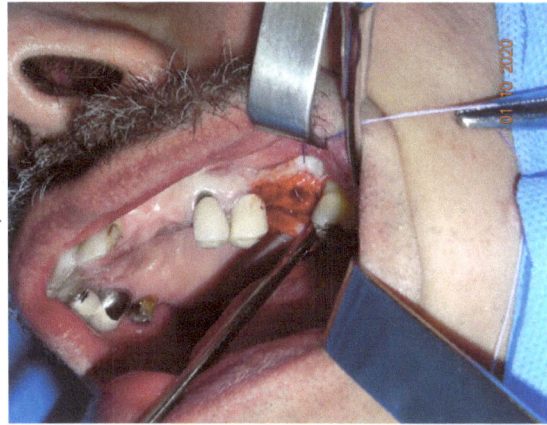

Figure 4.5 Buccal flap stabilised by suture and sutured to the buccal vestibule or clipped by needle holder and by retraction of the lip, the buccal flap is raised, and the bone is accessed, which the left hand can be used to stabilise the handpiece or other instruments. The surgical suction tip is placed palatal for removing blood or saline, providing the dentist with a better view of the field. A small light needle holder bites the suture with the weight of the needle holder and pulls the suture by the buccal retractor of the buccal flap; thus, the periosteum is sound.

Sutures are used to suture the edge of the keratinized labial/buccal flap to the palatal flap with interrupted and horizontal mattress sutures. Polyglactin 910 sutures with a 3/8 circle, reverse cutting, slim needle, 19mm or 26mm, are recommended. These are resorbable sutures with predictable absorption.

Generally speaking, three types of mucosa can be provided around dental implants: keratinized mucosa, non-keratinized mucosa, and non-mobile non-keratinized mucosa. There is no agreement over what type of mucosa is essential for the prevention of recession.

Buccal and vertical soft tissue augmentations are recommended to correct minor small-volume soft tissue defects around maxillary anterior implants and reconstruct the natural root eminence and ridge.

1. Modified Palatal Role techniques, which Scharf recommended to de-epithelialise any connective tissue pedicle from the palate into a prepared labial pouch.

2. Select an appropriate thicker abutment, placing it directly at the second stage of surgery of conventional implants or a thicker one-piece implant to bulge the soft tissue and give the look of natural root eminence and ridge (figure 4.6).

3. Provisional restoration placement before suturing around the abutment can be beneficial.

When a major bone graft is needed, the surface covering (mucosa) needs to be increased.

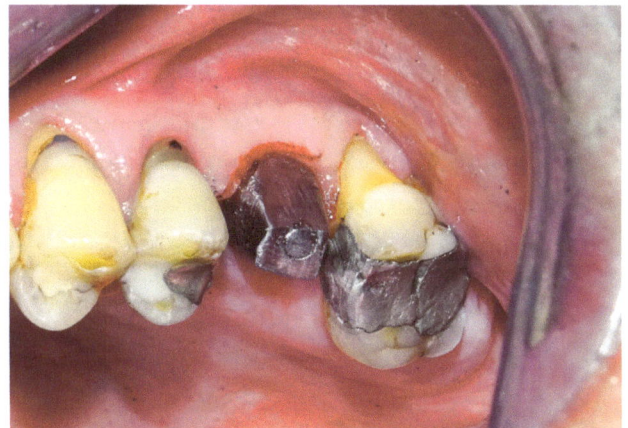

Figure 4.6 Placing a wide-diameter abutment can compensate for the soft tissue collapse.

In the maxilla, a dentist can use keratinized mucosa of the palate, which does not exist in the mandible. The partial/full-thickness flap is a method of choice that can be palatal-based and buccal/labial-based.

1. Labio/buccal based full thickness flap: A palatal para-crestal partial incision performed between the first molar regions. The incision is full thickness at the crest, and the flap retracted to the labial\buccal surface of the alveolar cortex. Releasing incisions were made in the second molar region, approximately 10 mm distal to the proposed distal end of the graft. The nasopalatine neurovascular bundle is incised to free the palatal flap.

After cortico-cancellous block graft placement, relieving incisions are made parallel to the alveolar crest to release the flap without perforating it. This permitted the flap extension over the graft, facilitating wound closure without tension.

2. For the palatally based partial/full-thickness flap: labial/buccal parasulcular incision (buccolabial mucosa) is made, and a mucosal flap is elevated to the mucogingival junction, where a full-thickness periosteal flap is elevated. The buccal flap is sutured to the depth of the buccal mucosa. The palatal full-thickness flap can be sutured to the palatal mucosa or around a premolar crown on the other side of the mouth to minimise the soft tissue and periosteum trauma using the mucoperiosteal elevators. Thus, the entire alveolar ridge, piriform fossa, and lateral wall of the maxilla to the zygomatic buttress can be exposed.

In the mandible, for the buccal/lingual-based partial/full-thickness flap, a split-thickness incision inside the lip between the premolars was performed. A submucosal dissection to a line 2 mm below the mucogingival junction is made. Electrosurgery or laser can be beneficial in reducing bleeding during surgery and post-operative discomfort.

At this position, the periosteum is incised using a new blade no 15, parallel to the mucogingival junction, and a full-thickness flap reflected and exposed the labial/buccal and lingual cortex of the mandible. A full-thickness mucoperiosteal flap is then retracted lingually and sutured around a premolar on the other side to reduce soft tissue trauma by mucoperiosteal elevators. A labial/buccal subperiosteal flap is also reflected buccally from the periosteal incision line. Thus, the entire alveolar ridge is exposed, and the mental nerve is identified if needed.

By transporting labial mucosa (mobile non-keratinized soft tissue) combined with a palatally based full-thickness flap of alveolar mucosa, a simultaneous vestibuloplasty can be performed at the time of bone grafting. The newly created base, a minimum of 3 mm clearance from the edge of the graft to the margin of the vestibuloplasty flap, the margin of the flap sutured in two layers, 3 mm behind the margin of the mattress sutured and the flap at the edge with interrupted or continuous sutures. This technique can reduce wound dehiscences (figures 4.7, 7.17, 9.15).

This technique can also be applied in the maxillae.

The advantages of each type of flap during bone grafting are as follows:

Palatally based partial-thickness flap:

• Simultaneous vestibuloplasty, which is almost always required in block bone graft cases, may be performed,

Labially based full-thickness flap:

• The periosteum covers the cortico-cancellous block,

• Minimise the ischaemic effect created by the vessels traversing dense tissue at the crest

• Primary closure of the soft tissue (less discomfort for the patient) is possible, whereas a palatally-based flap creates a mucosal defect, which subsequently epithelialises in the lip.

When the open sinus lift is necessary, two approaches can be recommended.

• A high buccal sulcus incision in the canine to the second molar region, the flap being reflected palatally,

• An incision is made at the palatal aspect of the crest along the alveolus with oblique releasing incisions anteriorly in the cuspid region and posteriorly in the tuberosity region. The author recommends this technique because there is a maximum distance between the incision line and the grafted area.

The flap is elevated, and the lateral surface of the maxilla is exposed approximately to the infraorbital foramina. If the lateral wall is thin, the sinus is visible as a translucent bluish appearance.

The incision should be made in the mandible so that at least 1.5 mm of keratinized gingiva is included in the lingual flap. A lack of keratinized gingiva in the lingual abutment will promote bone resorption.

If a relieving incision is needed, the premolar area should be avoided to prevent mental paraesthesia. As the mucosa is thin, the flap should be elevated by detaching the attachment to the occlusal ridge, thus preventing mucosal perforation. Using a rigid flat plastic to elevate the lingual flap and study the mylohyoid attachment and the undercut in the lower molar region is highly recommended.

There is a belief that immediate implant placement provides a better aesthetic, but delayed implant placement does not hinder the aesthetic outcome for the papillae when compared to immediate implant placement.

Allogenic and xenogenic tissues have been introduced, which reduce patient morbidity while increasing available tissue volume. The acellular dermal matrix (ADM) is collected from the human dermis, but the advantage gained from a keratinized

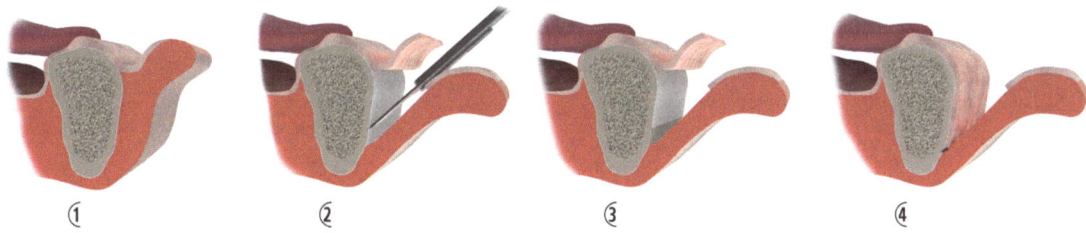

Figure 4.7 Vestibuloplasty provides a non-tension closure of the bone blocks and increases the vestibular depth or an ideal coverage of bone block graft.

mucosal graft is greater than that gained from ADM. Collagen matrix (CM), which is pure porcine collagen, can be safely used. A volume-stable collagen matrix (VCMX) provided results similar to those of connective tissue graft [8].

Most of the abutments have a round cross-section and cannot provide an ideal aesthetic profile. Suppose a one-piece implant is placed and an immediate provisional crown cemented, or, at the second stage of 2 piece implant surgery, instead of Gingival Former. The abutment is placed and prepared in that case, and the immediate provisional prosthesis is cemented. During the healing phase, the peri-implant mucosa will adopt the provisional emergence profile of the provisional prosthesis - as long as this stays stable or as long as the embrasures are not modified. The sutures guide the flap edges into occupying the embrasure spaces at the interproximal areas.

Factors such as the thickness of the keratinized mucosa, the suturing technique used, and the opening up of the provisional embrasures can affect the final shape and position of the mucosal contour. The implant shoulder should be slightly below the mucosal level to allow the provisional prosthesis to scallop the peri-implant mucosa.

The gingiva biotype strongly affects the outcome and crestal bone loss around the dental implants. There is less bone loss in thick gingival biotypes compared to thin [9].

THIN SCALLOPED GINGIVAL BIOTYPE:

The bony and soft tissue architecture is highly scalloped, the soft tissue is thin, and the cervical area of the crown is flat with a flat emergence profile.

THICK GINGIVAL BIOTYPES:

The bone and soft tissue architecture are flat, with short interdental papillae supported by a dense, thick band of attached soft tissue. This type of soft tissue will react to insult by pocket formation instead of gingival recession,

The teeth are square with long contact areas,

The emergence profile is pronounced,

The use of a pedicle graft with a blood supply should be the first choice,

The recipient surface should be uniform and immobilized.

Three non-invasive methods for estimating gingival biotype in maxillary aesthetic zones have been recommended: visual, proven transparency and soft tissue cone beam computed tomography (CBCT).

The hu-Fried Colorvue Biotype probe can help classify gingival biotypes. The system has three coloured tips, white, green and blue; whichever is visible in the gingival sulcus has a thicker biotype (figure 4.8). Haemostasis should permit adequate adaptation of the graft to the recipient bed.

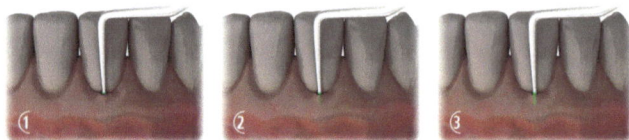

Figure 4.8 Insert the probe in the gingival sulcus with less than 30 gr of pressure, and the white probe first, insert it in the gingival sulcus with < 30g of pressure. The biotype is thin, if it is visible, meaning you can see the colour through the gingival tissue.

Gingival Recession:

The implant diameter, the gingival biotype (thin or thick), and the surgical technique will influence the gingival recession observed at a 5-year follow-up.

Most recession occurs within the first three months between implant placement/temporisation and the fitting of the definitive restoration. When placing a wide implant in a lateral incisor position, it is recommended that an implant with a maximum diameter of 3.5 mm should be chosen [10].

Increased gingival recession can be expected in the thin gingival biotype. The emergence profile of the abutment at the buccal surface should be under-contoured.

4.3 Hard Tissue Management

Bone Preparation for Dental Implant Placement

Drilling is an important skill which needs to be mastered. A major aspect of this skill is the ability to drill effectively without producing excessive heat.

Factors which affect heat generation during implant site preparations can be considered under:

a) Drill: factors such as drill sharpness, drill pressure, drill speed, drill time, drill movement, drill design, and the irrigation system.

b) Recipient: site anatomy and soft/hard tissue preparation design

Using a standard electrical dental implant micromotor is important – not an air motor. Using an air motor for oral surgery can be fatal because of the potential creation of an air embolism in the facial and pterygoid plexus veins, superior vena cava and right atrium [11].

Heat

Excessive heat production can have a number of consequences: it can cause denaturation of enzymatic and membrane proteins, decreased osteoclastic and osteoblastic activity, and dehydration and dryness. All of these may contribute to cell death [12].

During bone drilling, ischaemia can be detected immediately adjacent to the drilled holes, and it may be this response to thermal changes which lead to protein coagulation and vascular or lymphatic blockage. This blockage may also result from fine drill debris accumulation or regional vasoconstriction [13].

Besides potentially leading to thermal injury, drilling may also cause micro-damage (microcracks) in bone. It is proposed that micro-damage may also produce osteocytic apoptosis, and this acts as a signal for osteoclast activation and, thus, bone resorption [12].

Bone is a poor conductor of heat. The thermal conductivity of fresh cortical bone is in the range of 0.53-0.58 W/mk [14].

One needs to determine the optimal feed rate (drill speed) so that the force applied is not excessive and the drilling time is as short as possible. This will minimise the duration of friction between the drill and bone.

There are controversies over how much pressure and speed are needed to restrict heat generation to less than 47 degrees Centigrade. However, some authors believe increasing pressure is more influential than increasing speed [15].

Abougia et al. found that drilling at high speed and with heavy force would reduce the temperature and be more favourable than previously thought [16].

Some believe that this proposed increase in pressure and speed reduces the overall drilling time, which reduces heat production [17,18].

Other studies showed that the higher the speed, the less heat was generated. These findings were true regardless of the site of drilling. Slower rotational speeds required more drilling time, which produced more frictional heat. The longer the drilling time, the higher the bone temperature was, [19-21].

When using Nik dental drills, we strongly recommend that you maintain a force of around 2 kg and a speed of 1400-1500 rpm. To this end, implantology training must include access to a digital force gauge for training purposes. That said, no settled agreement exists over the optimum bone drilling speed or the axial force to be applied. However, the majority of researchers recommend high speed with heavy force [22].

The serial drilling technique and an alternative, simplified technique (pilot drill + final diameter drill) have been used in orthopaedic and dental implant surgeries. The Branemark team recommended the former, and this procedure consisted of the step-by-step removal of small quantities of bone [23].

The disadvantage of this technique is that bone debris can rapidly clog the drill flutes and may lead to a rapid local rise in heat. Since the amount of bone removed is relatively small, and a second and third drill will be used, the overall degree of flute clogging will not significantly affect the final implant result. However, if this drill design is used in the simplified pilot + final drill technique, the result will not be acceptable as clogging and heat rise can affect the final result. It should be emphasised that the one-step technique requires purpose-designed drills.

One-step drilling in dental implantology has been recently advocated because of the shortened duration of surgery. However, more data is needed for this to be recognised as applicable in all cases.

Always remember that a dull or wide drill can also produce a local rise in temperature [24].

Drill design can influence temperature production during drilling. Conical drills produce significantly less heat than cylindrical drills in the apical portion of the drill. The difference can be up to 2.5 degrees [25].

Irrigation: Reparation is reached.

Irrigation is fundamental to bone preparation. There are two methods for irrigation – internal or external. Internal irrigation systems are more expensive than external and have not demonstrated any benefit [26].

An intermittent site preparation technique has been recommended. The initial depth cut is made with pressure being applied for, say, three millimetres of depth cutting, then withdrawn three millimetres to permit access for the irrigant and allow the escape of bone chips. Pressure is then reapplied for further depth cutting, followed again by retreat. This in-and-out process is repeated until the end of the site preparation is reached. The disadvantage of this approach is that the multiple re-entries dictated by the drill designs provided by most manufacturers will reduce the precision of the bone preparation itself. Even so, because of the intimate contact present at the bone-drill interface, the irrigating saline will still reduce the temperature along the width and length of the bony walls. Thus, proper irrigation with effective debris removal will be achieved at the expense of less accurate site preparation. Is there an alternative?

The alternative proposal is that a more accurate preparation would be achieved if continuous drilling were performed. The result would be a far more accurate site preparation with reduced drilling time. However, this approach has two disadvantages: it would lead to a rise in temperature not only because of the inability of the saline to access the tip of the drill but also because of the clogging effect of the bone debris on the drill's cutting edge. This clogging of the drill will also decrease its cutting efficiency and increase drilling time.

The fundamental problem lies in the design of most implant drills. A drill design incorporating a couple of straight flutes, however, can significantly improve irrigant access to the apex of the drill. This will allow continuous drilling, accurate site preparation, and effective temperature control [26].

How can the irrigant be controlled? The dental implant irrigation tube has a perforator for the sterile solution bag, an air filter, and an on/off switch. The micromotor has a digital irrigant flow control wheel.

External irrigation can be delivered by two methods – fixed or removable.

The external silicone tube is attached to the fixed water tube on the handpiece in the fixed system. In the removable system, the removable irrigation spray clip is presented as a right- or left-handed unit to be slotted into position on the handpiece. Points to watch out for are:

- The inadvertent displacement of the removable spray clip occurred while the surgeon was focusing on the surgery. This allows the saline to miss the point where the drill is as close as possible to the bone surface. This is more likely to occur over time as the spay clip deteriorates with repeated use.

- The silicone saline tube's attachment to the fixed tube can be loosened, disrupting saline delivery.

- The fixed saline tube can also fracture, though this is more likely due to mishandling during sterilisation. Heavy instruments placed on top of the handpiece can bend the fixed attachment towards the handpiece body, so bending it back into position several times can lead to eventual fracture.

- The silicone tube runs over the handpiece and can be inadvertently compressed by the dentist's finger, affecting saline delivery.

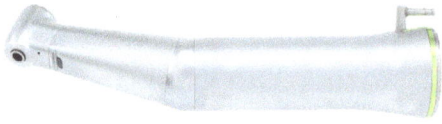

Figure 4.9 A handpiece via an external fixed irrigation tube at the rear of the handpiece.

The author recommends using a system where the saline enters the handpiece via an external fixed irrigation tube at the rear of the handpiece and continues with the inner independent water channel to exit through the external tube at the handpiece head.

This removes the need for any external silicone tube to interfere with the surgeon's handpiece control. It also obviates the need for any removable spray attachment. When the media-distal space is limited, and the handpiece head does not allow the drill to penetrate all the way, an extension drill is used. Latch-type chuck dental implant handpieces are narrower than push button type, and the need for an extension drill is reduced. A common mistake is that when the length of the shank of the drill is only 1-2 mm short, and the dentist thinks adding the extension drill is not necessary, the head of the handpiece tilted distally of the neighbouring crown and the tip of the drill is tilted toward the root and there is a chance of invading periodontal ligament of the neighbouring root.

The extension drill attaches to the drill and extends the shaft, and the elongated drill is used to access the drill between or near the tooth. The external irrigation can limit saline access to the drill-bone interface, especially in the maxillae. There are different types of attachments of the drill to the extension drill, and all the designs have their limitations. There is a push type which falls off during lower jaw implant placement. Screw type, which after a couple of times, opening and removal of the drill would be difficult. Tongue type, which, after a couple of times, the tongue may fracture.

Also, this cannot be done if there is a need to push the drill bodily toward a surface, such as palataly.

Stop drills

All the dental implant surgical kits do have stop drills. The stop drill aims to ensure precise, safe drilling, especially where there is reduced visibility and reading the lines of the drills is difficult,

like distal of the first molar.

The drill stop restricts drilling deeper than the predefined depth to be used in sensitive indications to avoid the mandibular nerve or sinus floor [28] (figure 4.10).

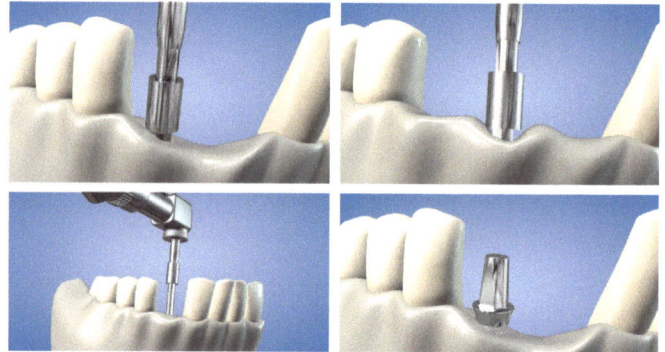

Figure 4.10 Stop drills may restrict drilling deeper than the predefined depth and prevent adequate irrigation at the drill bone interface, left (heated drill while using stop drill and extension drill), right (adequate irrigation by using extension drill only without stop drill).

There are two types of stop drills: fixed and removable. There is a wide variety in the market, and even the plug of an anaesthetic cartridge has been used.

However, there are limitations that are not indicated for extraction sites, where the bone cavity is often wider than the diameter required to hold the drill stop or the use of a drill guide template due to interference with the guide template. Also, on the angulated occlusal surface of the bone, it cannot be used in areas with limited mesial-distal space, like lower incisors.

When the soft tissue is thin and countersinking, the implant is wise, or when there is a peak of bone, it prevents the drill from going to the desired depth. The author does not recommend flattening the cortex. Removing the cortex reduces primary stability. If GBR is needed, one or two walls can help treat the dehiscence surface of the implant.

Regardless of the preparation method, a drill needs to be sharp. That sharpness depends on the material from which the drill is made, the number of times that drill is used, and the cumulative effect of repeated sterilisation cycles. A worn drill increases the local temperature.

It is thought that using a drill of more than 4mm in diameter may generate too much heat during preparation. If such a diameter site is required, supplementary irrigation will be required. The author recommends using extra irrigation with an irrigation syringe and the dental assistant's help.

Irrigant flow needs careful adjustment. It must not be so strong as to interfere with the operator's vision and should supply adequate coolant to the operative site. Additionally, it should not be so powerful as to prevent the collection of bone shavings in the drill flutes. The latter can be used to produce autogenous bone debris in GBR. The amount of cooling required is dictated by the design of the drill, the diameter of the drill, and the quality of the bone involved. There is no settled consensus on this.

Pilot drills may generate more heat than the larger diameter drills which may follow. This may lead the surgeon to compensate for the overheating by increasing irrigation. However, the pilot drills may also collect valuable bone debris, so any increased irrigation must be carefully controlled so as not to disturb the collected bone debris. In any case, the subsequent drills used will remove the overheated bone.

Poor bone quality bone sites prepared by either a drill or an osteotome were compared. It was found that both produced a similar temperature reading at the start of the operation (1mm depth) as well as at the end of the preparation (10mm depth). At the midpoint (5mm depth), the osteotome produced a lower heat reading than initially, while the drill heat reading increased significantly. At 10mm depth, both drill and osteotome approximate each other. Note that the osteotome readings reduce at each step [29].

Recently, however, there has been a proposal for a new method of bone preparation without irrigation.

Drills designed more recently may not generate detrimental heat and may be safe to use without irrigation in bone sites of lower density, but this requires a careful drilling technique [30].

This involves reducing the drilling speed to 50 rpm and tapping the bone. This approach should be treated with caution. You need to take into account different bone densities, drilling depths, and the likely extended time involved. This is especially so when the quality of the bone is hard. Because of the vertical forces involved, the dental handpiece cartridge, the surgical instrument that rotates the implant, or the internal aspect of the implant itself will be damaged. It is difficult to see how eliminating irrigation can benefit either the dentist or the patient [31,32].

Flapless surgery does not result in increased heat production during bone preparation when compared with flapped surgery [33].

Position of the dentist relative to the operative site

It is essential that the dentist have the best view of the operative site, both mesiodistally and bucco-lingually; thus, the surgeon needs to be able to move around the chair.

To enable this, the recommended seating position for each region is:

upper anterior: 11 – 1 o'clock
upper right: 9 – 11 o'clock
lower right: 7 – 9 o'clock
upper left: 1 – 3 o'clock
lower left: 3 – 5 o'clock
lower anterior: 5 – 8 o'clock

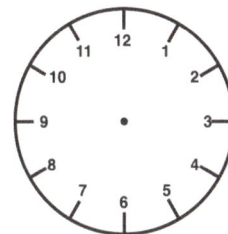

Stability of the drill during bone penetration,

The grip of the handpiece is one of the most important successes of dental implant placement. There are two schools of thought: one hand and two hands gripping.

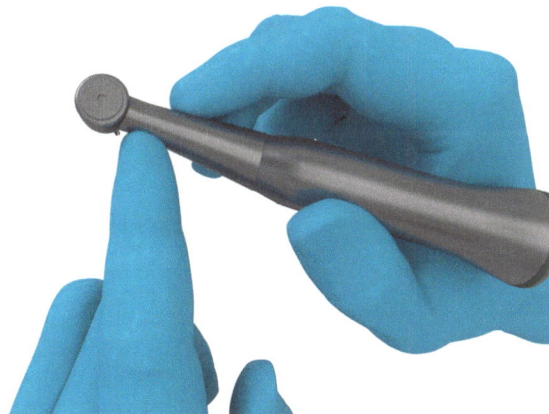

Figure 4.11 The dental implant handpiece can move in different directions (left); two-hand gripping is recommended by the author to have three-dimensional control of the handpiece (right).

Once drilling starts, with the vertical pumping manoeuvre, the quality of the bone will exert its influence on the position of the drill and, hence, the handpiece. If the drill meets palatal or lingual cortical bone, the bone will tend to push the handpiece away and out of position to the right or left. If the tip of the drill engages cortical bone, it can force the handpiece to alter position by pitching movement without the surgeon noticing. If the pilot hole is placed too mesially, the surgeon may decide to reposition it distally. When the drill is re-introduced, it is pushed bodily towards the distal wall by back, right or left movement without removing any bone from the mesial wall.

This approach has the potential to be successful, but it requires a sharp drill; however, it could strain the bearing and shorten its lifespan since the handpiece is designed for downward or upward movement. The drill must be sharp because the lateral force can cause it to fracture.

When the drill is withdrawn, the weight of the micromotor and handpiece may cause the surgeon to inadvertently tilt the handpiece by rolling movement and reshape the cavity previously created.

Good grip with two hands reduces the chances of these sorts of mistakes.

Bone-level Implant Placement

Consider two implants with different surface treatments, one where the entire surface is roughened from its occlusal level to its apex and the other where, at the occlusal edge, the first 0.5-1.0mm is polished. The advantage of the polished surface (collar) is that connective tissue will attach to it, but crestal bone will not. If the fully roughened implant is countersunk by 1.0mm, bone resorption may occur over the ensuing year. If the implant with the polished collar is countersunk in a similar fashion, then shear stress is transmitted to the crestal bone, and this, in turn, causes bone resorption. However, other factors may intrude during the healing phase and reduce the potential advantages. The most frequent problem occurs when the patient has a provisional prosthesis overlaying the implant site. Conventional use of the provisional removable prosthesis (flipper) can punch through the connective tissue around the polished collar of the implant. For this and other reasons, the author recommends the use of implants with a fully roughened surface treatment. In any event, a successful implant may still be subject to up to 1.6mm resorption. If the biological width that results is less than 3.0mm,

then even more bone resorption occurs, and the connective tissue will replace the bone lost.

Crestal bone resorption is initiated at the time of implant placement.

Biologic width formation during early osseointegration can also initiate bone resorption. To ensure normal sulcal depth formation along with junctional epithelium and a connective tissue seal, a minimum of 3 mm of biological width is needed. When the implant is placed too close to the oral environment, it invites plaque accumulation, and there may well be increased difficulty with flap adaptation. This may be accompanied by thinning the soft tissues, pulling off the periosteum, suture loosening, and disrupting the blood vessels.

When an implant without a polished collar is placed deep into the prepared socket (countersunk), less bone resorption is expected on the rough surface of the implant [34].

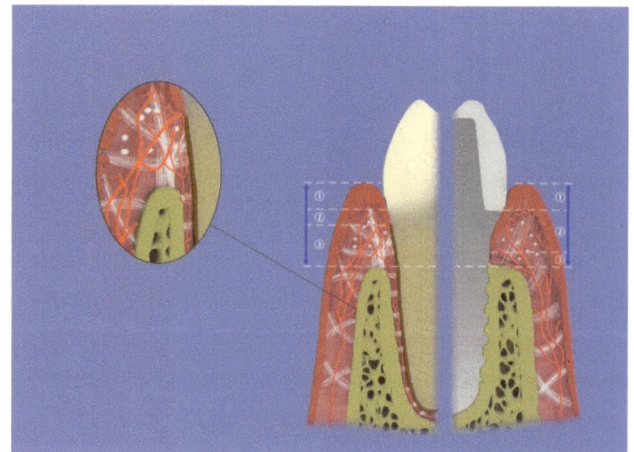

Figure 4.12 The difference in biological width between tooth and dental implant. 1) sulcus, 2) junctional epithelium, 3) connective tissue attachment, which is about 1 mm.

Hazards Related to the Position of Implant Placement

MAXILLAE:

In this area, the thickness of the soft tissues can deceive the dentist.

Usually, but not always, the palatal cortex is thick and dense, and it can be a reliable source of frictional grip that provides adequate primary stability.

After exposing the alveolar ridge, the dentist should monitor its

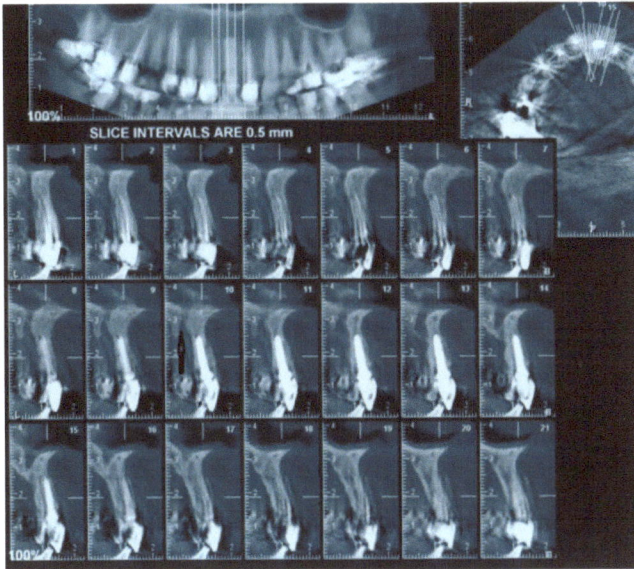

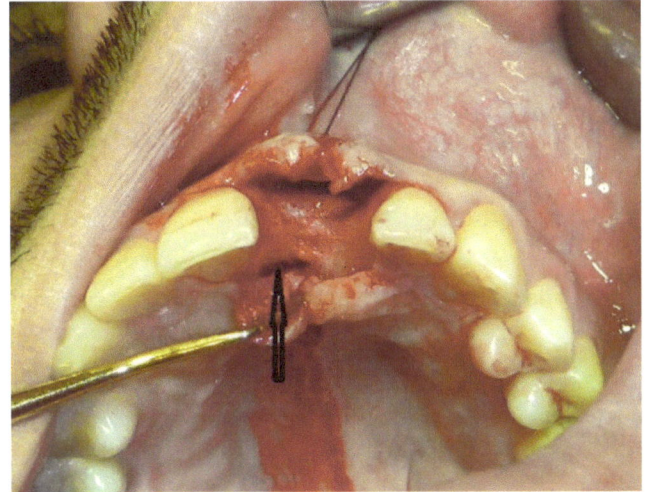

Figure 4.13 The nasopalatine canal needs to be identified during implant placement, replacing upper Central Incisors; the black arrows in the CBCT (section 10) and the photo demonstrate the opening of the nasopalatine canal.

width and carefully note the undercuts. The pattern of bone resorption influences the surgical technique that is adopted. Bone resorption of the alveolar ridge begins at the buccal/labial surface and is then followed by vertical bone loss.

• THE ANTERIOR REGION:

In the upper central incisor region, the nasopalatine canal is the most critical anatomical feature to be identified. It is pear-shaped, expanding as it is traced apically. The volume of the canal increases towards its apex, and the chance of invading it increases accordingly.

CBCT of the Upper Central Incisors region. The Nasopalatine canal reduces the width of the alveolar bone, and the dentist must ensure the prepared dental implant cavity does not invade the soft tissue and its anatomic structures.

Because resorption of the alveolar ridge starts from the labial surface, the implant may need to be placed palatally. This can make the placement more difficult.

In cases where an implant is positioned palatally, sufficient space must be allowed for the final porcelain crown. However, if the tilt of the palatal cortex of the alveolar bone is significant, it may necessitate angling the abutment obliquely to achieve proper alignment and support.

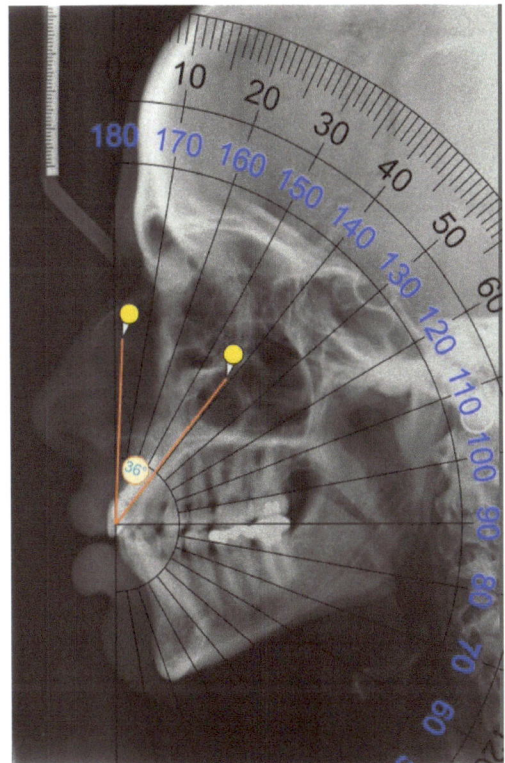

Figure 4.14 True lateral cephalometric demonstrates the axis of the alveolar ridge and, consequently, the dental implant, abutment, and crown, which in an average clinical scenario is 36 °.

96

Thus, placing one-piece screw implants in this situation can limit the position of the final crown unless it is designed with an angulated abutment.

If compensation is needed, the dentist has two options: augment the alveolar ridge to increase the width. The disadvantages of bone augmentation are that it is complicated, which means more expensive, painful, and less reliable. The better approach is ridge expansion with serial osteotome application.

Using serial osteotomes presents a better option because it avoids the unnecessary loss of bone (hence no drills) and works well in the upper anterior region because the bone is relatively soft. Furthermore, it provides greater stability and compresses alveolar bone.

In this technique, after the round drill and pilot drill (usually with a 2 mm diameter) are applied, the osteotome is placed to length using a surgical mallet. Now grasp the handle of the osteotome and swivel it bucco-lingually so that the tip in the alveolar bone is moved buccally while the handle is moved lingually. This will stretch the buccal alveolar bone without fracturing it. This will leave the site oval in shape. This may change the potential implant angle by a further 10-20 degrees. The next osteotome or drill will be placed in the corrected position to reshape the site further (figure 4.15). This technique is applicable for upper single-rooted tooth replacement. There are dental implant systems that, with counter-clock drilling, can expand the bone without removing it. Due to the use of a contra-angle handpiece, pushing the handpiece and the drill toward the palatal is more governable than using the osteotome after changing the angle of the alveolar bone.

It is crucial that after each bone preparation, the surgeon checks the depth of the prepared cavity with a thick, blunt periodontal probe. If a softness at the apical end can be felt, accompanied by much bleeding, then this indicates that the nasopalatine canal has been breached. However, if the probe feels bone rather than soft tissue at the apex but still has a lot of bleeding, this could indicate lateral stripping.

Reduce the bleeding using compression. The next step depends on the size of the breach, and the probe indicates this.

If the breach is minor (less than 2mm), it can be plugged using bone debris or autogenous bone if available. This is carried to the breach point using a small flat plastic and compressed laterally. Use an endodontic hand plugger, a hand-held drill, or

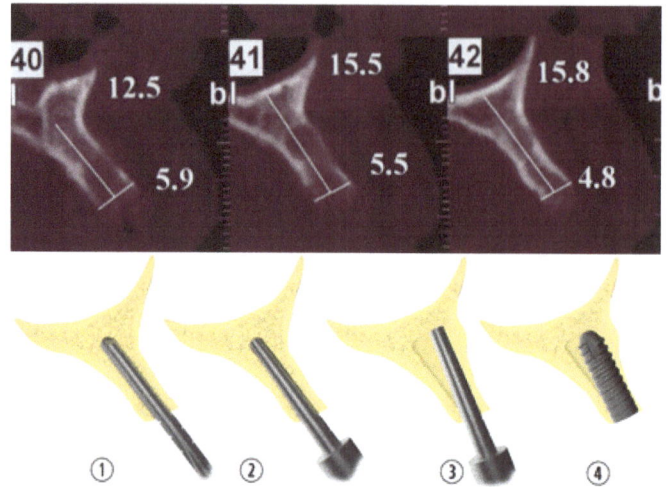

Figure 4.15 Stretching the buccal alveolar cortex by using serial ostetomes can Improve the angle of implant placement, especially in the upper anterior region.

an osteotome to apply the compression.

If the breach is greater than 2mm, then the contents of the nasopalatine canal beyond the breach need to be cured. Access to this curettage is gained through the oral palatal soft tissue.

The order in which these two breaches are dealt with is essential. The breach within the implant preparation site must first be filled with bone debris or autogenous bone to ensure that natural bone is in immediate contact with the titanium implant when placed. The secondary access point through the oral palatal soft tissue now fills the curetted site with bone substitutes. This bolsters the real bone initially placed within the implant site and prevents its collapse.

The implant should now be placed into position.

One other option is to change the drill's angle if possible. The section dealt with the anatomical restrictions imposed by limited bucco-palatal bone width. In the upper anterior region, the surgeon may often be faced with limited bone height and bone of poor quality. However, the floor of the nose has a thick cortex. There are reports that the floor of the nose can be pushed upwards, but the mucosa should not be ruptured. If it is ruptured, it should be sutured back in two layers.

Placing an implant in the incisive foramen (naso-palatally) is not practicable due to the difficulty in placing a restoration. Nevertheless, it can offer a practical answer when providing a maxillary overdenture, and if not enough bone is available to place an implant in an ideal position.

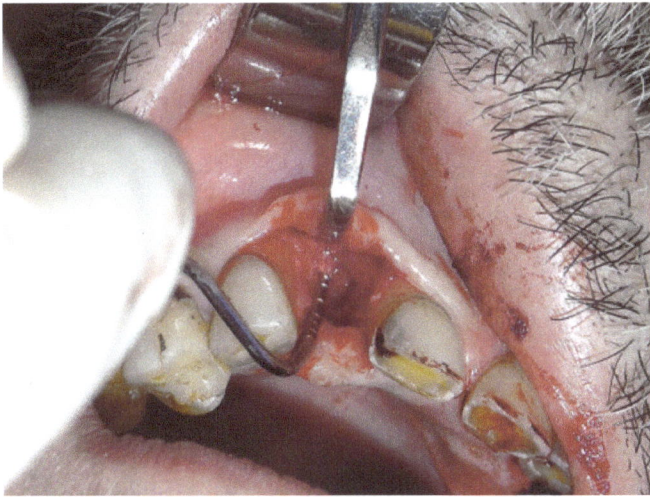

Figure 4.16 A blunt periodontal probe is used to check if the nasopalatine canal has been invaded during drilling.

THE POSTERIOR REGION:

An unwelcome consequence of tooth extraction can be the collapse of the sinus floor, along with apical bone resorption. Such a collapse, along with any accompanying bone resorption, can lead to the formation of an exudate within the sinus. Such an exudate can accelerate the coronal expansion of the sinus – and remember that the sinus can extend as far as the canine fossa. The bone palatal to the sinus can be thick enough to allow the use of a longer implant, which can increase the primary stability of a dental implant. The bone at the buccal aspect of the sinus is thin, so implant placement here is impractical.

In order to place an implant using an intra-socket sinus lift, three conditions need to be met: a minimum bone height of 4 mm, a minimum bone width of 5mm, and bone quality that is medium to hard (types A1-2, B1-2). It should be accompanied by immediate implant placement. In these cases, an intra-socket lift can increase the height by 50%. Extra height can be gained if there is a minimum of 3 mm of extra-bone at the palatal of the sinus,The cortex of the alveolar bone at the occlusal surface is usually up to 2mm thick, but there is also a cortex on the sinus floor. If the thickness is available, engaging the floor and the palatal cortex of the sinus to as little as 0.5mm can help increase primary stability in this controversial area. The maxillary tuberosity can be another area for implant placement. However, the bone quality here is poor (figure 4.20). Indeed, trabecular bone is sometimes absent, and the tuberosity itself can consist solely of fatty tissue.

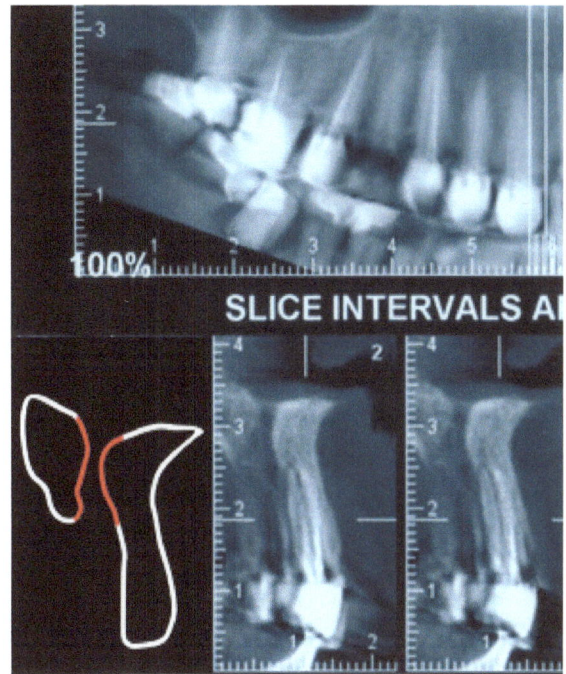

Figure 4.17 The window at the apical region of the prepared cavity must be grafted (bordered red) using autogenous bone debris after curettage of the nasopalatine canal.

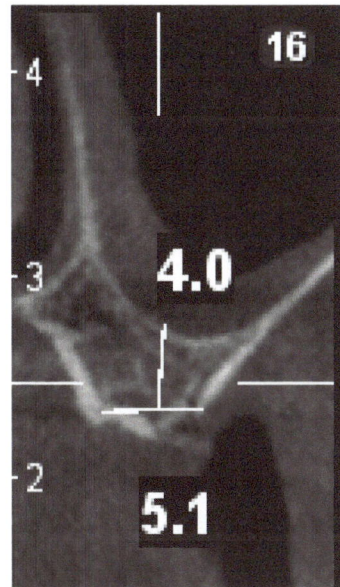

Figure 4.18 The above CBCT demonstrates the height available is 4.0 mm; however, if the implant is parallel to the cortical cortex, the height would be 8.0 mm, and maxillary sinus mucosa thickening is evident.

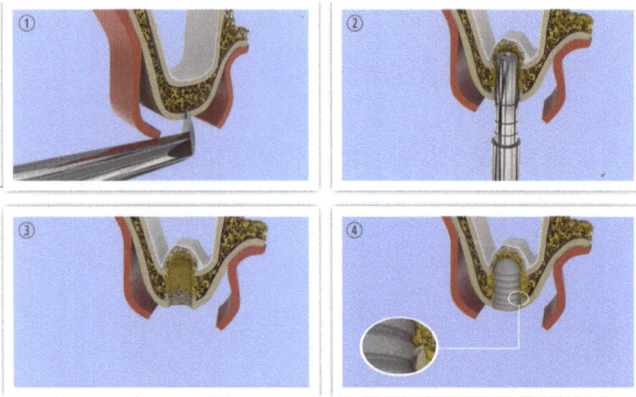

Figure 4.19 Application of non-rotary instruments for intra-socket sinus lift. 1) Apply the Mitchel trimmer instead of a round drill, and 2) use only the final osteotome size, one size smaller than the diameter of the dental implant. This manoeuvre will push the cortex inside the prepared bone cavity and increase the cortical bone-implant interface. 3) final cavity, 4) implant placement.

In these circumstances, placing a long implant, even as long as 20 mm, and engaging the cortical region from the inside can provide acceptable primary stability. Even so, the implant should be placed no closer than 3 mm from the distal surface of the tuberosity due to the risk of tuberosity fracture. Since the implant will be angled mesially, the future abutment needs to be able to compensate. Furthermore, the gingival height will likely be from 4 - 6 mm, so bear in mind that the implant system in use must be able to cater to the relevant gingival height.

MANDIBLE:

Generally speaking, the cortex of the mandible is thick and has low resilience. The intra-foraminal zone has been traditionally taught as being the "zone of safety". But beware, complications associated with implant placement in the anterior mandible indicate that the highest morbidity, and even mortality, can occur from improper implant placement in this area.

The intra-foraminal zone has traditionally been referred to as the "zone of safety."

But beware, complications associated with implant placement in the anterior mandible indicate that the highest morbidity, and even mortality, can occur from improper implant placement in this area.

In the anterior mandible, inadequate assessment and preparation for implant surgery have, on occasion, led to the patient's admission to the hospital because of suffocation, and even death has been reported. Such cases have occurred following haemorrhage within the floor of the mouth, with the consequential haematoma leading to the closing off of the airway.

The initial diagnostic mistake lay in the failure to assess accurately the shape of the lingual face of the mandible. Failure to detect the presence of an angle or concavity in the lingual cortex can lead the operator to inadvertently breach this cortex, causing the drill to penetrate into the lingual soft tissues. This error underscores the importance of careful examination and awareness of anatomical variations to ensure safe and effective dental procedures.

The Mylohyoid muscle is an incomplete septum; there is communication to sublingual, submandibular, and anterior and central muscle fascicles [35].

If the drill tip invades the lingual cortex above the genioglossus and mmes even more threatening when the drill breaches the distal of the mylohyoid muscle, invades the submandibular muscle, and closes off the pharynx too (figure 4.21, 4.22).

If the tip of the drill invades the lingual cortex below the genioglossus and mylohyoid muscles, a haematoma can form in the submental space, and with the latter's connection to the submandibular space, this may close off the pharynx. This may happen either when the mandible has suffered major vertical bone loss and/or when long implants are to be considered. (figure 3.13, 4.21, 4.22).

In these circumstances, it is best not to place the implant. Swallow your pride and explain to the patient that it is better not to stop the bleeding when the implant is not placed; the surgical hole provides a haemorrhage escape route and reduces the risk of suffocation.

The sublingual artery penetrates the genioglossus muscle and enters the lingual cortex through a single foramen or, sometimes, multiple foramina and does so above the muscle. Entry of the artery through a single foramen presents a greater risk for the surgeon than entry through multiple foramina. The presence of a single foramen carrying a relatively large artery of about 3mm diameter can be the source of significant haemorrhage if breached. It connects with the incisive artery in the incisive canal close to the lingual foramen. This anastomosis occurs

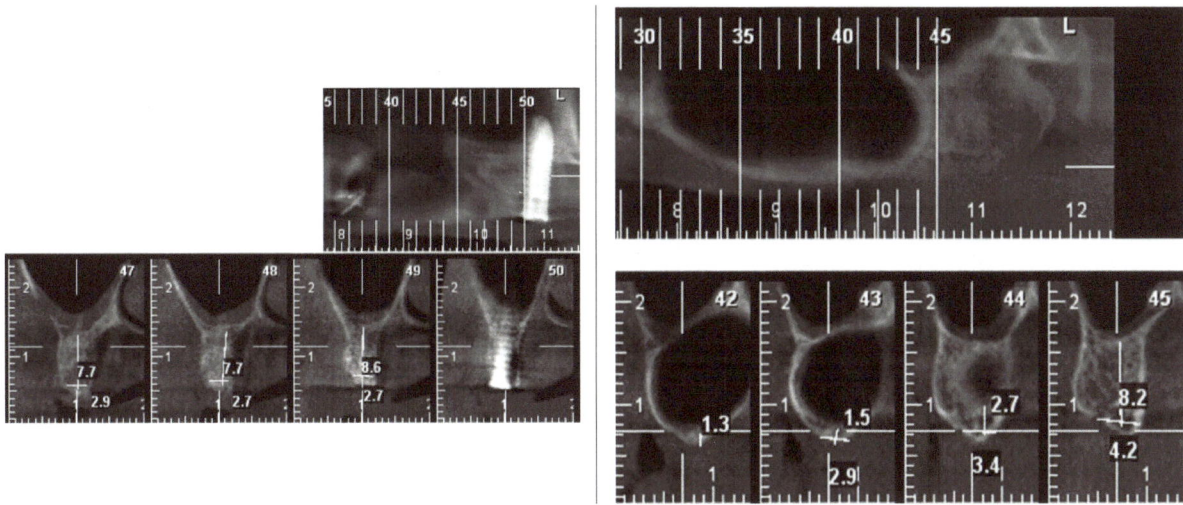

Figure 4.20 CBT of the upper left tuberosity with the major maxillary sinus enlargement. The right photo demonstrates placing a long implant.

either at the genial tubercle or at the adjacent midline symphysis; thus, breaching the incisive artery means the bleeding may occur from the incisive, sublingual and submental arteries with subsequent consequences.

If the incisive canal in the mandible is assaulted without piercing the lingual cortex, the cutting of the blood vessels will lead to the artery prolapsing back into the floor of the mouth. The subsequent haematoma in the sublingual space will have the consequences already described.

The traditional presence, almost by default, of the spiral drill design in standard dental implant kits seems to ignore the drill's effortless ability to snag and drag soft tissues and blood vessels in an expanding column of destruction. This is especially so for the sublingual and submental arteries and veins. The engagement of their contralateral increases the potential for danger. Non-spiral drills will only graze the blood vessels and are far less threatening (figure 4.23).

The mandibular incisive nerve is a terminal branch of the Inferior Alveolar Nerve and provides innervation to the lower anterior teeth and canines. The incisive nerve and canal are located in the interforaminal area.

Sensory disturbances such as neuropathic pain related to mandibular incisive nerve damage, incisive canal and nerve perforation should be considered as a complication of implant surgery in the anterior mandibular region.

The locations of the mandibular incisive canal, mental foramen and associated neurovascular bundles can vary. Their precise locations need to be identified before any surgical plan can be finalised. In deciding upon the appropriate surgical approach for any individual, the surgeon needs to consider the individual patient's anatomy, gender, age, and race, along with the degree of edentulous alveolar bony atrophy. All these factors will influence the surgical approach [36].

After branching off into the mental nerve that exits the mental foramen, the inferior alveolar nerve continues anteriorly within the mandibular incisive canal as the incisive nerve, providing innervation to the mandibular first premolar, canine and lateral and central incisors. The mandibular incisive nerve either terminates as nerve endings within the anterior teeth or adjacent bone or may join nerve endings that enter through the tiny lingual foramen.

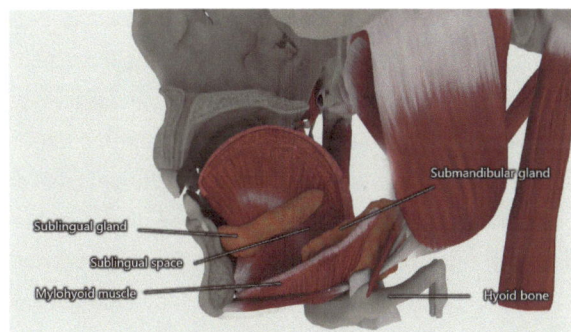

Figure 4.21 The Mylohyoid muscle separates the sublingual space and the submandibular space.

100

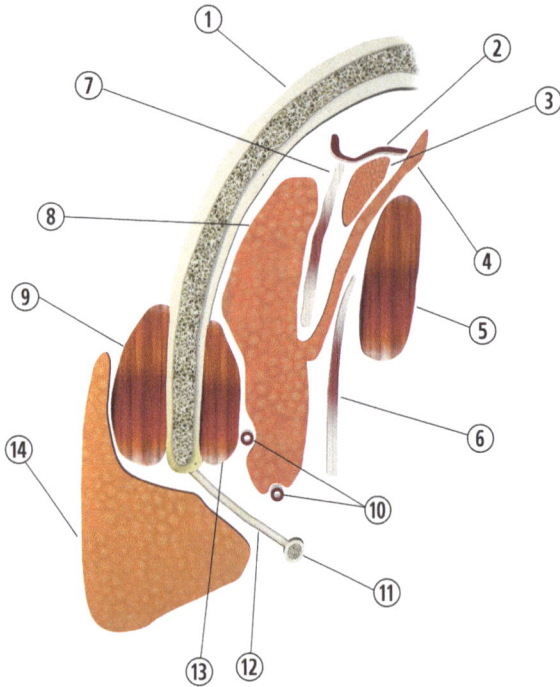

Figure 4.22 Horizontal cross-section of the mandible and major anatomic features.

1) Mandible, 2) Mucous membrane of mouth, 3) Sublingual gland 4) Submandibular duct, 5) Genioglossus, 6) Hyoglossus, 7) Mylohyoid, 8) Submandibular gland, 9) Masseter, 10) Facial artery, 11) Styloid process, 12) Stylomandibular ligament, 13) Medial pterygoid muscle, 14) Parotid gland.

The incisive canal is typically found within the middle third of the mandible in an apico-crestal direction, reaching the midline 18% of the time [37].

Now that most clinicians are using CBCT scans, the true complexity of the anatomy of the anterior mandible has become clearer. If the bone is dense, reducing or limiting the local blood supply can encourage resorption. Larger medullary spaces have collateral blood supplies, but close to the mental nerve, there is a risk of Wallerian degeneration of the proximal of the mental nerve with the consequence of dysesthesia or burning sensation. Paraesthesia is unlikely due to the few branches that supply the lip or chin. This complication should be considered during free chin graft harvesting.

POSTERIOR MANDIBLE:

The inferior dental canal extends from the lingula of the mandible, within the cortex of the body of the mandible, then diverts towards the buccal aspect below the border of the first molar or the second premolar. Its greatest convexity comes as it slopes upwards towards the crest while simultaneously moving toward the buccal surface until it reaches the mental foramen.

The dentist must bear in mind that double Inferior dental or accessory canals and double mental foramina have been reported.

It is crucial that the dentist take cautious note of the exact length of the drill with and without the addition of the tip length. This needs to be checked against the system's stated drill length. Some systems include the tip length as part of the whole length of the drill, while some do not. The former systems have the disadvantage of reducing the height needed of 1mm of the bone, which sometimes may change the treatment plan (Figures 2.12 and 4.24).

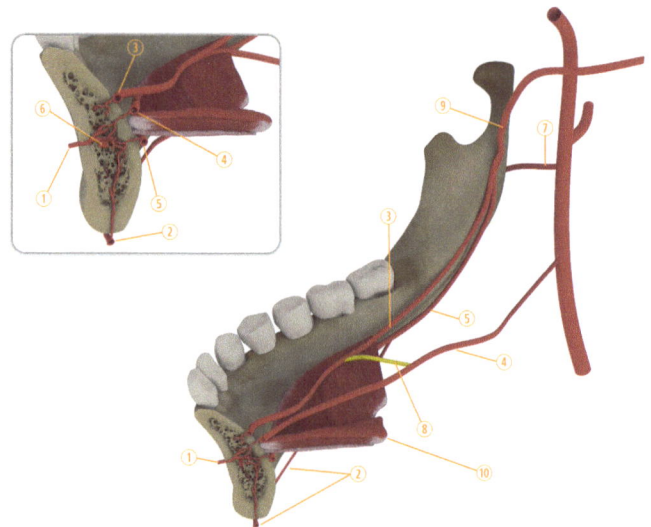

Figure 4.23 During drilling procedures, it is crucial to be mindful of the sublingual and submental arteries and veins, as if they lie in the drill's path and can be inadvertently damaged.
1. Mental branch of ID artery, 2. Submental artery, 3. Lingual artery, 4. Deep lingual artery, 5. Facial artery, 6. Anastomose of arteries, 7. Facial artery branch from external Carotid, 8. Lingual and Deep lingual artery anastomosis (10%), 9. Inferiore Dental artery.

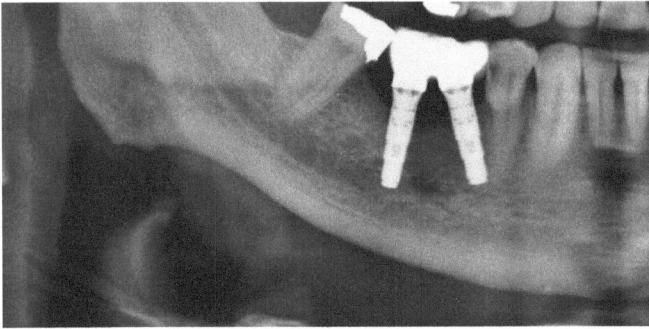

Figure 4.24 The length of the drill, including the tip: the dentist needs to know if the tip of the drill is longer than the dental implant, even though in the X-ray, the implant has not invaded the ID canal, but the drill has done it—for example, Noblebiocare vs Southern dental implant drills.

The surgeon needs to distinguish between cortical bone and cancellous bone. Usually, the cortex is more than 2 mm thick, and while the hardness of cancellous bone can approach that of wood, poor cancellous bone can be encountered. The surgeon must also distinguish between poor cancellous bone and lingual cortical perforation.

However, a panoramic radiograph (DPT) may be misleading by failing to reveal previously referenced undercuts. Drilling inadvertently through the bone can result in damage to the underlying soft tissue, including the lingual nerve, artery and vein.

As noted before, this is especially important when using spiral drills. Spiral drills can entrap the soft tissues and produce even more damage. If, after pilot drill application, there is any suspicion of perforation, a thick, blunt-ended periodontal probe can be applied to make sure that the lingual cortex has not been perforated. If it has been, you must do one of the following:

1. Reduce the length of your next drill.

2. place harvested cortical bone inside the cavity and pack it into place to prevent the soft tissue from entering and proliferating within the cavity. The latter can occur because the ability of the soft tissue to proliferate is greater than that of the bone to regenerate around the implant. In other words, the ability of the soft tissue to attach to the protruding tip of the implant will allow it to infiltrate the implant cavity before osseointegration takes place. This can lead to implant failure.

3. Another option is to change the angle of the drill in an oblique apico- buccal direction.

You need to determine the position of the mylohyoid ridge and, therefore, the point from which the lingual surface of the mandible slopes buccally or presents an undercut. Unless you know how deeply the lingual mandibular surface extends before any undercut, you will be blind cutting your implant site. To determine the vertical depth of the lingual mandibular surface, you need to make a small crestal incision with rigid flat plastic and using the end, which is at right-angles (bin-angled) to the shaft, reflect the soft tissue vertically downwards while initially keeping the edge of the flat plastic firmly in contact with the bony surface. When you contact resistant soft tissue, you will encounter the mylohyoid muscle.

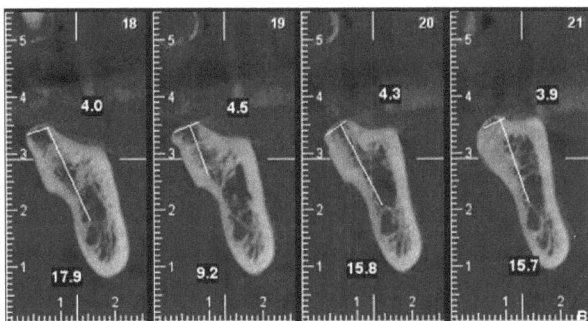

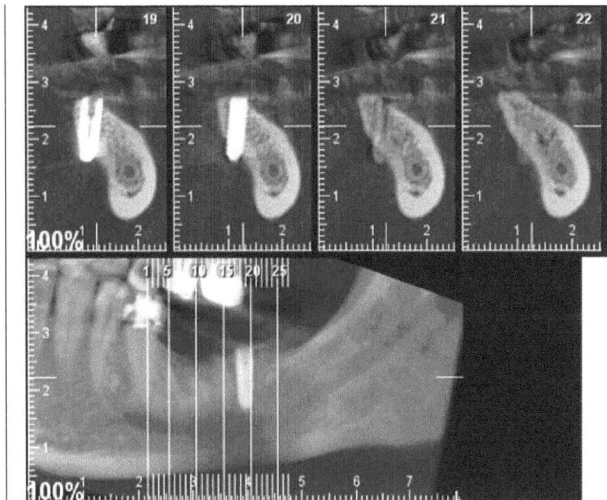

Figure 4.25 The dentist needs to bear in mind the different lingual cortex curvature in the posterior mandibular region. The danger of perforation of the floor of the mouth needs to be considered.

Using the scoop end of Mitchell's trimmer (sharp end), separate the muscle from the ridge to allow further vertical exploration of the lingual bony surface. Continue palpating the lingual surface until any undercut is found. Measure it.

If less than 9mm is found, other routines need to be employed to solve the problem.

The author believes that the best initial approach is to respect the bone's anatomy by allowing the cortex's inner surface to indicate the preferred pathway of the pilot drill. The surgeon should now, in the mind's eye, the final position of the implant and relax the grip on the handpiece to allow the tip of the drill to divert buccally. This means that the new angle adopted by the surgeon in response to the cortical 'nudge' will allow continued drilling to the required depth. Once the drilling is stopped, the pilot drill is removed from the handpiece and re-inserted into the prepared cavity. The angle of the drill can now be measured to indicate the degree of compensation needed for the crown. Any angle up to 40 degrees is acceptable. Any angle beyond that requires other surgical approaches.

Another option is available if drilling at the preferred angle has been carried out to some 7mm and resistance is felt. This will mean that the cortex is being penetrated. Since the cortex is 2-3mm thick, it can be penetrated for one further millimetre to provide a depth of 8mm.

When contradictory conditions are present - thick cortex and poor cancellous bone:

REDUCING THE RESISTANCE OF THE THICK CORTEX TO IMPLANT PLACEMENT:

In areas where there is soft cancellous bone and a thick cortex, typically seen in the posterior mandible, it is advisable to tap the cortex before placing the implant. Failure to do so can potentially result in complications. This is because the inherent resistance of the cortex may allow the implant to be placed but not to its entire length. Forcing the implant can lead to unpredictable outcomes. While you may succeed in screwing the implant to the desired length, there is no guarantee of this outcome. If the implant cannot be fully screwed to the intended depth, attempting to unscrew it may become difficult or impossible. This can result in the implant being exposed above the crest of the bone, potentially damaging the internal structure of the implant and preventing proper placement of the abutment.

For these reasons, it is important to measure the thickness of the cortex and tap only to the depth of the cortex. Subsequently, you can proceed to place either a one-piece screw implant or any self-tapping dental implant.

Ideally, cortical tapping should be limited to the thickness of the cortex alone, but if the cancellous bone is accidentally tapped, it should not materially affect primary stability, provided only about a millimetre of cancellous bone is involved.

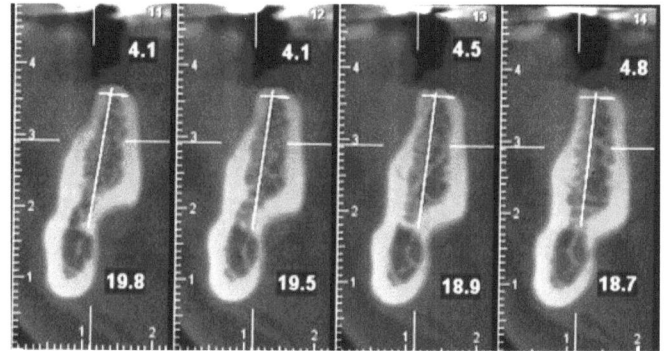

Figure 4.26 Thick cortex and poor cancellous bone, CBCT of the posterior mandible.

Placing a dental implant in the posterior region, distal to premolar or molar, there is an inherent tendency to "drift distally" with the starting point for the drill, and this can get increasingly more distal as larger drills are used so that the final channel is not centred where you would like it to be. It can be a good idea for the dentist to change his position and sit precisely right next to the patient after using the round bur. If the position of the implant is needed to move mesially, it can do so; it is helpful even with the application of the surgical template, as the surgical template can be displaced without noticing.

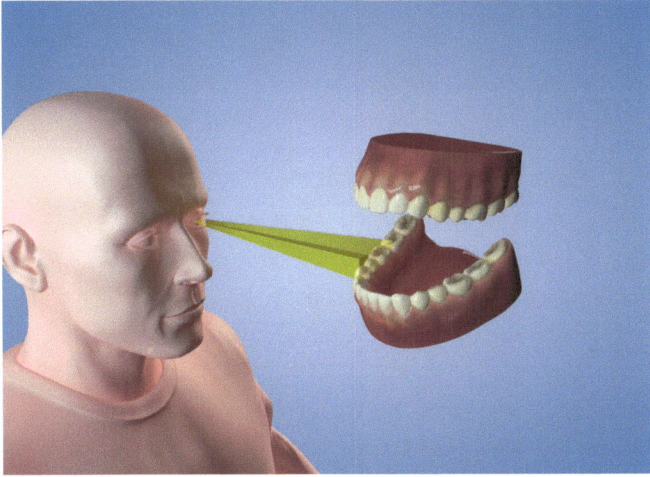

Figure 4.27 A direct perpendicular view will eliminate placing the implant distally.

Improving the mechanical quality of cancellous bone:

The implant's primary stability and osseointegration quality will be adversely affected if the quality of the cancellous bone is not improved.

In order to improve the quality of the cancellous bone, you need to be able to access it by breaching the cortex, usually with either an osteotome or a drill. However, the osteotome is contraindicated where the cortex is thick because its use may be traumatic for the patient's TMJ and may fail to breach the cortex.

This leaves the special drills, which rotate counterclockwise. The body of the drill can compress the cancellous bone or penetrate the cancellous bone without removing debris, but the tip can penetrate the cortex as the instrument of choice, both to breach the cortex and to compress the cancellous bone. The latter requirement, the compression of the cancellous bone by drill, can be provided for by a few implant manufacturers.

This technique will be new to most surgeons and is carried out as follows: the round drill is used to perforate the cortex, and the pilot drill is inserted and drilled to length. This is where the technique breaks new ground. Succeeding serial drills are now used but must be rotated counter-clockwise. The combination of specially designed drills capable of compressing the cancellous bone by counterclockwise rotation differentiates this technique. The drill, during rotation, will condense the bone by centrifugal force following Newton's second law.

Please note: this technique can only be used if the system you use makes provision for it.

Other ways to improve primary stability are by placing biocoral, bioglass, artificial bones (rocky), and lateral condensation in the prepared cavity. Artificial Bone substitutes can release Ca in ion exchange to infuse natural bone in the prepared site. Strontium ranelate may also be released to strengthen adjacent bone.

Osseodensification has been recommended in poor-quality bone to promote self-impaction of the bone, which increases the primary stability of dental implants due to the viscoelastic behaviour of bone [38].

Unpublished research by the author investigated the methods by which primary stability might be increased in bone of poor quality. The research compared different preparation techniques in artificially softened bone using a pull-out test of the 3.4mm diameter Nik cylindrical dental implant. The bone was softened by immersing it in dilute hydrofluoric acid. The experimental preparation was initiated by the round bur followed by the 2mm pilot drill. A 3.4mm Nik cylindrical dental implant was inserted into the test site. The pullout test was performed with an axial traction force toward the long axis of the dental implant (1.0 mm/min) through a device with a load cell of 100 Kgf (Kilogram-force).

The pull-out forces produced by the different preparation techniques were compared, as shown below:

1. Application of standard serial drilling, 92.2 N
2. Application of reverse drilling (counterclockwise): 130.6 N
3. Application of standard (clockwise) serial drills placing one size larger implant:201.2 N
4. Application of standard serial osteotomes with a surgical mallet: 221.6 N
5. Application of only the pilot drill (2 mm diameter) and placing a 3.4 diameter cylindrical implant: 418.8 N

The result of this research strongly recommends that when faced with soft bone, you should apply only the round bur, followed by the 2mm pilot drill, and then immediately place either the 3.4 or 4mm diameter cylindrical dental implant.

This technique is only recommended when using Nik cylindrical dental implants.

What do you do when facing a ridge width that has reduced width? Can it be widened, and if so, how?

While many likely methods are available, we focus on ridge expansion at this juncture. A ridge expansion is a method by which a ridge of limited width can be expanded to accept an implant of suitable width, and where the expansion is achieved by compacting the alveolar bone and stretching and microfracturing the cortical bone. This is an instance where unexpected benefits can appear where you least expect them.

If the ridge presented has a width of 4 - 6.5mm, then ridge expansion can work surprisingly well. Use the round and pilot drills to prepare the initial osteotomy site and drill to length. There are now two possible routes to completion: drill or osteotome.

Completion of expansion by drill: use serial drilling with reverse rotation to the required width. Completion of expansion by osteotome: use osteotomes of requisite width to expand the initial cavity.

The process of site expansion, by either method, starts by compressing the cancellous bone until no further compression is possible and then transfers its force to the expansion of the cortical bone by microfracturing. The implant will gain primary stability from its intimate contact with the contact with better compacted cancellous and bone cortex along much of its length. Added to these sources of stability are the collective elastic rebound forces of the affected cancellous and cortical bone, plus that of the associated periosteum and muscles.

A final benefit is that in contrast to the rectangular site left by ridge splitting, the site left by ridge expansion will be round.

As noted above, unexpected benefits can appear when you least expect them.

To make an informed surgical choice you need to understand how cortical and cancellous bone will respond to any given technique. Osteotomes are at a disadvantage when used to prepare implant sites as they will respond to the pressures of cortical bone but are much more difficult to control. They also demand great cooperation from the patient.

During in-vitro practice in the acrylic model, the consistency of the 'bone' presented is uniform, but inside the natural alveolar bone, the consistency is not uniform. Not only is the actual cortex covered by the periosteum, but there is an inner surface to the cortex of which, in some cases, a lower apical segment of

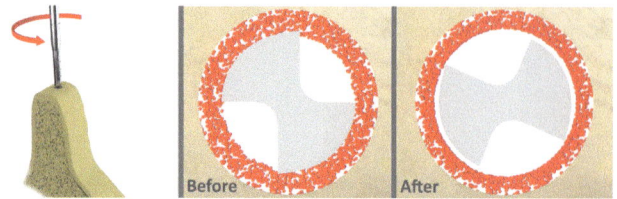

Figure 4.28 Today, there is a technology that some systems have; the drill can be used counterclockwise to compress poor cancellous bone. It is essential not to try the technique with any system which will have serious consequences.

bone can be engaged. This can assert its presence by pushing the drill in unanticipated directions, both buccally and palatally. Cancellous bone has differing-sized lacunae into which the drill tip can fall unexpectedly, this way or that. It can be advantageous for the drill to be rotated counterclockwise as this can afford greater control. The surgeon needs to control the drill while being fully aware of what direction it may be being forced to move.

Site Assessment and Method of Drilling:

Using a surgical stent to fix the position of the implant site is widely recommended. Its use is held to be twofold: to identify the initial crestal location of the implant site and then to assist the pilot drill in setting the subsequent angle of the implant site. The problem with this approach is that no stent can tell you how much bone is present at the site at the time of site preparation, and no stent accounts for the adjacent teeth' root angles. The stent can tell you the actual crestal point of entry, which may also need to be checked.

The digital surgical guide has been on the market and is prepared using scanned intraoral cavity and CBCT images. A study demonstrated that even though it was clinically acceptable, there were significant differences between the CBCT scans and cast deviations, especially the angle deviation 39 to 40, which can be concluded is useful but unreliable in sensitive cases.

The approach advocated here uses the round drill and its dimensions to help you fix the implant site's position yourself. The round drill is used first.

In use, the axis of the round drill should be held at almost 45 degrees (figure 4.29), as this angle stops the drill from sliding during bone preparation.

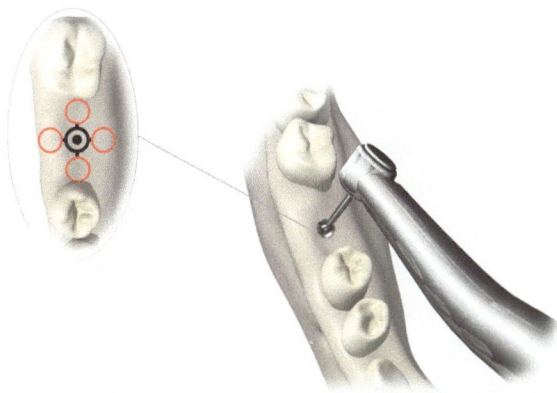

Figure 4.29 A round drill with a known diameter can be used as a gauge. The axis of the round drill should be angled to prevent sliding during bone preparation.

ASSESSING THE POSITION OF THE IMPLANT STEP BY STEP:

Initial assessment is made using the tip of the round drill. The round drill tip, without rotation, is placed on the alveolar crest and contacts the distal aspect of the root mesial to the implant site. Since the round drill will have a given diameter (usually 2 – 2.2 mm), the space filled by the drill tip denotes the space that the implant site cannot invade. Repeat the exercise at the distal of the implant site. The space between the second and the third areas is now selected as the implant site. Between the second and third circles, which touch externally, is the point at which the middle of the 2 mm round bur will penetrate the crestal bone (figure 4.29). Thus, the 2mm round bur is used as a gauge. The care taken to avoid any intrusion on either 'No Entry' area will help to prevent potential bone resorption in the future.

Measuring the ridge width:

To gauge or measure the thickness of the alveolar ridge, the diameter of the round drill's head can again be used. Noting the buccal bone's vertical axis, place the round drill tip on the ridge. Note the distance covered by the drill tip and reposition the drill tip more palatally or lingually. This now tells you that the ridge is either two tips wide or greater than this. An alternative method is using dental callipers, but this is more difficult to do with the more posterior site. The Iwansson Wax callipers can help - not the pointed callipers designed for crowns, as these can pierce

bone. An alternative is the Castroviejo Caliper, a straight dental, orthopaedic measuring instrument.

ASSESSING THE POSITION OF THE IMPLANT STEP BY STEP 2:

Following the procedure outlined in Step 1, the round drill is again used, but this time to gauge the bucco-lingual or bucco-palatal position of the implant site. The planned position of the implant site – mesio-distally and bucco-lingually or bucco-palatally – will have now been gauged. So, using the round drill, now make an initial pit. If the initial assessments have been correct, then you can now exchange the round drill for the pilot drill.

The diameter of the pilot drill is from 2mm to 2.2mm, so as noted before, you need to maintain the equidistance of the pilot hole from the adjacent distal, mesial, and bucco-lingual. If any adjustment is needed, it can be made before using the next drill.

What could go wrong, and how do I deal with it?

You have used the round drill and realised that the position is not equidistant as intended. Correct this by using the round drill to reposition the site. There are now two intersecting circular cavities. Place the round drill in the correct position and cut with great care.

The Initial drill position is correct, but you realise there is only 2mm of bone on either side. This means that only a 3mm implant can be placed if the treatment plan allows this. If it does not, then surgery needs to be cancelled.

You have made an initial 2mm hole and realise that the remaining bone adjacent to its buccal and lingual margins is less than 2mm wide. Bone-grafting is indicated.

If, as noted previously, the deficit is asymmetrical, it is essential to check that, at least on the buccal aspect, you have a minimum of 2mm of bone. This is because it is buccal bone, which tends to resorb more than lingual bone. In fact, 1.5mm of bone would be enough, but only in experienced hands. Therefore, the author prefers the presence of 2mm of bone. This rule may not apply to the palatal aspect only if the bone is rock hard.

Once the pilot drill is used, the surgeon's visual appreciation is altered because the black of the hole can be better distinguished from the yellow of the bone. The surgeon needs to appreciate the contour of the bone from the outside and imagine it from the inside.

The outer surface of the bone can be studied by CBCT observation and flap reflection, while the inside can be revealed by CBCT and the surgeon's manual feedback during bone drilling. The manual feedback has particular significance if the surgeon ever feels that the drill's direction is suddenly dictated by the bone, not by the surgeon. It will indicate immediately that the inner surface of the cortex is in danger of being breached. As noted below, you need to adjust the angle now imposed by the cortex's inner surface and compensate for this at the prosthetic stage (figure 3.9).

The next drill is the 2.2 mm pilot drill with the parallel or taper body. The length of the drill is pre-determined using a DPT or Computed Tomography. The need for the drill tip to be included in the total length depends on the dental implant system, but it provides a precise measure of the needed length.

If, during preparation, the tip of the drill contacts the internal surface of the cortex, the surgeon will feel resistance. The surgeon should not use extreme force because it will increase the temperature and may also lead to the perforation of the external surface of the cortex. Any such perforation can damage the soft tissue and adjacent anatomical structures (vein, artery, nerve, gland duct). If the tip just touches the inner cortex, it might indicate that the implant may not screw in all the way. Even worse, the drill may start to rotate in a frozen position. If this is allowed to continue, it will enlarge the bone cavity and make it too loose for the implant. In this case, it is recommended that you over-drill by 1mm in order to provide extra space. This avoids the rotation of a frozen drill and a subsequent loose implant. However, give it time and ensure the drill's angle does not change.

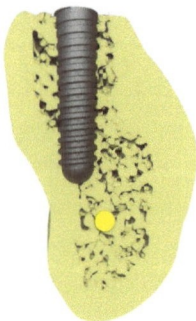

Figure 4.30 If the tip of the drill touches the inner surface of the cortex, over-drill by 1mm to provide extra space. This avoids the rotation of a frozen drill and a subsequent loose implant.

The relationship between the length of the drill, including the tip, and the length of the implant is different in various implant systems. It is essential when the surgeon is drilling near the vital anatomical structures. This is an important feature which is often not mentioned in the catalogue. Always check before you use (figures 3.15, 4.24).

If the ridge platform is not flat, some surgeons prefer to flatten it with an acrylic bur, while others prefer to drill and use the lowest point as the reference for the bone margin. The author agrees with this latter approach because the bone changes which may follow can be advantageous. Firstly, the inner depressed area may well fill up with bone, further protecting the implant, and secondly, any outer ridge resorption will not affect the already-protected implant.

For an implant with a diameter of 3.5 mm, a ridge width of 6.5 mm is needed.

Catering for different ridge widths

A. If the ridge width is between 4- 6.5 mm, then ridge expansion is acceptable. After using the pilot drill, the rest of the drills should be used counterclockwise if the drills are designed for such a task or serial of osteotomes - unless the cancellous bone is minimal so that the bone will not expand. There is a potential for buccal bone loss because of the resultant thinning of the buccal bone in the presence of poor vascularisation.

B. If the ridge width is between 3-4 mm, use a ridge split plus the placement of a wedge, which is a modification of a blade implant or blade implant. Some recommend a mixture of ridge split and ridge expansion and screw implant placement. Guided bone regeneration remains another option (figure 4.31, 4.42, 4.43).

C. A bone block is the main choice if the ridge is less than 3mm. Alternatively, ridge expansion can be performed without placing a dental implant. You will need to wait 3-4 months for the bone to heal and then repeat the procedure with simultaneous implant placement. Within the opening, the author considers autogenous bone as the material of choice, but others recommend different types of bone substitutes.

D. A bone block graft is the only method if the bone width is less than 2mm.

Mini-implants: Mini-implants form part of the armamentarium and are available to the implant dentist. The implant's diameter is between 2-3 mm, and the 2 mm are one-piece implants only.

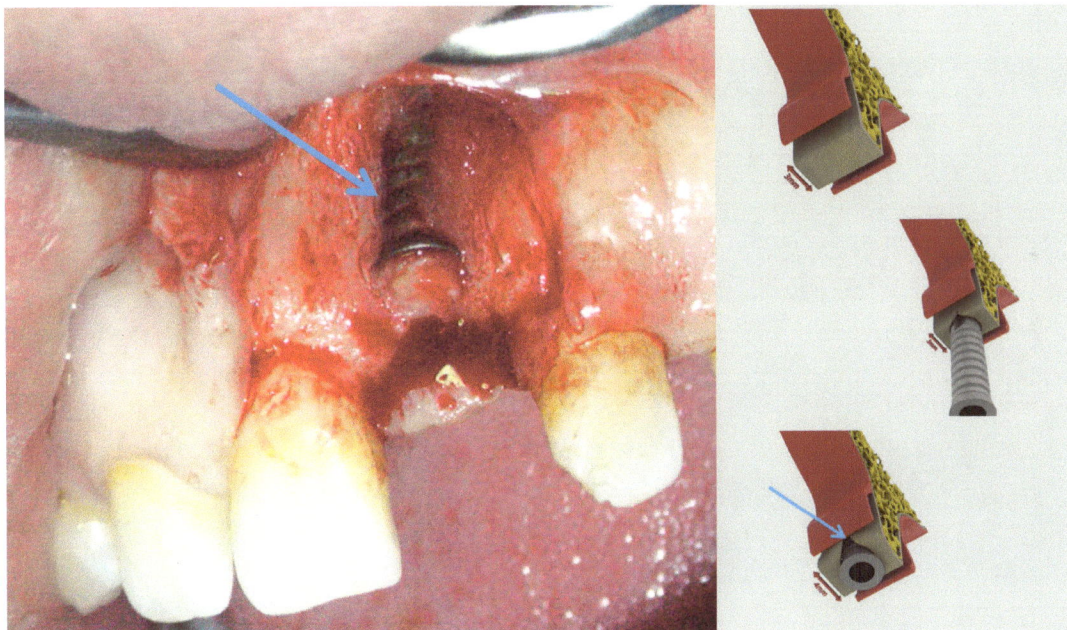

Figure 4.31 After ridge expansion, if the buccal bone is thin (less than 1.5 mm), bone loss can occur due to poor vascularisation.

You are not recommended to use them independently, except in the lower incisor region or in place of an upper lateral incisor with favourable occlusion. They can be used with standard-diameter dental implants that need to be splinted together.

In overdentures, the fracture risk increases significantly and is not recommended. A minimum height of 10 mm is suggested. It is highly recommended that only a fixed resin (e.g. BIOHPP) prosthesis be used in these cases.

Flapless surgery and osteotomy

Extra irrigation is recommended during flapless surgery because of the lack of direct access to the coolant from the drill-bone interface. After the pilot drill, it is recommended that you use serial osteotomes instead of a series of drills to reduce the probability of the drill tip's perforating the cortical bone and penetrating the soft tissues. This can promote soft tissue invasion around the implant from the apical area, followed by the implant's loosening and extraction.

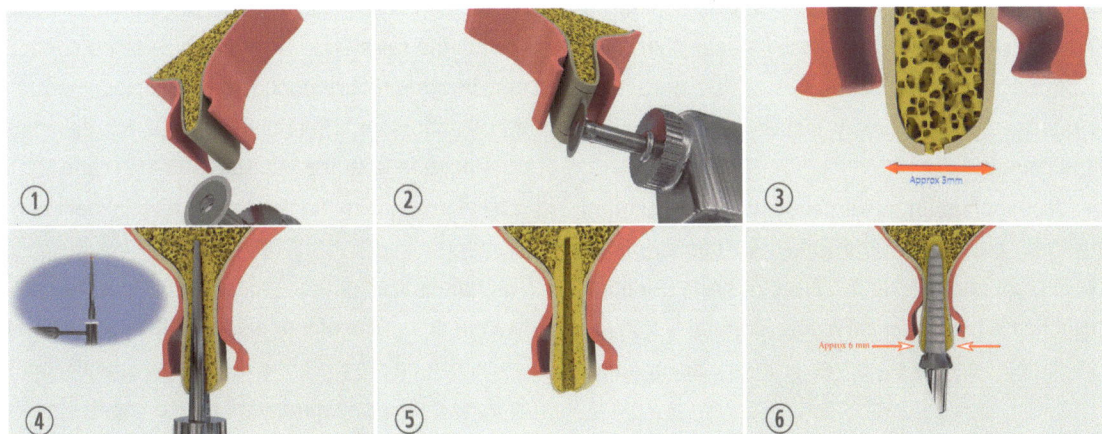

Figure 4.32 Ridge split and placing a dental implant is a good option when the ridge width is between 3-4 mm.

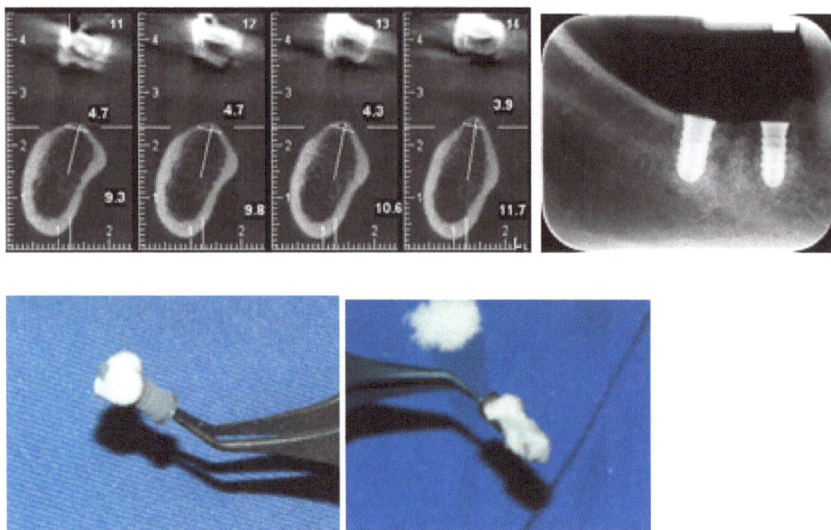

Figure 4.33 Bone substitutes may increase the quality of the cancellous bone, and the types with rocky structures can help increase the dental implant's primary stability. In the upper left, CBCT has poor cancellous bone, and in the upper right, the DPT after placing bone substitute in the socket and immediately implant placement after three months of healing. Lower left, the ½ apical is covered with bone substitute and lower right: the entire surface of the implant is covered with bone substitute prior to implant placement in the prepared bone cavity.

For this reason, you are strongly recommended to pick up a thick periodontal probe between each drill or osteotome application and ensure that no soft tissue is exposed. It would be best if you did this 3-dimensionally, especially in the apical region.

The author believes flapless surgery is indicated only if one one-piece implant is applied. With conventional two-stage surgeries, flapless surgery is not going to help the patient.

Poor bone quality:

Osteoporosis is a disease where decreased bone strength is observed. Osteopenia is a low bone mass or low bone mineral density. While it is not a disease, it may turn into osteoporosis. Bone scans from the hip and vertebrae can determine bone density but do not seem directly related to the mandible or maxillae.

Poor bone quality reduces primary stability and the potential healing of the bone cells.

The author recommends, in these cases, the application of a hybrid screw with parallel threads (press fit) dental implants. This type of implant is placed in the alveolar bone using a rod on the implant and a hand surgical mallet (preferably 250 gr) to press the implant inside the bone, rather than placing a nail in wood.

The dentist must bear in mind that the application of a hand-held surgical mallet while the patient's head is extended may provoke Benign Paroxysmal Positional Vertigo (BPPV) due to displacement of otoliths, which migrates into one of the semicircular canals and the posterior canal is most common. Applying an electric (magnetic) mallet provides a faster and more accurate method, which, through the axial and radial movement at the tip of the surgical rod of 90 daN/us, provides

greater comfort for the patient. Even though the force of application is four times higher than that of the manual mallet, the application period is only 0.1 seconds intermittently, and the patient cannot discern the impulse and interprets it as acceptable, almost inert. In these cases, bone compression and the use of bone substitutes inside the prepared cavity can increase primary stability by promoting bone formation.

When the bone quality is poor, but the implant has osseointegrated, the resistance to torque is reduced so that the implant may become mobile during abutment placement.

Whilst there are different techniques for the management of poor bone in both the maxillae and the mandible, the author's clinical experience has led to the development of a simple protocol:

To standardize the bone quality from just feeling to quantitative numbers. The author designed the pilot drill with two flutes, which can entrap the bone debris and quantify the bone quality to bone debris entrapment into three segments of the depth of the drill entered the bone. The first third is poor bone, the second third is medium-quality bone, and the last third is hard bone.

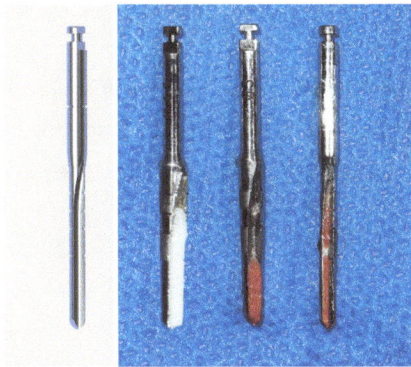

Figure 4.34 Left to the right: the pilot drill has a diameter of 2 mm with two flutes. Hard bone quality, in which the bone debris is white (no bleeding(and more than 2/3 of the depth of the cavity is filled; middle bone quality, in which the bone debris is between 1/3-2/3 and poor bone quality < 1/3 of bone debris in the flutes.

Maxillae:

1. Place the longest and widest implant possible unless it prejudices the final positioning of the crown.

2. When the bone is so soft that after final drilling, the drill flutes are covered either to less than 1/3 of their length by bone debris or even not at all, you must apply osteotomes. Osteotomes with a 2.5, 3, 3.4, 4 and 5 mm diameter can be used. Bone compression techniques are applied in conjunction with using the longest and widest diameter implant available, and they are considered suitable. But first, you need to address the following three questions:

a. How poor is the bone? What is the mechanical quality? What is the cortical thickness? What is the spongy trabecular bone? Which needs to be rectified, increasing the thickness of the cortical bone or compressing the cancellous bone?

b. How much increase in height is needed?

c. How much increase in width is needed?

The dentist will not likely find simultaneous solutions for all of the above three requirements at the same visit, and if there are such, one or two or all may be compromised.

If the height and width of the alveolar bone are acceptable, then you need to address only the quality of the bone in order to provide higher primary stability. Therefore:

1. Apply osteotomes,

2. Drill to one size less than the diameter of a dental implant,

3. Under drill a few sizes than the diameter of the dental implant,

4. Drill to one length shorter than you need,

4.4. Ridge expansion and ridge split

A narrow dentoalveolar ridge remains a severe challenge for the successful placement of endosseous implants. Reduced alveolar width may require an implant of reduced diameter, which can adversely affect the aesthetics of the final crown. This possibility can indicate a need for major ridge-width reconstruction to allow the placement of the smallest size of a three-piece implant, usually 3.3 or 3.4 mm.

Alveolar Bone Contour

Three types of alveolar bone contour can be observed:

Triangular cross-section:

These cases are more forgiving and give the best results. This is because there is good cancellous bone and nutrient irrigation from the apical region, and the chances of buccal bone fracture are minimal.

Triangular cross-section, but with a deep undercut, usually buccal:

This type has a greater potential for alveolar bone fracture, and during ridge split or ridge expansion, the instrument's tip should be angled as much as possible away from the concavity. If this is not done, ridge splitting/expansion with simultaneous implant placement will not be possible. Alternatively, the concavity can be grafted with a mixture of autogenous bone and artificial bone substitute with membrane placement. As the defect would be a space-making defect, the success rate will be high.

Be warned: To split or expand the ridge, you need to first have a minimum width of 3mm at the deepest point of the concavity and, secondly, contain flexible cancellous bone of at least 1mm width.

The buccal and lingual cortices of the alveolar ridge are parallel:

There is limited availability of nutrients and irrigation from the apical region, and the potential for bone plate fracture will be high. Where a single tooth replacement is needed, the likelihood of fracture is even greater. A complete bone plate fracture will significantly worsen the site and render it almost irretrievable.

Blade implants can be a better choice, and you will need to discuss this with patient so that patient can make a suitable choice.

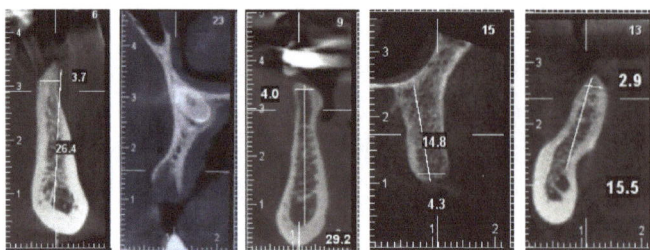

Figure 4.35 Types of alveolar ridge cross sections. Left to right: Triangular, triangular with deep buccal undercut in maxillae, triangular with deep buccal undercut in the mandible and parallel alveolar ridges.

Several techniques, such as guided bone regeneration and block grafting, may be considered to deal with this scenario. GBR creates a barrier to epithelial migration before the completion of bone healing and filling the defect.

Unfortunately, the downside of these procedures can be the membrane's premature exposure and bone block, which will likely lead to bone resorption. If there is no premature exposure of the membrane, then the likelihood of bone resorption is significantly reduced. This may be avoided by gaining experience, respecting sterilisation vigorously, and stabilising the alveolar bone membrane by mini-screws or tacks and sutures without tension and a perfect seal to the oral cavity.

The surgery needs a generous flap, and post-operative discomfort is inevitable, as is loss of depth of the vestibule. This will have a negative effect on both aesthetics and dental hygiene.

Most importantly, if the surgical procedure fails, the patient's status will be rendered even worse.

The splitting or expanding of a thin ridge of bone is done mechanically to make the ridge wide enough to allow an implant or bone graft to be placed between the two altered sides of the bone.

Ridge expansion or splitting can provide a faster method by which an atrophic ridge can be predictably expanded. It can then be grafted with autogenous bone or allograft or implanted with a one-piece or conventional implant. This avoids the need for a second (donor) surgical site.

The surgery can be performed using manual or motor-driven instruments, such as piezo surgery or any combination.

Bone graft material can be placed and allowed to mature for a few months before placing the implant. However, the implants are placed simultaneously with the ridge expansion in most cas-es. With this technique, the alveolar height will not be reconstructed.

Ridge expansion aims to increase the width of the alveolar bone and produce a round cross-sectional bone preparation, while the ridge split technique produces a rectangular cross-section. More details are in chapter seven.

Removing as little bone as possible is essential, ideally by pushing aside adjacent flexible bone and compressing the remaining bone.

In the maxillae, usually, due to the quality and rigidity of the palatal and lingual cortex, only the buccal cortex is expanded. However, on rare occasions, the palatal and lingual cortexes will be expanded, too.

The author classifies the width of the alveolar bone as follows: α = 6.5 mm and above, β = 4.0 - 6.5mm, γ = 2.5 – 4.00mm, δ = less than 2.5 mm.

While this technique for ridge expansion is more applicable in the maxilla, it can still be used in the mandible. However, its use in the mandible depends on the presence of a minimum 1mm width of cancellous bone between the buccal and lingual cortex. This is more likely in the posterior mandible.

This expansion technique is most applicable when the bone width is between 4.0 and 6.5 mm. The added advantage of using this is when the bone width is in class β (4- 6.5mm) because it will allow a wider implant. The increased bone-implant contact (BIC) ensures greater primary stability, plus, after healing, added long-term stability provided by the deep cortical support along the entire length of the implant.

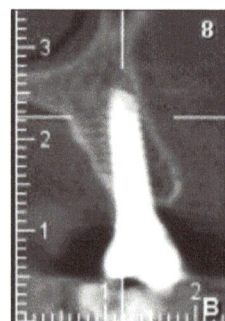

Figure 4.36 Prosthetic-driven implant placement requires adequate width ridge and angle, which dentists often do not have the luxury of. The cross-section of the CBCT demonstrates placing the implant in an ideal position.

Ridge expansion with immediate dental implant placement

Patients most suitable for this procedure will have:

β), ridge width between 4.0 - 6.5mm

(note: If conventional (two or three pieces) implants are to be placed, the patient should not be allowed to use a partial removable denture without a buccal/labial flange post-operatively).

1. Soft tissue quality around the future dental implant should be fixed and keratinized,

2. the minimum bone height available should be 8.5 mm.

SURGICAL TECHNIQUE:

The patient is preferably treated under I.V. conscious sedation (Midazolam only) and local anaesthetic.

When a conventional 3-piece implant is to be placed in the maxillae, a palatal para-crestal incision is made. When a one-piece implant is to be placed, a crestal incision is made, with a buccal reflection which includes the periosteum.

The periosteum is reflected in order to assess the width of the alveolus. Use a rigid flat plastic to expose and observe the buccal and palatal cortex. Using a round bur and the pilot drill, create an intra-bony cavity at the intended site of the implant placement and then Use either a surgical mallet plus a series of osteotomes or drills capable of running counter-clockwise, he pilot hole's width is gradually increased in the direction of the long axis of the proposed implant. Gradually increasing the diameter, the labial cortex is sequentially displaced labially, thus increasing the overall ridge width by plastic deformation or green stick fracture and warning that the most buccal segment twill be thinned (figure 4.3, 4.39).

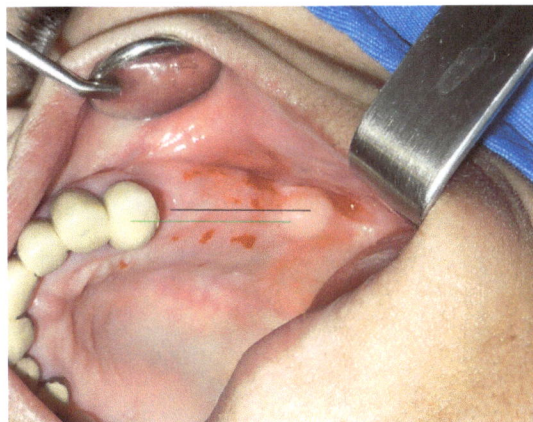

Figure 4.37 The black line shows the crest incision, and the green line para-crestal incision.

However, due to the high mechanical resistance of the palatal cortex, there is a tendency to push the drill or osteotome towards the buccal.

Bear in mind that when the maxillary bone is being enlarged, the pressure exerted by the surgeon's determined maintenance of palatal pressure will push the patient's head down. The surgeon and the surgical assistant must ensure that the patient's jaw is stable during this manoeuvre. It is recommended that the assistant's finger be placed in the premaxilla region (when the operative site is the anterior region) or on the cheek (for the posterior region) in order to counter the surgeon's manual pressure.

Failure to do this could lead to the bone cavity's oval cross-section. During screw implant placement, some bone will be grazed from the inner surfaces of the cortex. Where the cortex is thin, it is best to use a cylinder (hybrid screw) implant, which is placed

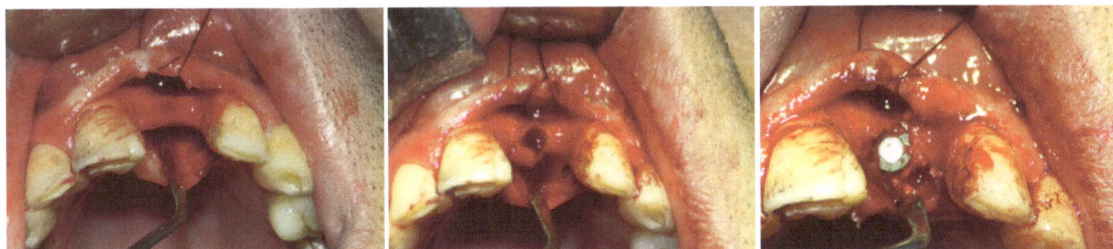

Figure 4.38 The ridge expansion technique is a valuable means to increase the width; however, there is a hazard of thin buccal and/or lingual cortex, which may fracture during implant placement or resorbed during the healing period.

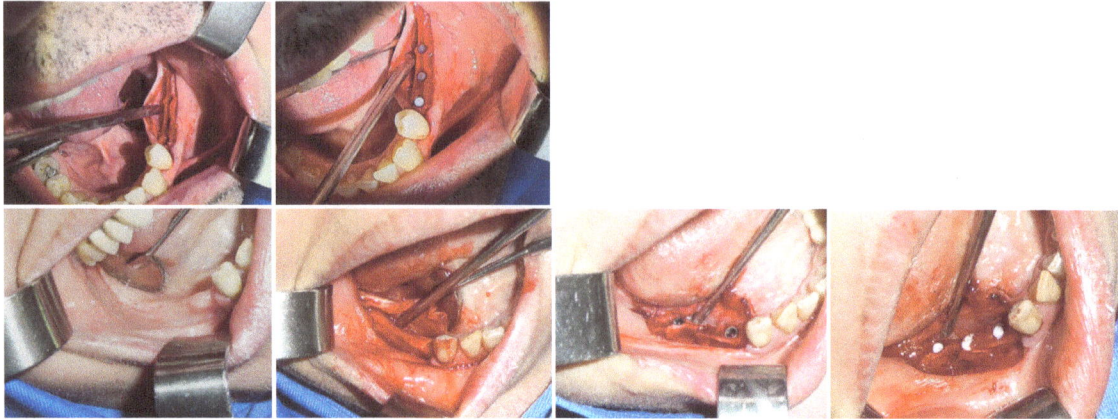

Figure 4.39 Simultaneous ridge splitting and then ridge expansion are effective, especially in the lower posterior region. Upper row: left to right; ridge split and expansion prior to implant placement and after dental implant placement. Lower row: left to right; demonstrate incision, flap, ridge split and then ridge expansion with the green stick fracture but stable buccal bone and dental implant placement.

like a nail, in order to reduce the risk of dehiscence of the thin buccal plate.

When the bone is soft (C3), it means reduced thickness of cortical bone and poor concentration of thin trabecular bone. The dentist can immediately place any self-tap implants. But using an implant which is inserted like a nail, parallel-threaded, called a Hybrid screw or cylindrical implant, is more reliable. The main reason behind it, sometimes there are tiny but thick cortical buds in the inner surface of the cortex that can prevent the threads of the screw implant from cutting through, and it may act like spinning screw and enlarging the cavity and lose the primary stability and not going through the whole length. The nail type of implant can dislodge the small bud and find itself in its final position.

When the thickness of the cortex is about one millimetre, and the quality of cancellous bone is poor, a self-cutting one-piece or conventional cylindrical dental implant can be placed immediately after the use of the pilot drill. This technique, called the "single drill technique", reduces the number of osteotome taps and increases primary stability. With this technique, higher stability and less bone resorption can be expected. Fracturing the cortex inside the cavity will increase the cortical thickness of the BIC surface.

In those cases where the ridge width at the implant site is between 2.5-4 mm, and the thickness of the cortex is more than 2 mm, the dentist does not have the intention to place a blade im-plant, and where between the buccal and lingual cortices there is still some cancellous bone, simultaneous ridge splitting and ridge expansion is recommended (figure 4.39), if not applicable than blade implant is an option.

The dentist should try to conserve bone as much as possible, and the pilot drill should not be used as it removes bone.

The knife edge of the crest with a height of less than 3mm is cut and preserved using a 0.25 mm thick diamond disc and pre-el-evator (figure 4.40, 4.42). Using the diamond-coated osteoto-my saw is not recommended, as controlling the handpiece is complex and can damage the surrounding hard and soft tissue aggressively.

The 0.25 mm double-sided diamond disk should be used to cut through the cortex and access the cancellous bone. As the cortex has more resistance to cutting than cancellous bone, this will reduce the surgical time and the patient discomfort.

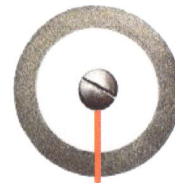

Figure 4.40 The screw top of the mandrel prevents the placement of the full radius of the diamond disc. The red line demonstrates the maximum depth it can penetrate to the crest of the alveolar bone.

Surgical stops should be provided at the proximal ends of the alveolar ridge to prevent crack expansion toward the PDL neighbouring spaces using a disc, pre-elevator, or number 15 blade. The stops should be at least 1.5 mm from the neighbouring (mesial and distal) root or PDL. It is preferred that the stop be perpendicular to the alveolar crest cut.

The perpendicular stops can be made using piezosurgery tips, Low-Speed Dental Contra Angle 4: 1 Interproximal Stripping Handpiece Sets or blade 15 and or fine chisel (as pre-elevator), which is less comfortable for the patient as short and light mallet blow is necessary, the last option is using round or fissure (1/2 mm) diameter fine burs.

If a rotary disc is the instrument of choice, and vertical cuts are not achievable by a disc, especially in the posterior region. For this manoeuvre, only small-diameter double-sided diamond discs with a diameter of about 5mm are recommended. However, a 45° rotation will enable the application, which consequently, another 1 mm distance from the buccal from the neighbouring teeth will be observed, and sometimes it can affect the ideal mesial-distal position of the implant.

It is crucial to remove a minimum of bone width for splitting the bone; on the other hand, the rigidity of the disc is necessary. The diamond discs are attached to an RA latch-type mandrel at the crest, cutting through the disc with a thickness of about 0.15-0.25 mm. The screw top of the mandrel has a diameter of 5 mm; thus, the dentist needs to understand if using a 10 mm diameter of a disc, the diameter of the screw top of the mandrel is 5 mm, and thus the active and the maximum penetration of the disc (the red straight line) is 2.5 mm only (figure 4.40). Cutting through the cortex using a disc is necessary as other means, like piezo surgery tips, remove more bone. It is essential to arrive at the cancellous bone using the diamond disc. It is quick and reliable; however, using a tongue retractor to protect the tongue is essential. That is why ridge split in single tooth replacement is the most challenging.

Using 10 mm discs means that about 6.5 to 7.0 mm to the neighbouring teeth, the cortex has not been cut in-depth, and using other means like smaller diamond discs, blade 15 and or a chisel (e.g. pre-elevator) can cut through the region.

Cutting through the cancellous bone with a blade number 15 and/or pre-elevator and tapping it to the predetermined depth is an option.

If the cortical buccal and lingual plates are stable, the dentist

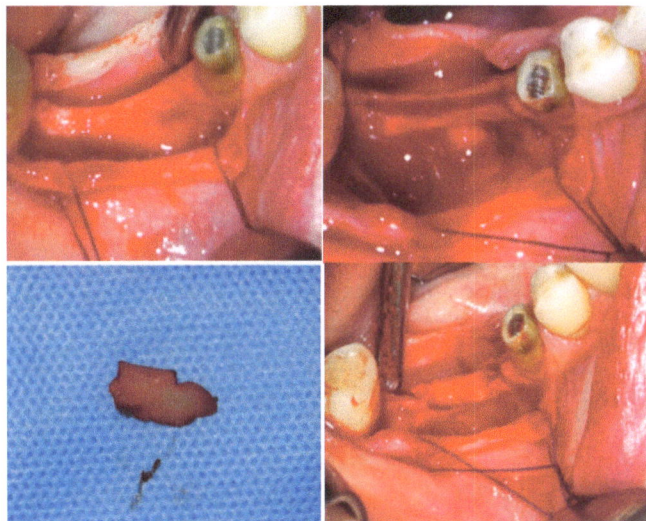

Figure 4.41 Ridge split in the posterior mandible, when one of the cortex walls is unstable, or the dentist feels it cannot be stretched more, a piece of thin bone plate can be harvested from the ridge or any other region and fit inside. It may need a push to enter the piece, providing a high stability that does not need other means to stabilise it. The dental implants can be placed after three months—a safe and predictable technique.

can continue to place a blade implant or use a series of counterclockwise drilling or osteotome and mallet to prepare the recipient cavity for a screw or cylindrical implant. Tapping the bone before implant placement requires caution, as removing any bone from the inner side will reduce the buccal or lingual wall, which is already a minimum.

Usually, the dentist is more in control using counter-clockwise drilling and is more comfortable for the patient than osteotomes and mallets, especially in the posterior mandible region.

If, for any reason, axial stability of the implant cannot be achieved, but the buccal and palatal bone is still intact, it is recommended that the preserved pyramidal shape harvested bone placed on the occlusal surface of the gutter and suture the flap and re-enter in 3 months (figure 4.41).

If either the buccal or palatal cortical plate is not stable, a rigid, non-resorbable membrane should be placed, even though there would be a need to strip the bone from the periosteum to place the membrane. Usually, membrane fixation with tacks or screws is not necessary or is not possible due to the potential damage to the neighbouring tooth or lack of stability of the fixator (pin or screw).

Expanding the cortex is not applicable in the mandible, where the cortex is thick. A mixture of ridge splitting and ridge expansion is recommended (figure 4.39).

After ridge splitting, with or without implant placement, it is recommended to close the opening with a small membrane or cortical bone, but only on the defect.

A disc with a thickness of less than 0.25 mm and a diameter of 4mm or less is used to remove the alveolar crest's 1-2 mm tip. This can only be done if the remaining bone height is 8.5 mm. The excised cortical bone of the triangular cross-section needs to be preserved in a moist, sterile area.

Section the newly created ridge along the mid-line (mesiodistally) to a depth of 1.5mm and within 1.5 mm of any neighbouring root. A surgical stop must be provided at 1.5 mm proximal to each root to prevent the cracks from running into the sound alveolar bone of the adjacent roots. If a disc is used, the cut cannot be made perpendicular to the sagittal bone split as it would be oblique. Using a pre-elevator with the mallet or tapping the blade handle (no. 15 scalpel) can provide a better perpendicular cut; the use of a bite block or mouth props is highly recommended, or the surgical assistant to push the chin upward and backwards to prevent damaging the TMJ complex.

After the final bone preparation is completed, the primary stability of the implant can be analysed by positioning the final drill in the prepared cavity. The axial stability is now checked. A conventional or one-piece screw implant can be placed. Conventional implants should be placed when simultaneous GBR is needed or when the axial stability of the final drill is more than 15 degrees off the ideal angle.

Ridge splitting is usually mono-cortical, but it is sometimes possible to apply bi-cortical displacement in the maxillae when palatal bone resistance has been reduced.

Microfixation has been used when the cortical plate is not stable.

Ridge splitting is a reliable and predictable technique and presents an alternative method for placing implants in narrow ridges. This technique has a high success rate and fewer complications.

4.5. Blade dental implants:

The main indication of the blade implants where there is not enough bone width (3-4 mm) with other options, GBR, block graft, and there is no minimum of 8.5 mm height, especially in the posterior mandible, which GBR, block graft or nerve repositioning is not a priority due to the medical history, risks and potential complication during the surgery. Bear in mind that the other options are applicable after a failed blade implant and would not put the patient in an inferior position.

In the 1970s, Linkow introduced the blade implants, and even though the surgeries were not the same as today, touching and bending the titanium surface and dental implant surgery without sterile gloves still had an acceptable success rate. He emphasised not wearing a sterile surgical glove does not increase the infection rate. Of course, touching or pressing to bend the rough titanium surface today is unacceptable. In 1980, the FDA classified the blade implant as Class III. This followed the results of extensive preclinical studies. In 1998, root-form implants were classified as class II, but they did not reclassify blade-form dental implants due to insufficient clinical information.

In January 2013, the FDA proposed reclassifying blade-form dental implants from class III to class II based on many reports, including that of Roberts,1996, which demonstrated a high success rate after 25 years as the applied forces are transferred over a large area of bone. Blade-form implants are an acceptable alternative for atrophic ridges because of the reduced need for bone grafting or nerve repositioning with the ensuing repercussions 41. At least the option should be given to patients; complicated surgeries could be the second option when the blade implant is unsuccessful (Figures 4.43 and 4.44).

There are two types of blade implants: portrait and landscape. The landscape type is used in the posterior mandible with a mesiodistal dimension of more than 6 mm and an occlusal-apical of 4-5 mm.

The blade landscape implants need to be placed by a rod hit by a surgical mallet. With the thick cortex in that region, the osteotomy should be meticulous to prevent patient discomfort, TMJ injury, and fracture of the non-resilient cortical bone. When the bone width is limited to 3-4 mm, bone removal is hazardous, and ridge splitting with minimum bone removal is the option.

The thick cortex is the first obstacle that needs to be passed, and access to the cancellous bone is needed. It is recommended that cortical bone be cut with a motor-driven diamond disc. The cutting instruments should have a minimum thickness, usually 0.25 mm, to minimise bone removal and maximize bone preservation. Remember that the mandrel's radius prevents the cutting radius when measuring the disc's active radius. This

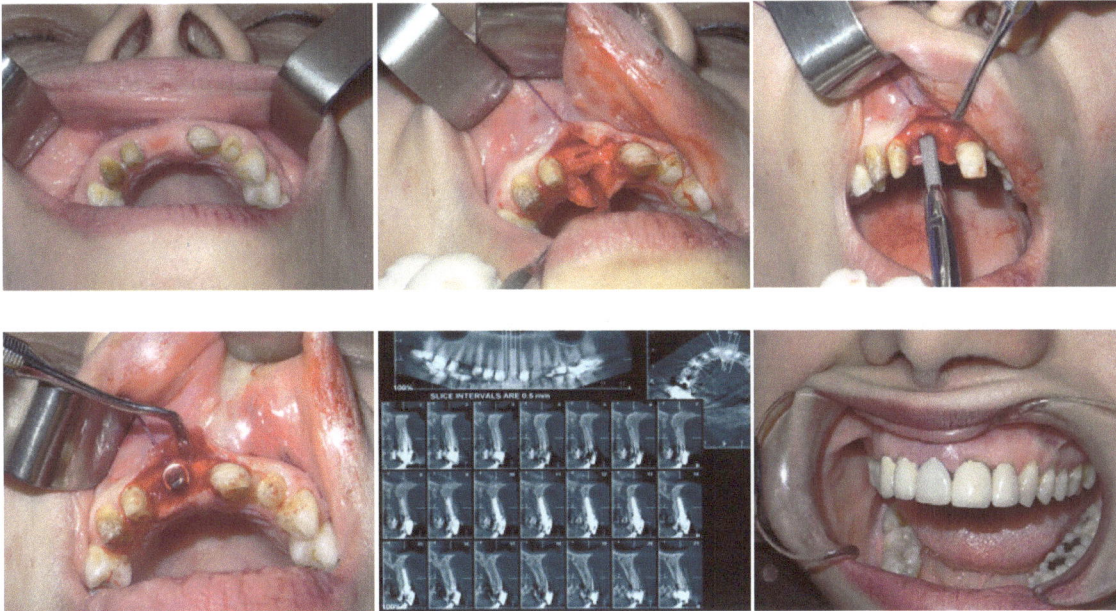

Figure 4.42 Replacing UR1, instead of a big flap and traumatic surgery, an envelope flap and atraumatic ridge split one-piece blade implant is placed, and an immediate provisional crown is cemented.

maximizes the available alveolar bone. Saw discs are not recommended; they are thick and have the potential to skid and damage the soft tissue, especially the mental nerve. Piezoelectric surgery is useful, especially in this area. The piezo surgery inserts(tips) of the osteotomy kit are more than 0.25 mm; thus, if the dentist wants to be conservative, it is recommended to cut through the 0.25 mm thickness disc and then continue with the piezo surgery insert.

After providing access to the cancellous bone, use a pre-elevator to penetrate the bone like a wedge and split the buccal and lingual plates. The final opening of the alveolar bone should be rectangular, and the blade implant with its rectangular cross-section and a thickness of 2.5 mm opens the bone. The landscape blade implant needs 2 mm distal and 2 ml mesial space, and the mesio-distal length cannot be curved. High stability is guaranteed, and a one-piece blade implant can be placed.

If you access the mouth from the 11 o'clock position, the bar that drives the implant inside the bone barely touches the buccal surface of the upper premolars or molars. The reason for adopting this access position is that the distal side of the blade implant in the lower posterior region lies more apically than the mesial side, which must be rectified by applying more pressure towards the mesial side of the implant.

Blade implants are a good option for treating complex cases and afford a straightforward approach. The author designed a modified blade implant. This type of blade implant is self-cutting and provides high stability.

The blade implant is modified with the triangular cross-section, which provides better primary stability like Nik one-piece wedge implants and the Rex system, which, after many years of the author wedge implants, introduced the three-piece wedge implants. Both are wedge-shaped and have a rectangular cross-section at the crestal level. However, there is a difference between them: the Nik dental implants, the one-piece implant is countersink, and the bone grows on its occlusal surface, increasing BIC and more resistance to torque and pushout forces. Two types of blade implants are available: the landscape blade implant and the portrait blade implant.

After the ridge split of the alveolar bone and the implant placement proximal to the implant, bone cavities would be left almost like a uniform triangular pyramid (tetrahedron). The base of each cavity is the titanium implant; the faces are the cavity's buccal and lingual cortex floor. The other is the opening of the cavity. The rectangle base, with a length of about 1.5 mm, defines the cavity's depth, and the 2mm width of the rectangle base is the opening of the defect. If not treated, up to 50% of the bone defect will heal due to the triangular morphology. Filling

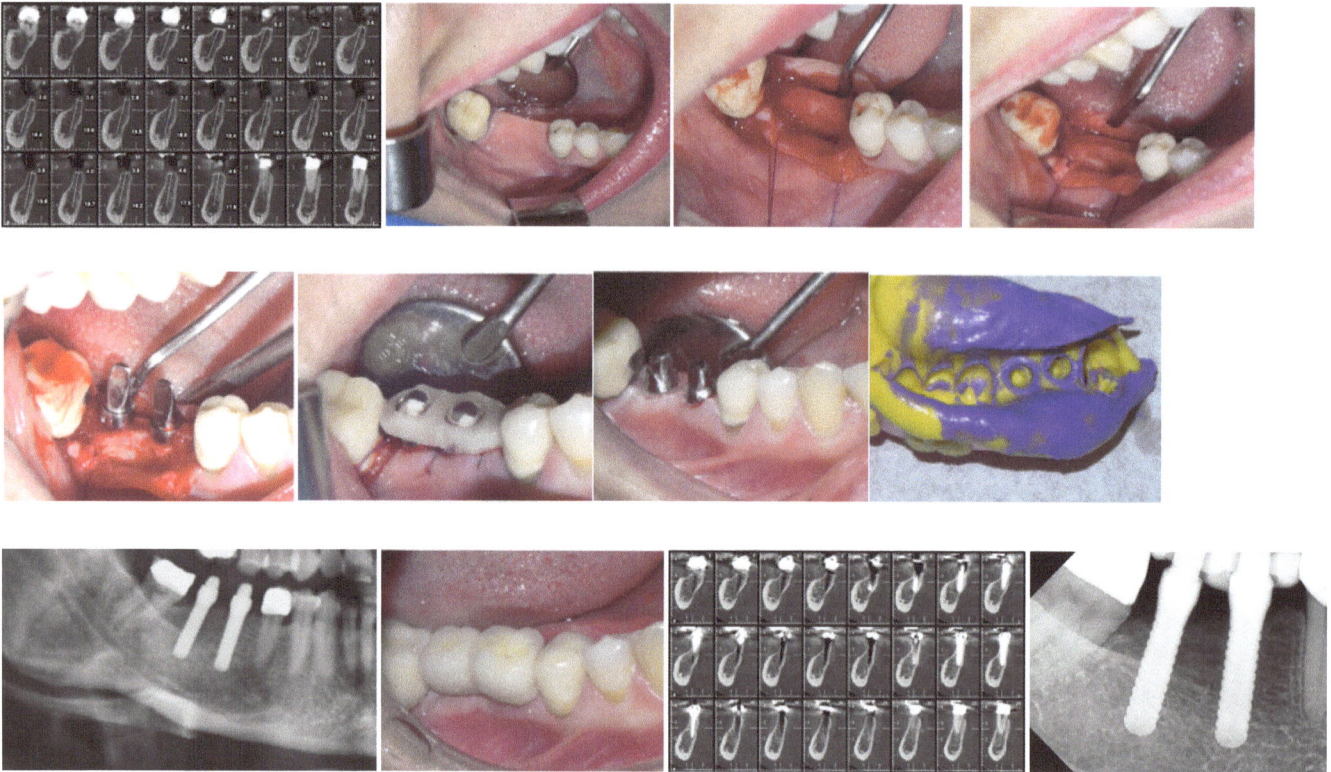

Figure 4.43 The CBCT prior to surgery demonstrated an alveolar ridge width of 3.0-3.4 mm, ridge split and placing one piece blade implant, which was splinted with composite and the abutment was clear off occlusion of 2 mm. After three months, the splint was removed, and a conventional impression was provided after final abutment preparation. The final splinted PFM crowns and CBCT demonstrated the osseointegration. The final photo is the periapical after ten years.

the defect with autogenous bone debris would have a better prognosis.

There is always the option to place a one-piece blade implant, but the dentist must believe in them and the requisite training.

Some patients have previously had ridge augmentation using iliac crest bone, and this has suffered from bone resorption that left a final thickness of less than 6.5 mm. However, the quality of iliac crest-grafted bone is such that ridge expansion can be used efficiently and safely, even when there is not enough bone to insert an implant of the desired diameter.

If, during bone expansion, a crack is produced in the labio-buccal bone surface, implant placement may still be done as long as the periosteum is intact and the primary stability of the implant has been achieved. Some recommend that where (a) the remaining cortex is thin and/or (b) the bone is soft, you should not reflect the soft tissue flap extensively and so denude the labio-buccal and/or lingual-palatal cortex.

If this has been done, then matters can still be retrieved using bone debris and applying a non-resorbable barrier membrane. The success rate of ridge expansion using this technique appears to be high, but Its limitation seems to be simply the degree of expansion that can be achieved.

Above all, it is imperative that the basic principles of dental implant surgery are adhered to, namely:

(i) that an implant of adequate size in relation to functional and aesthetic requirements is used,

(ii) that primary stability of the implant is achieved,

 iii) that adjunctive methods of ridge augmentation are employed,

iv) that tension-free soft tissue closure can be achieved.

The fabrication of crowns on 3 mm diameter implants causes aesthetic problems in some cases, and the temptation to insert a narrow implant into an inadequately expanded ridge must be resisted. It is preferable to place a conventional implant where the abutment is chosen with reference to the size of the final crown rather than the implant. This means that all abutments with different diameters are matched with implants of different diameters.

With this in mind, at implant exposure, the mesiodistal width of the proposed future crown should be measured pre-operatively, and the implant diameter should be decided upon that basis. If ridge expansion cannot be achieved to a degree that permits the placement of the chosen diameter, then ridge expansion and augmentation should be performed rather than inserting a narrow implant, which would satisfy neither functional nor aesthetic demand.

After preparing the final bone cavity and inserting an implant, it is essential that the future implant's vertical position is assessed by inserting either a depth gauge or the final drill.

THE BUCCAL AND LINGUAL ALVEOLAR RIDGES ARE PARALLEL:

Even though these cases can be treated successfully, there are a couple of issues which need to be highlighted:

Great care is needed so as not to fracture the bone at the apical of the bone cavity preparation; the buccal-lingual position of the implant needs to be determined only by the angle of the ridge (Figures 4.15 and 4.25).

If there is a resulting discrepancy, you can sometimes correct this, at least to a degree, during osteotome application by pushing with the handle towards the palatal (figure 4.15), but in this type of bone is not recommended as there is the potency of fracture of the bone plates and put the patient in a worse position to be treated.

γ group alveolar bone: where the bone width is between 2.5-4 mm, ridge expansion can be hazardous; the labial bone may become too thin (less than 1.5mm), and bone resorption can result in a fracture

In the maxilla, where the cortical bone is thin, and the alveolar bone is flexible, the bone can expand, and a round cross-section of bone will be available. However, at the peak of the circle, the bone is thinner, has less vascularisation, and is prone to resorption.

The cortex is too thick in the mandible to expand, so a ridge split is recommended. In the posterior mandible, ridge splitting is more applicable than bone block or GBR. The single tooth replacement is more limited and predictable as the number of teeth replacements increases. The alveolar bone resorbs from

the buccal surface, and the lingual segment is the bone that will split. As there is an undercut at the first and second molars at the sublingual fossae, an acute angle between 10-40 degrees can manifest as the limitations of ridge splitting. The dentist has a couple of options, but the least complicated treatment plan is the ridge split, leaving it to heal for three months and going back and repeating the same procedure and simultaneous implant placement. It is the second time that there is a better chance of correcting the angle of the implant.

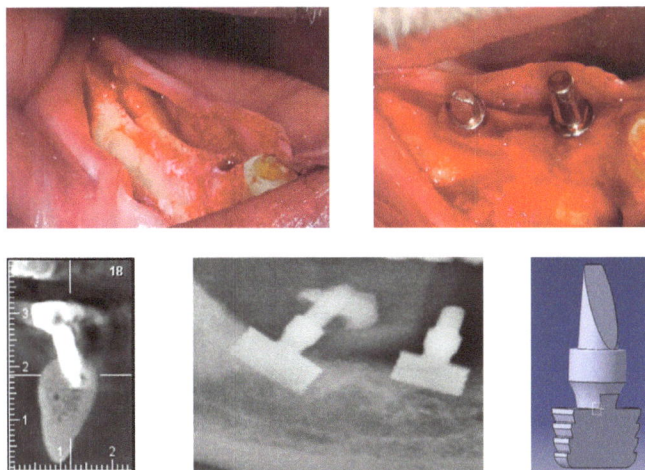

Figure 4.44 Horizontal blade implants with a height of 4-5 mm can be a good option for implant placement instead of complicated other options such as bone block graft or nerve repositioning.

For multiple implant placement, where there are defects between the blade implants, the best approach is to close the opening with autogenous bone and leave the depth. Alternatively, a rigid, non-resorbable membrane can be applied instead of the cortical bone chips. However, cortical bone chips are more reliable.

The portrait blade implants are more indicated in the maxillae between premolars, and it is indicated when the bone is between 3-4 mm and the dentist or the patient does not want to proceed with the more aggressive surgeries. However, the author had a high success rate in the posterior mandible when the 8.5 mm bone height was unavailable.

Even though porcelain fused metal Prosthesis achieved a high success rate, it is more logical to apply the BIOHPP prosthesis. It is lighter and absorbs the functional forces that can prevent the fracturing of the blade implants.

Complications:

Mallets with osteotomes are uncomfortable for the patient despite the surgical benefits compared to other surgical techniques involving major flap reflection.

Benign Paroxysmal Positional Vertigo (BPPV)

Dizziness or vertigo can occur immediately after maxillary osteotomy. During maxillary osteotomy, as a result of hyperextension of the neck and the transmission of the percussive forces of the osteotomes, heavy inorganic particles (otoliths) detach from the otoconial layer of the utricular macula and free float into the endolymph of the semicircular canal as well as, usually, the posterior semicircular canal. A Dix-Hallpik test needs to be conducted to establish a diagnosis of vertigo by making the patient change rapidly from the sitting position to the left or right head-hanging position. Medical treatment is not indicated and is used only to suppress symptoms if they are severe or intolerable. Different types of drugs have been recommended as antihistamines (Meclizine), dexamethasone, Carbamazepine, tricyclic antidepressants, diazepam, Clonazepam, Meclizine which is anti-emetic. The guidelines of the dental council are different between countries, and the dentist needs to respect the diagnosis and prescription.

TMJ post-operative discomfort following mandibular surgery.

During blade implant placement in the mandible, it is crucial to protect the TMJ by biting the bite block and or by the hand of the assistant by pressing the chin upward.

Guided implant surgery is a major advancement in dental implantology, using digital technology to improve precision, predictability, and aesthetic results. This method involves meticulous planning and computer-generated surgical guides to ensure that implants are placed accurately according to each patient's unique anatomy. However, the increasing use of guided implant surgery by general dentists (GDPs) brings both opportunities and challenges.

4.6. Guided Implant Surgery

The process starts with detailed digital planning. Cone Beam Computed Tomography (CBCT) scans provide a 3D view of the patient's oral structure, including bones, nerves, and sinuses. This data is then used in specialised software to plan the virtual placement of implants with high precision. This planning phase ensures optimal implant positioning, angulation, and depth, which are critical for both function and aesthetics.

A surgical guide is created once the digital plan is complete, often using 3D printing. This guide fits over the patient's teeth and directs the surgical tools to the exact planned locations. Using these guides minimises errors during surgery and ensures that implants are placed precisely as planned.

Increasing Use by General Dentists

More general dentists are now placing dental implants. These dentists, who might have less experience in oral surgery, rely on advanced technology to bridge the knowledge gap. This trend is similar to orthodontics, where systems like Invisalign have simplified the treatment process.

For general dentists, guided implant surgery enhances precision and confidence. Digital planning and surgical guides help ensure accurate implant placement, reduce complications, and improve patient outcomes. However, this technology requires continuous education and training to be used effectively.

Aesthetic Considerations

Aesthetic outcomes in implant dentistry depend heavily on managing the soft tissues. Guided surgery helps preserve the natural gum contour by enabling minimally invasive techniques, which is particularly beneficial in flapless surgery. Guided surgery ensures implants are positioned to support the final restoration, aligning well with adjacent teeth and maintaining a harmonious smile. This precision helps maintain proper gingival architecture and avoid asymmetries.

Dynamic Considerations

Accurate implant placement also contributes to better bone preservation and regeneration. It avoids critical anatomical structures and places implants in the most suitable locations. Guided surgery's precision reduces complications such as misalignment of dental implants.

Static Guided Surgery

Static-guided surgery uses pre-made surgical guides based on digital plans. These guides, created from CBCT scans and virtual implant placement, fit onto the patient's teeth, mucosa, or bone, guiding the drills to the exact positions for implant placement. The data for static guides comes from patient impressions (conventional or optical scans) and CBCT scans, which are converted into STL files for 3D printing.

There are three types of surgical guides:

1. Teeth-supported (most accurate and least invasive)

2. Mucosa-supported (less accurate and less invasive)

3. Bone-supported (accurate and most invasive, requiring a large flap for stabilisation pins)

Static guides need metal sleeves for implant drills, which limit irrigation unless the drills have internal irrigation. A good mouth opening is essential due to the drill length. Poor planning or fit can lead to significant deviations.

Dynamic Guided Surgery

Dynamic-guided surgery, or computer-assisted surgery, uses real-time navigation systems. These systems track the patient and surgical instruments, providing real-time feedback on a monitor to help the surgeon place the implants precisely according to the digital plan.

Optical tracking systems are crucial for dynamic guided surgery, using stereo vision to determine object distances. These systems are either passive (reflecting light) or active (emitting infrared light tracked by cameras). Both offer similar functionality, but active systems provide real-time tracking of CBCT files. Thermoplastic guides with fiducial markers are used in dynamic surgery and updated through trace registration, which aligns the virtual plan with the surgical site. Tracking arrays (tags with reflective spheres) attached to the patient and dental handpiece allow precise navigation.

Literature reports a 3% increase in success rates for dynamic-guided surgery compared to freehand surgery. This success may also stem from avoiding riskier surgeries requiring less bone removal. While guided surgery offers clear advantages, proper training in dento-alveolar surgery remains essential.

Conclusion

Digital technology promises to improve dental implant procedures, potentially replacing manual techniques with robots. Dentists must balance improving traditional surgical skills with mastering guided implant surgery. This balance depends on expertise, patient needs, and practice goals.

Traditional techniques hold value, especially for experienced practitioners who have honed their skills over the years. These methods offer flexibility that guided surgery might not replicate in some situations. Additionally, investing time, money, and effort into learning classic hands-on surgery may be more beneficial than focusing on high technology. Of course, with the future arrival of robots in dentistry, the use of expensive high technology will become essential, but that time is not now.

Guided implant surgery requires significant equipment, software, and training investment, which may not be feasible for all practices, especially smaller or less affluent ones. Ultimately, while guided surgery offers many benefits, dentists must assess each case individually to determine the best approach, considering both traditional and innovative methods.

ROBOTIC SYSTEM

Robots using artificial intelligence have entered the medical field. Visual, audio and tactile feedback position the drill in the correct position. The robot resists movement away from the pre-determined position. The only FDA-approved dental robot is the YOMI robot, which uses tracking arms connected to the intra-oral splint and uses CBCT and a series of landmarks. Then, the handpiece is locked in the axis of the implant placement. However, the dentist still remains in control of the advancement of the drill [42]. The robotic system is safely used for autogenous bone block osteotomy in the chin [43]. There is no doubt that robots will be used in the future for dental implant surgeries.

References:

1. Øystein Fardal 1, Christopher A McCulloch: Impact of anxiety on pain perception associated with periodontal and implant surgery in a private practice. J Periodontol 2012 Sep;83(9):1079-85.

2. Corbett IP, Ramacciato JC, Groppo FC, Meechan JG: A survey of local anaesthetic use among general dental practitioners in the UK attending postgraduate courses on pain control. BDJ 2005,199,784–787.

3. Nagao H, Munakata M, Tachikawa N, Shiota M, Kasugai S: Clinical study of risk management for dental implant treatment--changes of blood pressure and pulse rate during implant surgery under local anesthesia. Kokubyo Gakkai Zasshi, 2002 Mar;69(1):27-33.

4. Aravena PC, Barrientos C, Troncoso C, Coronado C, Sotelo-Hitschfeld P: Effect of warming anesthetic on pain perception during dental injection: a split-mouth randomized clinical trial. Local Reg Anesth 2018 Feb 22;11:9-13.

5. Etoz OA , Nilay Er, Ahmet E Demirbas: Is supraperiosteal infiltration anesthesia safe enough to prevent inferior alveolar nerve during posterior mandibular implant surgery?, Med Oral Patol Oral Cir Bucal 2011 May 1;16(3), e386-9.

6. Esposito M, Maghaireh H, Grusovin MG, Ziounas I, Worthington HV, 2012, Soft tissue management for dental implants: what are the most effective techniques? A Cochrane systemic review. Eur J Oral Implantol 5(3):221-38.

7. Schrott ARM, Jimenez. 2009; Five year evaluation of the influence of keratinized mucosa on peri implant soft tissue health and stability around implant supporting full arch mandibular fixed prosthesis. Clinical Oral Implants Research 20(10):1170-77.

8. Clem DS, McClain PK, McGuire MK, Richardson CR, Greg A Santarelli GA, Schallhorn RA, Scheyer ET, Gunsolley JC, Thiago Morelli T. Harvest graft substitute for soft tissue volume augmentation around existing implants: A randomized, controlled and blinded multicenter trial. J Periodontol 2023 Dec 9. doi: 10.1002/JPER.23-0305. Online ahead of print.

9. Akshaya K, Arvina Rajasekar A. Association between Gingival Biotype and Crestal Bone Loss in Implants Placed in Anterior Maxilla. J Long Term Eff Med Implants. 2024;34(1):71-78.

10. Ross SB, Pette GA, Parker WB, Hardigan P: Gingival margin changes in maxillary anterior sites after single immediate implant placement and provisionalization: A 5-year retrospective study of 47 patient. Int J Oral Maxillofac Implants 2014;29:127-34.

11. Davis JM, Campbell LA: Fatal air embolism during dental implant surgery: a report of three cases. Canadian Journal of Anesthesia 1990, 37(1),)112-121,

12. Noble B: Bone microdamage and cell apoptosis. Eur Cell Mater 2003;(21); 6: 46–55.

13.   Field J.R., Sumner-Smith G: Bone blood flow response to surgical trauma. Injury 2002, 33, 447–451.

14. Davidson SR, James DF: 2000. Measurement of thermal conductivity of bovine cortical bone. Medi Eng Phys 2000; 22 (10), 741–7.

15. Brisman DL. The effect of speed, pressure, and time on bone temperature during the drilling of implant sites. Int J Oral Maxillofac Implants 1996;11:35–37.

16. Abouzgia MB, James DF. Measurements of shaft speed while drilling through bone. J Oral Maxillofac Surg 1995;53:1308–1315.

17. Abouzgia NB, Symington JM. Effect of drill speed on bone temperature. Int J Oral Maxillofac Surg 1996;25:394–399.

18. Abouzgia MB, James DF. Temperature rise during drilling through bone. Int J Oral Maxillofac Implants 1997;12:342–353.

19. Eriksson A, Alberktsson T, Grane B: Thermal injury to bone: A vital microscopic description of heat effects. Int J Oral Surg 1:115, 1982.

20. Eriksson RA, Alberktsson T: Temperature threshold levels for heat-induced bone tissue injury: A vital microscopic study in rabbit. J Prosthet Dent 50:101, 1983.

21. Reingewirtz Y, Szmukler-Moncler S, Senger B: Influence of different parameters on bone heating and drilling in implantology.Clin Oral Implant Res 8:189, 1997.

22. Pande RK, Panda SS: Drilling of bone: A comprehensive review. J Clin Orthop Trauma. 2013;4(1), 15-30.

23. Brånemark P-I. Osseointegration and its experimental background. J Prosthet Dent 1983;50:399–410.

24. Giro G, Tovar N, Marin C, Bonfante EA, Jimbo R, Suzuki M, Janal MN, Coelho PG. The effect of simplifying dental implant drilling sequence on osseointegration: An experimental study in dogs. Int J Biomater. 2013; Article ID 23-31-.

25. Scarano A, Piattelli A, Assenza B, Carinci F, Di Donato L, Romani GL, Merla A. Infrared thermographic evaluation of temperature modifications induces during implant site preparation with cylindrical versus conical drills. Clin Implant Dent Relat Res. 2011 Dec;13(4):319-23.

26. Bennington IC, Biagioni PA, Briggs J, Sheridan S, Lamey PJ. Thermal changes observed at implant sites during internal and external irrigation. Clin Oral Implants Res. 2002 Jun;13(3):293-7.

27. Watcher R, Stoll P. Increase of temperature during osteotomy. In vitro and in vivo investigations. Int J Oral Maxillofac Surg 1991;20:245–249.

28. Greenstein G, Greenstein B, Desai RN: Using drill stops on twist drills to promote safety and efficiency when creating osteotomies for dental implants. J Am Dent Assoc 2014 Apr;145(4):371-5.

29. Misic T, Markovic A, Aleksandar Todorovic A, Colic S, Scepanovic Miodrag S, Milicic B: An in vitro study of temperature changes in type 4 bone during implant placement: bone condensing versus bone drilling. Oral Surg, Oral

Med, Oral Path, Oral Radiol, and Endodontol, 2011, 112 (1), 28-33.

30. Flanagan D. Osteotomy irrigation: is it necessary? Implant Dent. 2010 Jun;19(3):241-9.

31. Kim SJ, Yoo J, Kim YS, Shin SW. Temperature change in pig rib bone during implant site preparation by low-speed drilling. J Appl Oral Sci 2010 18(5):522-7.

32. Calvo-Guirado JL, Delgado-Pena J, Mate-Sanchez JE, Mareque Bueno J. Delgado-Ruiz RA, Romanos GE. Novel hybrid drilling protocol: evaluation for implant healing-thermal changes. crestal bone loss, and bone-to-implant contact. Clin Oral Implant Res 2015;26(7):753-60.

33. Jeong SM, Yoo JH, Fang Y, Choi BH, Son JS, Oh JH. The effect of guided flapless implant procedure on heat generation from implant drilling. J Cranio-maxillofac Surg. 2014;42(6):725-9..

34. Al-Juboori MJ, Rahman SA, Hassan A, Ismail IHB, Tawfiq OF: What is the effect of initial implant position on the crestal bone level in flap and flap-less technique during healing period? J Periodontal Implant Sci. 2013 August; 43(4): 153–159.

35. Noguchi T, Morita S, Suzuki R, Matsunaga S, Hirouchi H, Kasahara N, Sugahara K, Abe S. Structural analysis of the mylohyoid muscle as a septum dividing the floor of the oral cavity for the purposes of dental implant surgery: variety of muscle attachment positions and ranges of distribution. Int J Implant Dent 2023 Dec 8;9(1):49.

36. Juodzbalys G, Wang HL, Sabalys G. Anatomy of Mandibular Vital Structures. Part II: Mandibular Incisive Canal, Mental Foramen and Associated Neurovascular Bundles in Relation with Dental Implantology. J Oral Maxillofac Res. 2010 Apr 1;1(1).

37. Greenstein, G; Cavallaro, J; Tarnow, D. "Practical Application of Anatomy for the Dental Implant Surgeon," J Perio 2008;79:1833-1846.

38. Fontes Pereira J, Costa R, Nunes Vasques M, Salazar F, Mendes JM, Infante da Câmara M. Osseodensification: An Alternative to Conventional Osteotomy in Implant Site Preparation: A Systematic Review. J Clin Med. 2023 Nov 11;12(22):7046.

39. Ma B, Park T, Chun I, Yuncorresponding K: The accuracy of a 3D printing surgical guide determined by CBCT and model analysis. J Adv Prosthodont. 2018 Aug; 10(4): 279–285.

40. Ku JK, Lee J, Lee HJ, Yun PY, Kim YK: Accuracy of dental implant placement with computer-guided surgery: a retrospective cohort study. BMC Oral Health. 2022; 22: 8.

41. Strecha J, Jurkovic R, Siebert T, Prachar P, Bartakova S: Fixed Bicortical Screw and Blade Implants as a Non-Standard Solution to an Edentulous (Toothless) Mandible. Int J Oral Sci, 2(2) 2010: 105–110.

42. Dibart S, Kernitsky-Barnatan J, Di Battista M, Montesani L. Robot assisted implant surgery: Hype or hope? J Stomatol Oral Maxillofac Surg. 2023 Dec;124(6S):101612.

43. Zhou L, Ding J, Xiao Y, Liu Y, Chen J, Dong Wu D. Autogenous bone block osteotomy in the chin using a robotic system: A clinical report. J Prosthet Dent 2023 Dec 11:S0022-3913(23)00764-3.

CHAPTER FIVE:

ASEPTIC THEORIES AND PRACTICE

5. ASEPTIC THEORIES AND PRACTICE

Aim:

To learn aseptic practices in dental implant surgery and restoration environments.

Assumed Knowledge:

It is assumed at this stage that you have a general knowledge of basic science related to dental implant surgery and soft and hard tissue management.

Learning Outcome:

After completing this chapter, the reader will have gained basic knowledge of radiographic and clinical assessments.

> The Health and Social Care Act 2008 requires healthcare providers to have a standardised aseptic technique in which education and audit can be demonstrated.
>
> Aseptic Non-Touch Technique (ANTT), standard and surgical, is the standard aseptic technique.
>
> Personnel must wear a hat, mask, and protective eye-wear, gowns and sterile gloves. Wash the hands from subungual areas to forearms, holding the hands directly above the elbows and work down from fingertip to elbow.

Infection must be prevented due to inadequate aseptic techniques in clinical procedures, which allow micro-organism contamination of surgical equipment and surgical sites.

Any liquid infusion from any part of the patient's body is high risk. The Health and Social Care Act 2008 requires healthcare providers to have a standardised aseptic technique to demonstrate education and audit.

Aseptic Non-Touch Technique (ANTT), standard and surgical, is the standard aseptic technique in the UK. Rowley introduced this in 2001 to reduce healthcare-associated infections (HCAIs). The ANTT for the operating theatre should be adopted for use in the dental surgery environment. This can only be accomplished through staff training in providing and maintaining a safe clinical environment. Such a training programme must cover the A-Z of the requirements for an aseptic environment. Effective hand hygiene and glove usage provide an example of one of the elements of such a programme.

But first, the words 'clean', 'aseptic' and 'sterile' need to be defined. They are not interchangeable but hierarchical in nature. In a restaurant, we accept a 'clean' knife and fork that would be thrown out the window in an operating theatre. Context gives the clue. We happily carry the food on a fork to our mouth after we have cut it with a knife that we would never use for an incision. Context: The fork is unlikely to infect us because of our relative immunity to everyday bugs. However, if that knife is to be used to make an incision, it must be autoclaved and demonstrably validated as such before we break the integrity of the skin or mucosa: context and hierarchy. You could call it the 'clinical safety' version of Maslow's Pyramid.

'Clean' is not a precise term in the context of invasive dental surgery procedures, 'Asepsis' means the absence of pathogenic microorganisms, and 'sterile' means the absence of microorganisms - which is impossible to achieve in dental surgery.

So, how do we go about providing for patient safety? Furthermore, the answer is to conduct a Risk Assessment. A patient's risk assessment needs one to assess potential risks from the patient themselves, the clinical environment, the healthcare workers involved, and the clinical procedure envisioned.

The surgical staff should not wear watches, bracelets, or jewellery on the hand, head, or neck.

Different types of handwashing methods have been recommended, and one of the most common is as follows:

1. Wash hands with tap water

2. Apply surgical soap and rub hands palm to palm

3. with fingers of each hand interlaced, rub palm-to-palm

4. With the back of the fingers of one hand opposed to the palm of the other and fingers interlaced, rub both hands together. Apply the reverse

5. Sweep hands from fingers, tForce the handpiece position to alter thumb.

6. Rub the tips of fingers in the opposite palm

7. Rub each wrist with the opposite hand

8. Rinse hands with tap water from hand to the wrist - without touching any surfaces,

9. Use the elbow to turn off the tap

10. Wipe each hand with different tissue paper and discard

Sterile gloves usage is an obligation, and the equipment is sterilised or covered with caps or covers after aseptic cleaning.

Different types of hand-cleaning techniques

The Surgical team: one nurse in the sterile zone and the other in the non-sterilise zone is needed. Only the necessary staff should enter the room. Different types of surgical scrubs can be effective. Waterless antiseptic surgical hand scrub (1% chlorhexidine gluconate and 61% ethyl alcohol) or waterless surgical scrub (Avagard) alone is effective as traditional surgical scrub (5-minute scrub with 4% chlorhexidine soap using a sterile scrub brush with water)[1]. (figure 5.1).

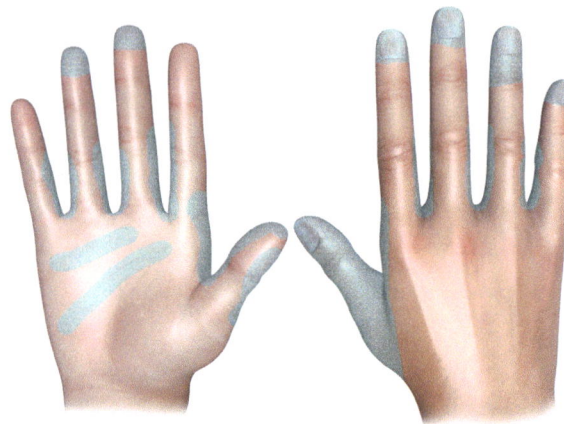

Figure 5.1 During hand cleaning, the areas that are most missed need to be emphasised.

The disinfection of the walls up to a distance of 1.2m is not applicable in dental surgeries with painted walls. The nails must be short. All hand washing must be in the dedicated hand-washing sink. Personnel must wear a hat, mask, protective eyewear, gowns, and sterile gloves. Wash the hands from subungual areas to forearms, holding the hands directly above the elbows and working down from fingertip to elbow. For each hand, use a sterile disposable towel to dry it. The area from the shoulder to the waist on the front is classed as needing to be sterile. The sterile nurse handles only sterile items. A chlorhexidine-soaked sterile gauze is wiped around the patient's mouth from the lip to the chin and nose. The patient is covered with a sterile drape from the face to the knees.

The circulating non-sterile nurse assists the scrub sterile nurse in setting the sterile field by opening the first layer of the double-layer package and does not contaminate any sterile instruments by handing them. He/she does not reach over or come nearer than 30 cm to the sterile field. The biomaterial and dental implants are also packaged in 2 layers, with an outer non-sterile container and an inner sterile vial. The circulating nurse opens the outer container and empties the sterile vial onto the sterile field.

The implants or any bone graft material should be opened only when it is immediately required for placement. This minimises the potential for airborne contamination. The violes should be open immediately before being used. The surgical stent must be disinfected and preferably autoclaved.

Note: cleaning problems associated with diamond drills have

been reported, and this potential problem should be considered in relation to diamond discs and diamond piezo surgery tips used in dental implant surgery [2].

A threshold value has not been defined as an acceptable residual value for protein left on surgical instruments after cleaning. Automated washer-disinfectors have been recommended, and manual cleaning by itself or manual cleaning plus ultrasonic cleaning with detergents does not affect the residual protein levels. Only best practices should be accepted [2].

The disinfection of the impressions by the laboratory on arrival and labelling of them by the dentists have still not been implemented. There is a lack of agreement between the practices and laboratories [3,4].

Training and audit of the dental nurse to disinfect the dental impression, abutments and abutment screws is important. The titanium abutments are contaminated after customisation [5].

Microparticles may activate osteoclasts and provide titanium wear and inflammation. Also, the abutment-implant fit may be jeopardised with increased mechanical stress on the connection. Plasma argon and ultrasound can effectively clean the titanium abutments, reducing surface tension and increasing wettability, promoting soft tissue attachment. The chair-side Plasma R appliance is on the market. It is triggered in a special vacuum chamber that generates ionic bombardment with Argon gas and detaches the microdebris [6].

Shafie from Washington Hospital Centre recommended the procedures below for cleaning and disinfection or sterilising the abutments [7].

1. Cleaning: brush the inner and outer surfaces and rinse. Immerse them in a solution that does not contain strong acids, organic solvents, or oxidizing agents such as peroxide and halogens and then rinse them three times.

2. Disinfection: soak them in the disinfectant solution, rinse them three times with purified water, air dry, and pack them.

3. Pack each abutment in a single-use sterilisation package suitable for steam sterilisation and sterilise them with the validated class B autoclave.

126

References:

1. Burch TM, Stanger B, Mizuguchi KA, Zurakowski D, Reid SD: Is alcohol-based hand disinfection equivalent to surgical scrub before placing a central venous catheter? Anesth Analg. 2012 Mar;114(3):622-5.

2. Vassey V, Budge C, Poolman T, Jones P, Perret D, Nayuni N, Bennett P, Groves P, Smith A, Fulford M, Marsh PD, Walker JT, Suttone JM, Raven NDH. A quantitative assessment of residual protein level on dental instruments reprocessed by manual, ultrasonic and automated cleaning methods. BDJ 2011 ,210(9),E14.

3. British Dental Association. Advice sheet A12: Infection control in dentistry. London: BDA, 2009.

4. Berry J, Nesbit M, Saberi S, Petridis H: Communication methods and production techniques in fixed prosthesis fabrication: a UK based survey. Part 2: production techniques. Br Dent J. 2014 Sep;217(6):E13. doi: 10.1038/sj.bdj.2014.644.

5. Canullo L, Micarelli C, Lembo-Fazio L, Iannello G, Clementini M. Microscopical and microbiologic characterization of customized titanium abutments after different cleaning procedures. Clin. Oral Impl. Res. 25, 2014, 328–336.

6. Canullo L, Tallarico M, Penarrocha M, Corrente G, Fiorellini J, Penarrocha D. Plasma of Argon Cleaning Treatment on Implant Abutments in Periodontally Healthy Patients: Six Years Postloading Results of a Randomized Controlled Trial. Int J Periodontics Restorative Dent. 2017 ;37(5):683-690.

7. Shafie HR: Clinical and laboratory manual of the dental implant abutment. Chapter 10, cleaning, disinfection and sterilization techniques for implant abutments, 2014. Chapter 10, 177-9.

CHAPTER SIX:

TIME SCALE

6. TIME SCALE

Aim:
This lecture aims to take the viewer through the different stages of the time scale between the extraction and the dental implant placement.

Assume Knowledge:
It is assumed that you have a general knowledge of basic science related to dental implant surgery and soft and hard tissue management at this stage.

Learning Outcome:
1. You will understand and can describe the advantages and limitations of delay-immediate and immediate fresh socket replacement.
2. You will understand and can describe the technique of the fresh socket with immediate implant placement.

> It is suggested that 'immediate' and 'delayed immediate implant placement have a higher failure rate.
>
> Implant placement in fresh sockets is technique sensitive, and primary stability is essential for treatment success.
>
> In cases where root removal is performed prior to implant placement, the Periotome or pre-elevator should be used to extract the roots of teeth.

Randomized clinical trials (RCTs), with a minimum of one year's follow-up, compared different implant approaches along with their time scales studied by the Cochrane Oral Health Group. Because too many of the trials studied were underpowered or had a high-risk bias, it concluded that there was insufficient evidence to determine the advantages or disadvantages of any particular time scale. However, they did suggest that 'immediate' and 'delayed immediate implant placement have a higher failure rate [1].

6.1. Delayed dental implant placement
Even though the soft tissue will have healed in a few weeks, the dentist must not be fooled - the bone underneath takes three months to heal, although it may take longer in sporadic cases. In other words, four months after surgery is the most predictable time to place a dental implant.

6.2. Delayed-Immediate dental implant placement
The fresh-socket immediate-implant placement has limitations as it is more difficult to achieve good primary stability. This is especially so when teeth are replaced with multiple roots or when severe periodontitis leads to extraction. There can be difficulties with primary closure due to unfavourable mucogingival conditions and the need for extension in the presence of adverse soft tissue contour. The dentist's inexperience can present further limitations. To avoid such impediments, the delay-immediate replacement approach is recommended. You need to be wary when either periodontal disease or bone infection has been the cause of tooth extraction. In those circumstances, the combination of guided bone regeneration and dental implant placement with the added difficulty of soft tissue closure provides a pathway for site infection.

The technique of delayed-immediate implant placement, where the timing of the implant placement is delayed between 6-12 weeks, overcomes a number of clinical problems. The actual number of weeks needed will depend on the clinical demands, primarily on the size of the defect. By the time the host tissue has eliminated the infection, the problem of wound closure will have become easier to deal with. After some 8-12 weeks, there will be osteoblastic activity. Delayed-immediate implantation preserves the height of the alveolar bone but with a small amount of attachment loss - probably due to the flap elevation and remodelling at the extraction site. Usually, clinically sufficient bone fill and bone growth will have occurred, rendering the need for any alternative bone-growth techniques unnecessary. However, the waiting period helps to narrow the socket.

6.3. Fresh socket and immediate dental implant placement

Immediate implant placement into a fresh extraction socket can reduce treatment time, as socket healing and implant osseointegration occur concurrently. Immediate implant placement can be combined with immediate restoration, which provides the patient with a fixed restoration immediately after tooth extraction.

Nevertheless, the buccal or labial alveolar bone may be missing or partially missing after extraction. The immediate post-extraction prospect may be missing, undermined, and/or diminished anterior facial bone in the maxilla.

The placement of implants in this situation poses increased aesthetic risks because of the unpredictability of bone contours after healing. Immediate loading of immediately placed implants would further increase the risk of aesthetic compromise.

Immediate implant insertion and membrane application have a higher complication rate than delayed replacement, which can be increased up to 50%, and membrane perforation of the soft tissue can be expected.

In cases where root removal is performed prior to implant placement, the Periotome or pre-elevator should be used to extract the roots of teeth. Following such an approach, and in the absence of periodontitis, chronic infection, mobile mucosa or socket defect, you can now carry out an immediate implant placement.

If not previously indicated, "delayed immediate" implant placement can be performed 8-12 weeks after tooth extraction. Placing an implant after 12 months is considered delayed implant placement.

After implant placement, the patient should be instructed not to use the provisional partial denture for at least one week. The labial flange is removed, the denture is rebased in the surgical area with tissue conditioner, and soft-liners like Viscogel are not recommended. Tissue conditioner minimises loading pressure on the mucosa, but a minimum of 2 mm thickness is needed and replaced every two weeks. Soft liners are too rigid and traumatic for non-healed mucosa. The occlusion is checked, and any premature contacts or interferences are removed.

There is a suggestion that immediate and immediate-delayed implants may be at a higher risk of implant failure and complications than delayed implants. On the other hand, the aesthetic outcome can be better when implants are placed just after tooth extraction. Can augmentation help here? There is not enough reliable evidence to support or counter the advisability of augmentation procedures in conjunction with immediate implants placed in fresh extraction sockets. Nor is there any evidence in favour of any particular augmentation technique [2].

Implant placement in fresh sockets is technique-sensitive, and primary stability is essential for treatment success. Bone-implant contact is reduced due to the lack of congruent morphology between them. The openings of the sockets are ovoid or trapezoidal, with a lesser line on the palatal surface.

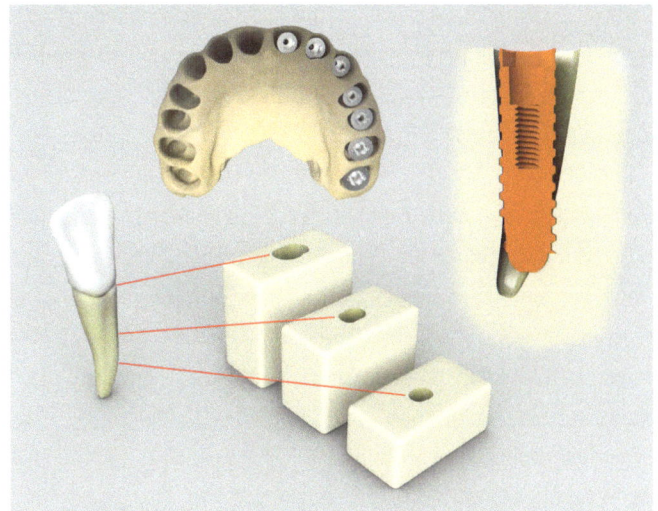

Figure 6.1 The discrepancy between the geometry of cross-sections of the alveolar bone and dental implant.

The dentist needs to prepare beyond the apex without perforating the buccal and lingual cortex or invading anatomic landmarks such as the floor of the sinus, floor of the nose or Inferior Dental Canal, and the coronal space can heal by the end of the healing phase. Bone mass must be sufficient for primary stability, with an adequate bone length of 3-5 mm in order to provide enough bone beyond the implant's apex. An alternative would be an implant wider than the existing alveolus [3].

Mineral-organic bone adhesive (Tetranite) was introduced in orthopaedic and oral surgery for clinically unstable implants immediately after extraction [4].

Simultaneous bone regeneration may be needed, making the procedure more complicated. Closure of the alveolar bone is one of the main downsides of fresh socket conventional implant placement. It is necessary to perform plastic closure. The soft tissue mucoperiosteal tissue is reflected on the buccal surface of the alveolar process. Releasing and relieving incision reduces the tension of the soft tissue and is undermined on the lingual surface. The buccal and lingual surfaces can then be approximated and sutured.

This procedure will result in the loss of the vestibule, post-operative bleeding, and pain. It is recommended that you do not place a membrane or any type of bone substitute on the lingual surface of the implant due to the increased chance of infection. A minimum of 3 mm is recommended between the grafted area and the incision line, which in these cases will be the lingual border of the extraction socket. If the root position is not in an ideal position, implant positioning will be compromised. These procedures at the molar surface will be more complicated due to the multi-roots of the teeth and the increased width of the exposed surface, which will need to be grafted and sealed by plastic closure.

Few studies have been reported on the extraction of periodontally affected teeth with immediate implant placement, and these demonstrated more failures. A lower success rate has been observed in the maxillae and in cases of single-tooth replacement. The lack of a uniform alveolar ridge highlights the need for ideal implant positioning in conjunction with the need for simultaneous bone regeneration. The limitations imposed by these requirements can lead to complications.

During the 2-3 months of the healing period, there will be pronounced bone morphology changes, which are not predictable. Bone resorption is usually on the buccal side, and this can expose the implant threads. The thickness of the alveolar bone can affect the amount of bone resorption, and the influence of the micro gap between the implant pieces, even before prosthetic loading, can influence the amount of bone resorption [5,6].

When a one-piece implant can be placed, or an abutment is placed immediately after implant placement and gains adequate primary stability, attention needs to be paid to soft tissue coverage. The one-piece implant covers the alveolar bone opening, lessening the need for aggressive soft tissue management, especially in single-root tooth replacement.

Patients are in high demand for a provisional fixed prosthesis in a fresh socket in the aesthetic area. It is highly recommended, in these circumstances, that an immediate replacement be carried out. The single-root replacement success is more predictable.

The future for customised zirconia implants is promising. Ideally, teeth should not be lost to periodontal disease. After extraction, the tooth's crown is prepared, and the whole length of the crown and roots are scanned. The zirconia implant is prepared, and the surface treatment is applied. The customised implant is washed, packed in 2 layers, and sterilised in a cleanroom environment. The manufacturing and sterilisation of the customised dental implant must be done within 7-10 days.

At another session, the socket is curetted under local anaesthetics, a specialised bur (figure 12.1) or ½ round drill provides a series of holes to promote bleeding, and the implant is placed. Even though it has been reported that excessively large horizontal and vertical gaps between the titanium surface and inner layer of the cortical bone would osseointegrate coronally at the implant-socket interface without primary flap closure, the author believes bone graft or a barrier membrane and primary closure is necessary to promote healing of the defect.

We recommend that immediately after root extraction, you check the internal surfaces of the alveolar bone with probe No.17 to determine whether the walls are sound and that acceptable stability can be achieved by internal bicortical engagement or drilling beyond the apices within the alveoli. Before selecting the implant, manually place the drill inside the prepared bone. If axial stability can be achieved, the assistant should remove the sterile implant from the box and place it into the sterile surgical tray.

Bacteria are present where there are signs of infection, and implant placement in a fresh extraction socket can acquire such infection. A saline rinse before and after bone preparation can reduce the level of bacterial contamination [8].

When immediate replacement coincides with immediate restoration, the patient can benefit from reduced treatment time, fewer surgical procedures, less traumatic surgery and the satisfaction of having a fixed provisional prosthesis placed immediately after tooth extraction. Nevertheless, you cannot ignore that soft tissue and hard tissue healing are unpredictable, with attendant problems that can affect the soft tissue and the aesthetics. In the anterior maxillary region, the treatment has a high success rate, one that is comparable to that achieved with traditional protocols [9].

Success and acceptable aesthetics rely on the integrity of the buccal socket wall. Soft tissue around a single-unit crown should be natural, and the height of the papillae, the embrasure fill, and the mid-buccal gingival margin judge this.

Many dentists believe that thick, soft tissue can prevent bone resorption, but enough evidence has not been found to support this. Nor does flapless surgery influence the aesthetics of immediate implant placement with an immediate restoration.

One study observed that where recession had been between 0.23-0.27mm, a year later, after the final crown placement, there had been a gain in the level of the interdental papillae through papillary rebound [10].

A connective tissue graft cannot be applied as a routine procedure but can be beneficial in advanced recession cases [11].

As limited studies utilise patient-centred parameters, a final conclusion can not be reached on whether or not immediate implant placement will benefit patients' aesthetics [12].

The placement of implants in fresh sockets requires certain conditions.

Intact alveolar bone: The buccal cortical bone needs to be at least 1.5 mm thick. If it is less than 1.5mm, extra support will be needed to prevent bone resorption. The implant will also need to be placed more palatally. This can be accomplished by imagining the buccal-lingual dimension of the bone socket opening divided into three segments, the first segment being at the buccal; the implant is then placed between the second and third segments.

As a rule of thumb, if the opening between the inner side of the buccal cortex and the outer side of the implant is no more than 1mm, and as long as there is a soft tissue barrier at the opening between the buccal cortex and the implant, then the alveolar bone will fill from inside without the need for grafting. However, soft tissue invasion inside the cavity can be expected if the gap between the inner cortex and implant is more significant than 1mm. Prevent this by grafting with autogenous bone.

If the buccal bone is thin, trying to gain primary stability from the inner surface of the cortical bone can be hazardous. In these circumstances, it is better to gain primary stability by preparing beyond the apical area by at least 0.5mm of the cortical bone, buccal, palatal or floor of the nose, sinus or the safest of all-palatal cortex.

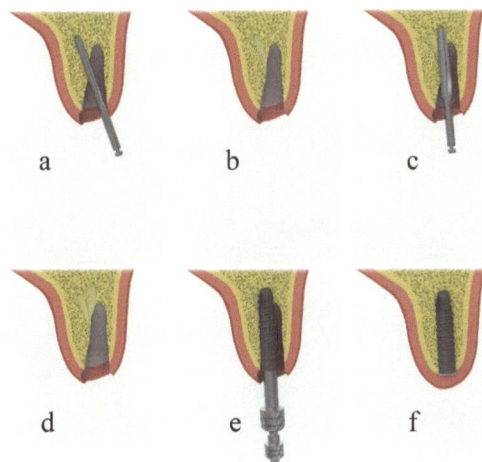

Figure 6.2 Immediately after root removal and three-dimensional observation that the alveolar bone is sound, the pilot drill with an angle of 45 ° penetrates beyond the alveolar bone to prevent slipping of the drill. The next drill can start with the same entrance; however, the angle can be corrected. Between the final implant placement and the inner alveolar bone is a gap which, if needed, is grafted, and the bone will heal.

Suppose the bone quality is poor in the maxillae, placing a one-piece cylinder (hybrid screw). In that case, the implant can be beneficial, as they achieve acceptable stability, first, through their macro design, and second, by being countersunk.

Alveolar bone is delicate, and you should not remove bone from the socket margins before placing the implant. By placing a one-piece cylinder implant with an angulated abutment and a gingival height of 4 mm, you should be able to countersink it. Bone chips can be produced with a no. 15 blade and a fine needle holder. The chips can be placed between the buccal surface of the implant and the alveolar bone. To reduce the number of bone chips needed, you can induce a predictable greenstick fracture of the buccal alveolar bone toward the implant. In this way, the surface opening will be reduced or eliminated (figure 6.3).

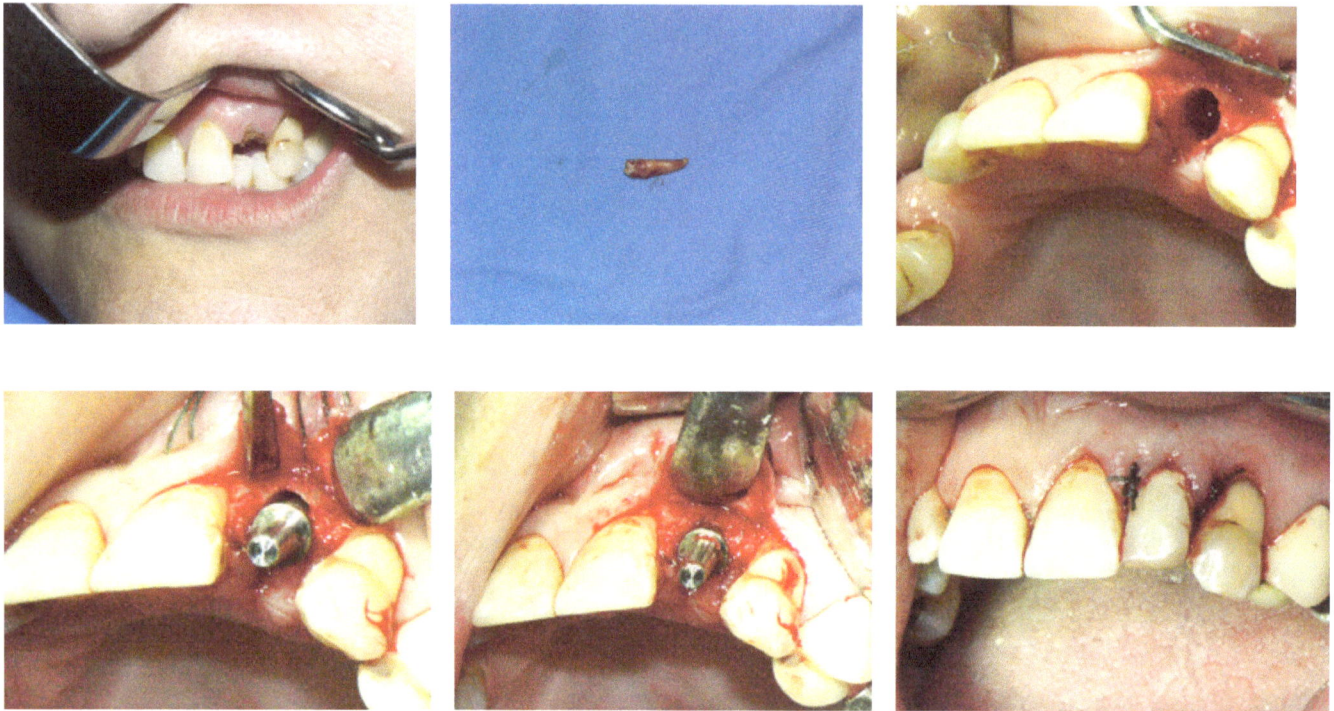

Figure 6.3 Immediately after extraction and implant placement, the gap between the one-piece implant and the labial alveolar bone can be treated by a 2-3 mm green stick fracture toward the implant. The gap entrance is closed by cortical bone and prevents soft tissue invasion, which the bone will heal inside. Immediate provisional crowns can be cemented successfully.

The green stick fracture toward the dental implant can be made just by pressing it and placing the thumb on the labial surface and the index on the lingual surface of the soft tissues. Suppose the labial/buccal cortex is thick. Get help using a new sharp no.15 blade or 1/4 round bur. The bur cuts through the buccal cortex and makes two stops at the proximal of the buccal bone. These two holes are joined through a horizontal apical cut, which only goes halfway through the bone. Now, push the rectangular bone wall toward the implant with your fingers or rigid flat plastic. You have now induced a controlled greenstick fracture of the buccal plate toward the implant.

Extraction with an anticipated immediate implant placement plus an immediate restoration needs a series of conditions:

Sound buccal cortex, axial stability, and, if the chronic infection exists, good curettage with irrigation is essential prior to any preparation. Before preparation, the position of the alveolar bone should have been confirmed as unlikely to jeopardise the implant placement or the final restoration. An example would be where the root is deviated mesially due to poor tooth positioning.

If a membrane is needed at the crest of the alveolar bone, the placement of a conventional 3-piece dental implant is recommended. The margin of a membrane should be 3mm away from the suture line. This will not be the case if a one-piece dental implant is placed.

In single tooth replacement, the occlusion of the provisional restoration must be clear of all contacts.

Animal studies have been undertaken to compare the immediate placement of implants in fresh sockets using a flapless versus a flapped approach. These studies aimed to compare the level of alveolar bone resorption resulting from each approach. These demonstrated that the flapless approach was no better at preventing alveolar bone resorption than when a mucoperiosteal flap was raised [13].

However, opposite conclusions have been reported that the potential for bone resorption was more significant when a flapless technique than when a flapped approach was chosen [14].

The decision to raise a flap should be made before osteotomy is undertaken. Bear in mind the possibility that, during the osteotomy, cracks can occur in the bone attached to the buccal periosteum. Raising a flap at this stage may detach the bone chips on the buccal surface.

133

Immediate Restoration and Loading:

'Immediate loading' is generally defined as the production of a load-bearing unit through the placement of a restoration on a freshly placed implant within 2-7 days of the implantation. Without the restoration, there is no load bearing. Single-tooth provisional restorations would typically be out of occlusion.

The trend towards shortening treatment times and reducing patient discomfort has pushed scientists and dentists to move beyond the boundaries of conventional implant treatment's hitherto predictable, high success rate. Immediate loading or restoration can help the patient to have a fixed provisional prosthesis within a maximum of a few days. Marginal bone loss has been shown to be similar to that attending conventional 2-stage loaded surgeries, and a few studies even reported better and faster osseointegration [15].

Primary stability has proved to be the most important determining factor for the immediate loading of the factors involved. If primary stability cannot be achieved, a conventional treatment protocol should be the method of choice.

Immediate loading of an implant bears a particular biological risk as the healing process has only just started. Early loading increases bone-implant contact and induces a faster remodelling process than unloaded controls when a short and low amplitude of mechanical strains is applied, which can enhance the biological fixation of implants.

There is evidence that Screw designs develop higher mechanical stability, but it is a false belief that the screw provides high stability in all types of bone.

A key element for implant success is the prevention of excessive surgical and thermal trauma to the bone. The most efficient cutting technique involves the simultaneous increase in speed with an accompanying increase in load. The amount of bone involved, the sharpness and design of the drill, the depth of the osteotomy and the cortical thickness - all these factors can affect success. The dentist's experience can affect the success or failure rate. If the dentist has placed over 50 implants, that dentist's success rate can almost double, reflecting the same for one-piece implant placement. Surgeons with little or no previous experience must expect a definite learning curve [16].

A fixed provisional prosthesis on a one-piece implant can be beneficial for two reasons: firstly, it can reproduce the patient's aesthetic appearance and phonetic ability, and through the restored occlusal height, enhance the patient's confidence level; and secondly, in conjunction with the cross-arch prosthesis, it can act as a splint to guarantee primary stability.

As the immediate-load technique gains more popularity than conventional implant placement, it is advisable to learn the application of one-piece implants.

Why 'one-piece'? When the three parts of an implant, the bone-anchoring part, the soft tissue attachment part, and the abutment, are all in one piece, it is called a one-piece implant. The absence of a micro gap between the parts is a clear advantage as it produces less bone resorption in comparison with multiple-piece implants [17].

Usually, the shoulder abutment is at the soft tissue level. It is accessible for dental impressions and removal of excess cement and provides a good base for a cement-retained dental prosthesis. The implants are placed more apically using the immediate implant placement and immediate restoration technique. Naturally, the length of the crown should be longer. However, as the soft tissue tends to have crepitation toward the incisal/occlusal, a better soft tissue outcome is expected in the one-piece dental implants. Thus, by placing a one-piece implant, a shorter and more natural-looking height is expected.

Immediate Implant Placement Following Tooth Extraction: A Step-by-Step Approach

Several critical factors must be addressed when considering immediate implant placement post-extraction to ensure optimal patient outcomes and implant success. This protocol outlines a cohesive approach to this procedure, encompassing pre-operative evaluation, surgical technique, and post-operative care.

Pre-operative Assessment:
1. General and Oral Health Evaluation:

• Ideally, the patient should be in good general health, without significant systemic diseases or smoking habits that could compromise healing.

• Oral health assessment should confirm good gingival architecture, adequate bone support (approximately 3mm from gingival margins), and absence of bruxism or parafunctional habits.

Day of Surgery Protocol:
2. Patient Preparation and Consent:

• If indicated, the patient's vital signs, including blood pressure, pulse, and ECG, are recorded on the day of surgery."

• The planned treatment is reiterated to the patient, acknowledging that immediate implant placement is contingent upon socket conditions post-extraction.

3. Medication Administration:

• Before surgery, antibiotics such as Amoxicillin 500 mg and Metronidazole 250 mg, along with painkillers like Paracetamol 500 mg, are given unless there are contraindications.

4. Local Anesthesia:

• Local anaesthesia (Mepivacaine 3%) is administered to ensure patient comfort during the procedure.

Surgical Technique:

5. Socket Preparation:

• A rigid, flat plastic instrument gently detaches the soft tissue from the bone, minimising trauma during extraction.

• A periotome or pre-elevator is strategically used to break down periodontal ligaments, facilitating atraumatic tooth removal with controlled luxation movements.

• Following luxation, extraction is completed using appropriate forceps to delicately remove the tooth or root without undue pressure.

6. Socket Examination and Management:

• Post-extraction, the socket is thoroughly inspected and probed for structural integrity or during curettage.

• If the buccal alveolar bone is compromised, appropriate flap techniques are employed: a. Large defects necessitate membrane placement, delaying implant placement. b. Medium-sized defects may require flap adjustments and membrane fixation, allowing for delayed or immediate implant placement with adjunctive bone grafting. c. Small defects may only require envelope flaps for optimal healing.

7. Osteotomy and Implant Placement:

• Osteotomy is performed to optimize implant positioning based on axial alignment, ensuring maximal stability and restorability.

• Implant size and shape considerations are made to address gaps between the implant and socket walls, with potential adjunctive bone grafting to enhance integration.

Immediate implant placement following tooth extraction demands a meticulous approach that integrates patient-specific considerations, precise surgical techniques, and post-operative strategies. This structured protocol aims to optimize treatment outcomes while minimizing risks associated with immediate implant procedures.

References:

1. Esposito M, Grusovin MG, Polyzos IP, Felice P, Worthington HV. Timing of implant placement after tooth extraction: immediate, immediate-delayed or delayed implants? A Cochrane systematic review. Eur J Oral Implantol. 2010 Autumn;3(3):189-205.

2. Esposito M, Grusovin MG, Poluzos IP, Felic P, Worthington HV: Timing of implant placement after tooth extraction: immediate, immediate-delayed or delayed implant? A Cochrane systemic review. Eur J Oral Implantol 2010 3(3):189-205.

3. Weng D, Nagatal MJ, Bosco AF, de Melo LG. Influence of microgap location and configuration on radiographic bone loss around submerged implants: an experimental study in dogs. Int J Oral Maxillofac Implant 2011;26:941-6.

4. Norton MR: First-in-Human Pilot Study to Assess Methodology for Using a Mineral-Organic Bone Adhesive for Optimization of Primary Stability and Implant Success for Implants Glued into Immediate Extraction Sockets and Immediately Temporized: Pilot Study. Int J Oral Maxillofac Implants. 2023 Dec 19;0(0):1-11.

5. Chrcanovic BR, Albrektsson, Wennerberg A. Dental implants inserted in fresh extraction sockets versus healed sites: A systemic review and meta-analysis. J Dent 2015(43)16-41.

6. Tomasi C, Sanz M, Cecchinato D, Pjetursson B, Ferrrus J, Lang NP. Bone dimensional variations at implants placed in fresh extraction sockets: a multi-level multivariate analysis. Clinical Oral Implants Research 201;21:30-6.

7. Tarnow DP, Chu SJ. Human histologic verification of osseointegration of an immediate implant placed into a fresh extraction socket with excessive gap distance without primary flap closure, graft, or membrane: a case report. Int J Periodontics Restorative Dent 2011, 31(5):515-21.

8. Manor Y, Alkasem A, Mardinger O, Chaushu G, Greenstein RB..Levels of Bacterial Contamination in Fresh Extraction Sites After a Saline Rinse. Int J Oral Maxillofac Implants. 2015 Nov-Dec;30(6):1362-8.

9. De Rouck T, Collys K, Cosyn J. Single-tooth replacement in the anterior maxilla by means of immediate implantation and provisionalization: A review. Int J Oral Maxillofac Implants 2008;23:897-904.

10. Slagter KW, den Hartog L, Bakker NA, Vissink A, Meijer HJ, Raghoebar GM. Immediate placement of dental implants in the aesthetic zone: A systemic review and pooled analysis. J Periodontol 2014;85:e241-e250.

11. Cosyn J, De Bruyn H. Cleymaet R. Soft tissue preservation and pink aesthetics around single immediate implant restorations: A 1-year prospective study. Clin Implant Dent Relat Res 2013;15:819-857.

12. Khazm N, Arora H, Kim P, Fisher A, Mattheos N: Systemic review of soft tissue alteration and esthetic outcomes following immediate implant placement and restoration of single implants in the anterior maxilla. J Periodontol 2015;86:1321-1330.

13. Caneva M, Botticelli D, Salata LA, Souza SL, Bressan E, Lang NP. Flap vs. "flapless" surgical approach at immediate implants: a histomorphometric study in dogs. Clin Oral Implants Res. 2010 Dec;21(12):1314-9.

14. Maló P, Nobre Md. Flap vs. flapless surgical techniques at immediate implant function in predominantly soft bone for rehabilitation of partial edentulism: a prospective cohort study with follow-up of 1 year. Eur J Oral Implantol. 2008 Winter;1(4):293-304.

15. Piattelli A, Corigliano M, Scarano A, Costigliola G, Paolantonio M. Immediate loading of titanium plasma-sprayed implants: an histologic analysis in monkeys. J Periodontol 1998;69:321-7.

16. Lambert PM, Morris HF, Ochi S Positive effect of surgical experience with implants on second-stage implant survival..J Oral Maxillofac Surg. 1997 Dec;55(12 Suppl 5):12-8.

17. Herman JS, Cochran DL, Nummikoski PV, Buser D. Crestal bond changes around titanium implants. A radiographic evaluation of unloaded non-submerged and submerged implants in the canine mandible. J Periodontol 1997;68:117-1130.

CHAPTER SEVEN:

AUGMENTATION

7. AUGMENTATION

Aim:

This chapter comprehensively explains techniques and considerations for augmenting soft tissue and bone in preparation for successful dental implant placement.

Assume Knowledge:

It is assumed that at this stage, you have a general knowledge of anatomy, hard tissue management, and management of systemic diseases.

Learning Outcome:

1. Defining and treatment of bone defects
2. Techniques of bone harvesting
3. Complications of augmentation and their treatment

> Mechanical separation of the soft tissue from the augmented area is sufficient to inhibit or delay the soft tissue invasion of the defect till the osteoblasts have enough time to migrate inside the cavity. Gore-tex membrane is a expanded polytetrafluoroethylene is non-resorbable material. Autogenous specimens demonstrate new bone formation with increased quantity and improved quality when compared to the specimens obtained from the sites grafted with allogenic bone.

After tooth loss, alveolar bone resorption occurs [1], which needs to be addressed and assessed.

There are different types of classifications for bone defects. We present one type here. This classification divides bone defects into non-space-making (I) and space-making (II).

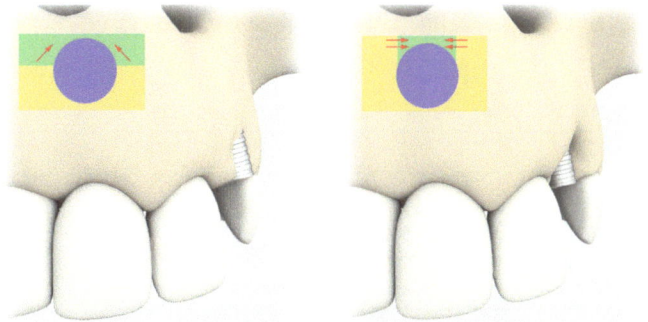

Figure 7.1 cross-section of a dehisced titanium dental implant. Left, non-space-making defect with minimum osteogenic source. Right, space-making defect with a better osteogenic source (red arrows).

- ▦ Bone host
- 🟩 Dehisced titanium
- 🔵 Titanium dental implant

Alveolar bone resorption can interfere with the correct positioning and, thus, placement of implants. Several bone augmentation procedures have been proposed to increase either the height or the width of bone - or both simultaneously.

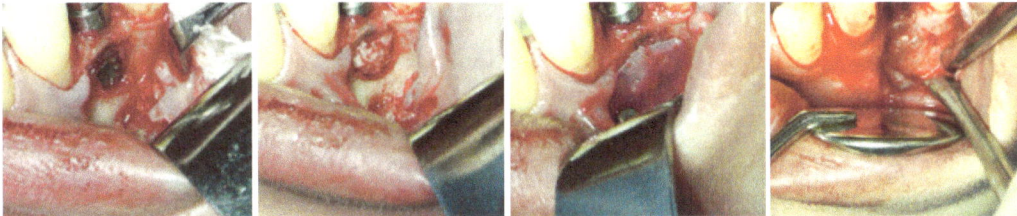

Figure 7.2 The space-making defect is filled with a mixture of allograft and autogenous bone and protected with a non-resorbable membrane. The membrane is fixed to the alveolar bone. The right photo demonstrates the healing defect and the tac and membrane removal after the healing period.

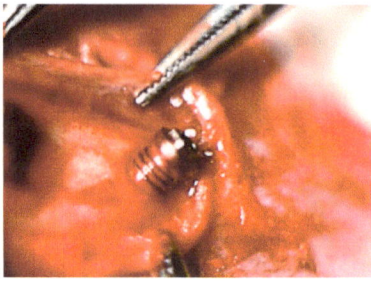
Figure 7.3 Non-spacing defect.

These techniques are Guided Bone Regeneration (GBR), ridge split, ridge expansion, bone block graft, osteotomies of the ridge, and distraction osteogenesis. Materials, including auto-grafts, allografts, xenografts, and alloplasts with different barrier membranes, have been recommended [2-5]. Bone substitute acquire terminology; osteogenic grafts contain living cells that differentiate into bone as autogenous bone grafts.

matrix of BMP (Bone Morphogenic Protein). Osteoconductive graft provides a scaffold for mesenchymal cells or osteoblasts to migrate and proliferate.

The process of bone promoted and ingrowth from local osseous tissue onto the surface of the scaffold as hydroxyapatite (HA). Osteopromotive grafts promote bone regeneration by stimulation of the biological or mechanical environment.

These processes are interrelated and not absolute terms. Autogenous bone grafts are osteogenic, osteoinductive and osteoconductive. Augmentation procedures can be performed either separately from implant placement or combined into a single operation.

The dentists' surgical approach should be based on the clinical assessment of the status of the surgical site, current evidence for dealing with the assessed risks and likely complications, and the dentist's training.

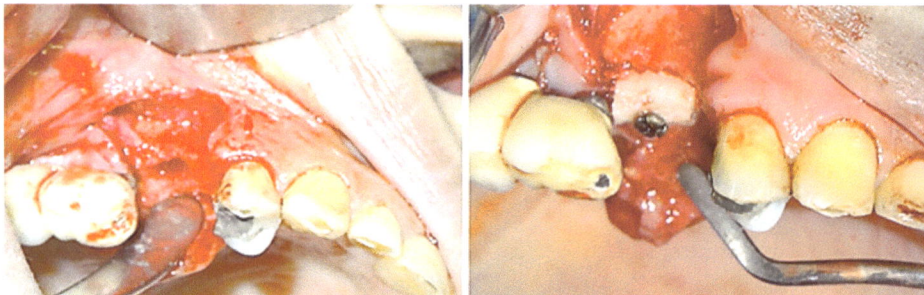
Figure 7.4 increasing the height with autogenous bone block and stabilising with one screw.

Osteoinduction is a process in which new bone formation is induced by undifferentiated stem cells into osteoblasts, where no bone formation will occur as autograft, demineralised bone

It may not be clear which procedure will have better short- and long-term success with minimum complications, but increasing the width is more predictable than increasing the height.

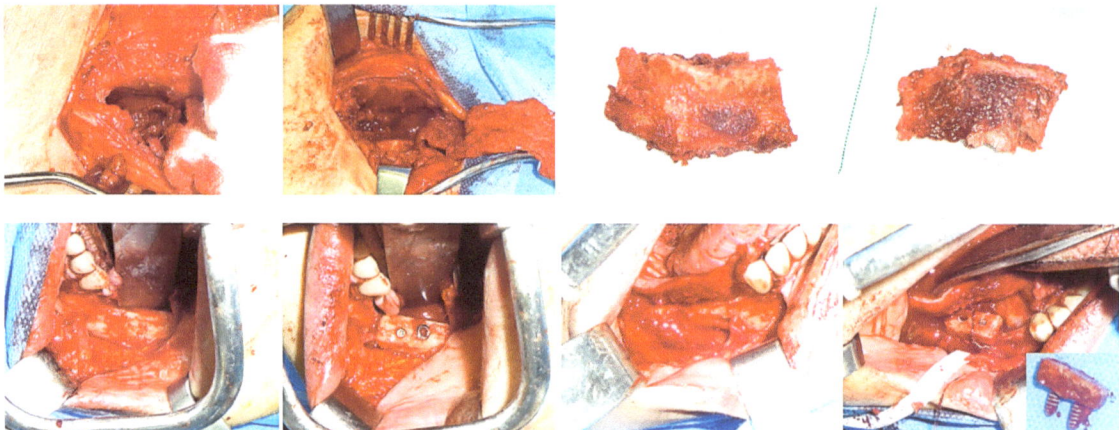
Figure 7.5 Increasing the height with the autogenous bone block from the medial surface of the iliac crest. Even though the surgery is more complicated than harvesting from the lateral surface, the cancellous surface curve coincides with the alveolar bone curve. Lower right: there is an option to place the implant in the cortical bone and simultaneously stabilise the block with the screws and or wires.

This book mainly concentrates on the one-piece dental implant, so ridge expansion or ridge split is the preferred means to increase the alveolar bone's width. There are many schools of thought, but the dentist must bear in mind that if a surgery has failed, the surgeon should have tried to keep the side effects to a minimum.

The factors which need to be considered in treatment planning are as follows:

QUESTIONS	ANSWERS
Type of reconstruction	a) Vertical b) Horizontal c) Combined d) Sinus area
Type of bone substitute	a) Autogenous bone (osteogenic) b) Non-autogenous bone (osteoinductive, osteoconductive)
Type of bone substitute	a) Block b) Particles
Timing, Procedural steps?	a) Simultaneous implant placement b) Separate procedures
Complications of the surgery	a) Back to square one b) Worsen the scenario before grafting
Type of environment of the surgery	a) Local anaesthetic b) Local anaesthetic and sedation/mindfulness meditation c) General anaesthetic
Types of defects	a) The defect is a space-making defect b) With ridge splint and/or expansion, the non-spacing defect can be transformed into a space-making defect c) It should be treated as a non-space-making defect.
The need for an additional site to harvest bone?	a) Yes b) No
Use a mallet in bone grafting? Alternatives?	a) Yes b) Other options like using the drill anti-clockwise c) Piezoelectric surgery,
Location of harvesting autogenous bone graft blocks	a) Mono-cortical apex of the implant region b) Third molar region c) Chin d) External oblique ridge e) Anterior nasal spine.
Is an attached bone graft possible?	Using a green-stick fracture to close the gap
Types of membrane	a) Resorbable b) Non-resorbable and rigid c) Cortical plate with a 1-1.5mm thickness.
Types of soft tissue flap	a) Envelope flap b) Triangular or two-sided flap c) Trapezoidal flap
Does it need relieving and releasing incisions? aggressive soft tissue management and post-operative swelling and pain	a) Yes b) No
What type of temporary? Patient's expectations regarding the dental prosthesis	a) Fixed - attached to the one-piece implant b) Fixed provisional bridge attached to neighbouring teeth c) Removable denture e) None

Maximising the initial bone cells-defect interface, which provides the nutrients, signals and primary cells to the defect and provides a space that is easy to protect, is favourable; thus, the space-making defect has a better prognosis (figures 7.1 and 7.2).

Guided bone regeneration (GBR) for horizontal augmentation, with simultaneous dental implant placement, has been successfully carried out.

Titanium mesh has been suggested as a membrane, although it is commonly used as a space-maintaining device for autograft particles [6].

To increase the chance of success, the author recommends that by using different techniques, the dentist should change the non-spacing defects to space-making defects such as ridge split or ridge expansion to increase the width and different types of sandwich techniques to increase the height.

Various materials have been used for GBR procedures. We should not be too optimistic that a particular bone graft material will be suitable in all situations, as the osteogenic potential of bone defects differs depending on the extent and morphology. Protecting the defect from soft tissue invasion is more critical. Time may also influence the progress of bone regeneration (figures 7.6, 7.21, 1.5).

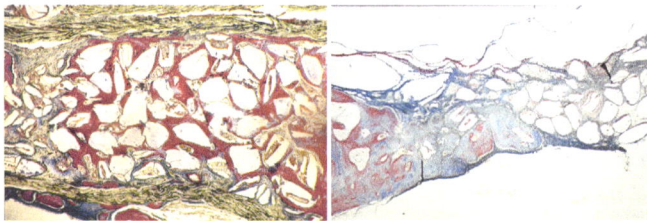

Figure 7.6 Using a rabbit's parietal bone in the calvarium and studying bone healing after placement of Bioglass, with and without a barrier membrane in the space-making defect, demonstrates when a barrier membrane has not been used, even though the cavity has healed, but it mainly consists of fibrous tissue and bone substitute particles (right). When the barrier membrane is used, bone has healed the defect (left).

The success of each surgery may depend on the dentist's experience and skills and the degree to which any technique requires a delicacy of touch. As a rule of thumb, an open sinus lift can gain an average of 5mm in subantral bone height. If more is needed, a simultaneous intrasocket (closed) sinus lift can increase the height during implant placement. A two-stage procedure, with a 5-6-month interval between bone grafting and implant placement, can follow it. Bear in mind that the efficacy of membrane placement to cover the lateral window is not fully established.

The technique of segmental osteotomy accompanied by interposition grafting has been reported as a practical and predictable procedure with a low incidence of complications and a high probability of success. This approach leaves the soft tissue on the oral side of the midcrestal incision attached to the crestal bone segment; thus, a linear incision is made 3 mm above the mucogingival junction. The mucoperiosteum is detached, and the vertical and horizontal osteotomies are prepared using micro-saws, piezo surgery tips or fine round and fissure bur. Piezo surgery has a good indication in these cases. Pre-elevator or a fine chisel and then chisel, finalise the osteotomies and mobilize the bony segment. Care was taken not to damage the palatal mucosa. The surgery proceeded to remove a bone graft block from the mandible's ramus and the adaptation to the recipient site, with the cortical portion facing the vestibular side. The bone segment or the interposed bone graft block is fixed using Y-type microplates and screws. Crushed autologous bone particles apply in any dehiscence.

Different techniques have been recommended to reconstruct alveolar ridge defects, such as:

1. Simultaneous implant placement can act as tent poles for the elevated sinus membrane, allowing the coagulum to occupy the space.
2. Particulate autografts from different donor sites,
3. Bone substitute alone,
4. Bone substitute mixed with autogenous bone particles,
5. Autogenous block grafts from the iliac crest,
6. Microvascular fibula flaps are designed for large segmental defects.

The downsides of autogenous bone graft include donor site morbidity, unpredictable resorption, and limits on the amount of bone available. Nonetheless, autogenous bone is the gold standard, especially in large defects, and because of second surgical site morbidity, some prefer it to alternative materials but with less predictability.

In selecting the most suitable grafting material for alveolar ridge augmentation, you need to consider the size and site of the defect, the quality and quantity of bone needed, potential donor site morbidity, and the cost before making your selection.

In minor defects, autogenous bone can be harvested and, if needed, can be mixed 50/50 with any bone substitute. If the bone substitute is used, the application of membrane is essential. Although surgical manipulation is more challenging, the non-resorbable membrane is more predictable. When high volume is needed, an iliac crest graft is indicated. However, the author prefers to avoid iliac crest grafts unless no other solution is available [7].

Space-making defects with a horizontal gap of 1.5 mm or more can be augmented with autogenous bone debris or particles without using a membrane.

In gaps of more than 4mm, a non-rigid membrane without bone substitutes cannot guarantee a perfect outcome. Support is necessary; any resulting collapse will decrease bone filling (figures 7.6, 7.21).

Based on the author's experience, the following protocol is recommended.

7.1. For space-making defects

1. use autogenous bone (no need for a membrane)

2. any other type of bone substitute is applicable, but the use of a membrane is necessary; a non-resorbable membrane has a better Bone Implant Contact (BIC) and minor collapse in the defect than a resorbable membrane.

When a non-resorbable membrane is used and dehiscence is observed, the dentist will realise that something is wrong and needs to implement remedial treatment. However, resorbable membrane dehiscence does not always have signs and symptoms till the exposure of the implant, and the dentist will be surprised. Also, replacing granulation tissue instead of bone formation will mislead the dentist. The dentist sees tissue surrounding the defect, a red colour, believing it is bone or immature bone, which it is not.

7.2. For non-space making defects

1. Autogenous bone, in this instance, needs a membrane-resorbable, which is acceptable, but non-resorbable with fixation is better.

2. any bone substitute (non-resorbable membrane but must be fixed to the alveolar bone by any means).

In cases where guided bone regeneration is carried out as a separate procedure prior to implant placement, the ridge defect is classified to permit accurate monitoring of surgical outcomes. The system of classification is described below.

A defect must be measured apico-occlusally, mesio-distal (a-b), buccal-lingual (c-d).

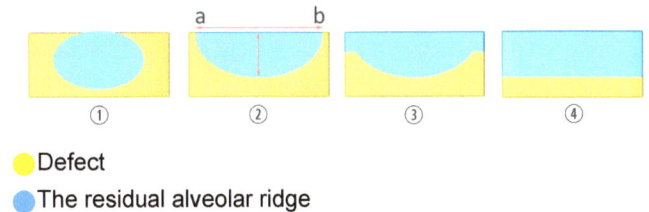

● Defect

● The residual alveolar ridge

Figure 7.7 The alveolar ridge from an occlusal perspective.

In cases involving simultaneous implant placement and guided bone regeneration, we classified the morphology of the exposed titanium surface of the implant concerning the bone. Each defect described below can be further sub-classified as space-making (SM) or non-space-making (NSM) defects, e.g. NSM/DE3.

- Oval/circular dehiscence (DE1),
- V-shaped dehiscence (DE2),
- Rectangular dehiscence (DE3),
- Fenestration with an osseous margin thickness of 1 mm or less (F1),
- Wedge-shaped intraosseous defect (WD).

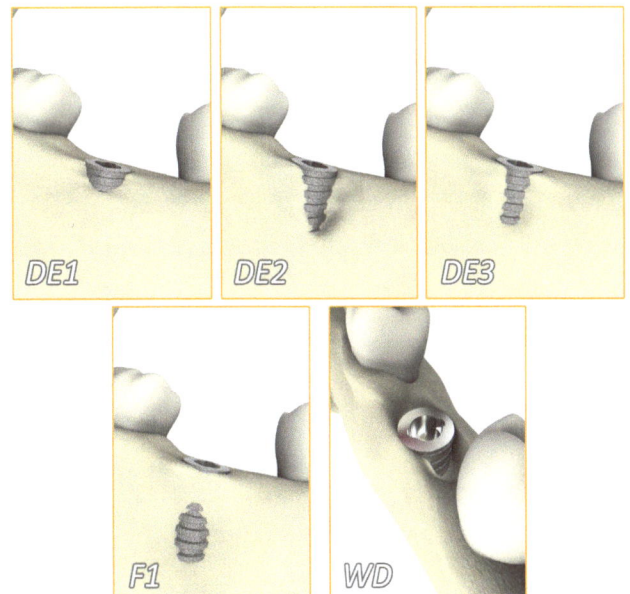

Figure 7.8 Classification of the morphology of the exposed titanium surface of the implant in relation to the bone.

The surgical procedure is as follows:

• Palatal/buccal for maxillae and buccal for the mandible, incision line approximately 3-4 mm from the mid crest, continued to the sulcular incision and if needed, the distal/mesial line angle releasing incisions,

• the flap is elevated palatally using Mitchell's trimmer to expose the crestal alveolar bone, and then buccally, by careful subperiosteal dissection, the papillae reflected by a rigid, Flat plastic,

• in cases of simultaneous implant placement and guided bone regeneration, the exposed titanium surface is measured, and the morphology of the osseous defect is noted,

• when augmentation is carried out as a separate procedure, the morphology of the dehiscence is noted, and the defect is measured using sterile callipers,

• in cases where augmentation is performed as a separate procedure, the labio-buccal cortex is perforated with a fine rose head bur to increase osteogenic contact with the allogenic material,

• the allogenic material is moistened, preferably with a blood clot, and placed on the buccal aspect to extend the ridge width; then, the defect/dehiscence is filled and supported by the membrane,

• the membrane is trimmed with sterile instruments, and if it cannot be stabilised by the defect's anatomy, with support given by the positioning of the soft tissue, the membrane must be stabilised by small pins or screws.

Tac pins are easy to use, but the downside of Tac pins is that they may bend or fracture during their placement or removal. The small screw is more challenging to place, but it does not bend or fracture.

• The membrane is placed so that it does not contact the adjacent tooth or lie on the incision line,

• the flap is closed, tension-free. Two types of tests can be made to confirm the lack of tension:

1. Use surgical tweezers to bring the margin of the flap to the incision line and see if there is any tension,

2. Confirm the absence of blanching in the flap when the margins are approximated. If the tension in the flap is observed, a releasing incision (to a depth of 1 mm) is made in the periosteum, parallel to the alveolar crest,

• the wound is then closed with interrupted and horizontal mattress sutures,

• Antibiotics are prescribed for seven days, followed by Chlorhexidine oral mouthwash for two weeks.

From the donor site, three kinds of autogenous bone can be harvested:
• puree
• chips or particles
• a cortico-cancellous block

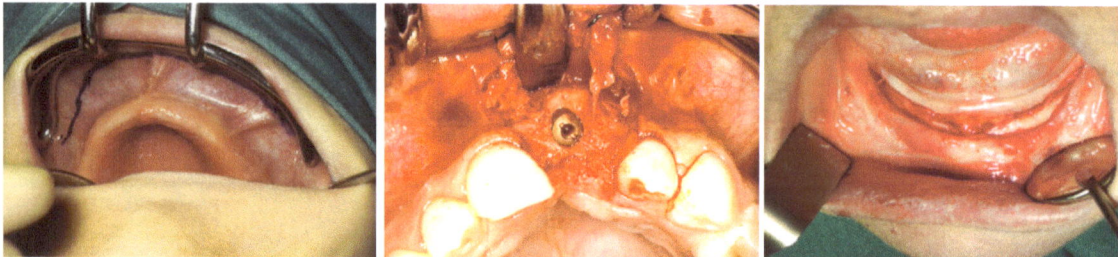

Figure 7.9 Left: in the maxillae incision in the depth of the buccal vestibule; middle: in the maxialle paracrestal incision with mesial and distal releasing incisions; right: mandible, the incision is made buccally.

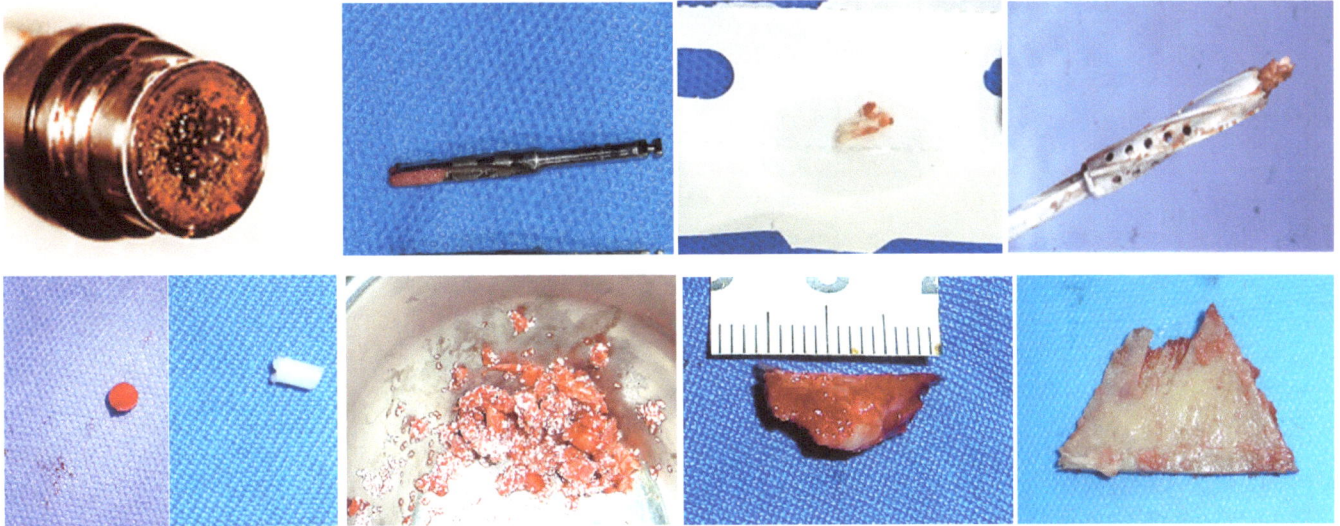

Figure 7.10 Upper left, puree from the bone filter or drill flutes. Bone tablet or core using trephine. Bone chips from the iliac crest are mixed with allogenic particles as volume expanders and bone blocks from the chin or iliac crest.

Where alveolar reconstruction is undertaken, a graft may be classified as:

• inlay graft

• saddle graft

• veneer graft

• onlay graft

• interposition bone graft (bone split technique)

• cylindrical filling (as dental alveolar).

• Bone ring technique (BRT)

• BRT is a one-stage approach to restoring vertical alveolar ridge defects. The bone block graft is stabilised with a dental implant inserted simultaneously.

• Inlay grafts are used when a graft is needed to restore the contour and volume of bone or facilitate the placement of an implant and give it a proper emergence profile. In the posterior mandible, the loss of bone height due to bone resorption may prevent the placement of dental implants due to the risk of nerve damage.

• A saddle graft will gain bone height and/or width. This technique can be applied in other selected cases.

• Onlay grafts are indicated when there is inadequate alveolar bone height and width.

• Veneer grafts are applied when there is an adequate height for the placement of dental implants but inadequate width.

• Ridge split with an interposition bone grafting technique needs only a little flap reflection. After mobilisation of the osteoperi-osteal soft tissue segment, harvested bone is inserted and sutured. The main advantage of the interposition technique in increasing the width and or height, it does not need screws for stabilisation of the bone, even though adding graft material application is not necessary in all cases [8].

7.3. Bone graft donor sites
Intra-Oral:

Same operative field:

The main advantages are that there is no need for a second surgical site, it is easier to place the grafted bone into the defect, and the recipient and donor site have the same quality of bone.

The Implant Bed:

When bone is drilled to prepare sites for implant placement, the surgical aspirator discards the cortico-cancellous particulate bone. Nevertheless, if you wish to save this bone, then it can be saved by any one of three methods (figure 7.10):

The first method is to use hollow trephine drills to remove a bone cylinder. Then, applying the classic implant drill sequence depends on the dental implant system. Cutting in pieces is not user-friendly, and placing and stabilising the cortical bone particles in the non-spacing defects is not easy as the pieces are rock hard and cannot be pressed and sit still in one place.

The second method – requires the use of two suction tips.

144

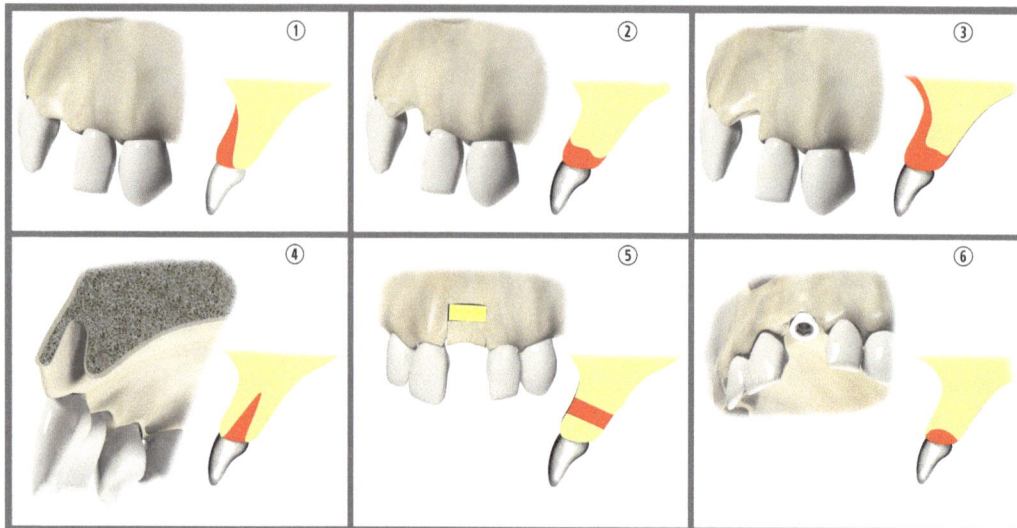

Figure 7.11 Different types of graft. Veneer, Saddle, Onlay, Inlay, Interposition, Cylindrical, Ring.

The first surgical tip is reserved for use only before and after bone collection. The second tip is used in conjunction with bone filters in the suction apparatus to collect bone dust as puree, sucked up during bone drilling and must be used only to collect bone, blood, and sterile saline from the surgical site. Bone puree has been used successfully to treat intra-bony pockets, but microbe entrapment remains a concern. The pores of the filters are different between the systems and affect the size of the collected debris and the amount of microbe entrapment.

Few systems have drills in which bone debris is entrapped inside the drill flutes. This entrapped bone, which has a puree (mashed potato) consistency, has an ideal texture for modelling, especially in the non-spacing bone defect.

The following points need to be borne in mind:

the quality of the bone to be drilled must be good enough to allow its collection by any of the above methods,

the trephine technique will be less suitable for any region where cracks need to be filled, bone filters have been found to have entrapped microbes along with bone debris.

Rongeurs have been used to remove bone chips from bony ledges and protuberances. By extending the flap laterally and in isolated areas, trephine drills can obtain bone tablets. Bone dust can be collected as puree by scraping the cortex with a Mitchell's Trimmer spoon or a bone scraper. A bone scraper consists of a blade body and a collection chamber. The hardened hollow ground blade makes point contact with the flat bone surface when it is held at an angle of 5-50 degrees to the surface. It is pulled along the cortical bone surface and shaves the bone. Bone chips advance into the storage chamber and are collected for storage.

If it is planned to harvest bone during bone preparation without exposing other areas, the table below provides guidelines for making the best choice.

Technique	Pre-request	Caution
Trephine drill	Adequate bone quality	Distance from anatomic landmarks (e.g. ID nerve, lingual soft tissue)
Bone filter	Adequate bone quality. Two surgical tips must be available	Smoker / any oral inflammation or infection
Bone scraper	Mandibular region where there is a thick cortex	It is not recommended in areas with a thin cortex
Rongeur	Availability	During bone removal, the buccal plate of the prepared bone cavity may fracture.
Special drills	Adequate bone quality	During drill removal from the bone cavity, the drill should not touch soft tissue or surgical suction tip as the bone debris may dislodge from the flutes.

Table 7.1 Summary of guidelines in using different techniques in harvesting bone from implant bed.

In those areas where flap reflection exposed dehiscences at graft sites, between 12-16% were found to have had resorbable membranes used, and 24% to have had non-resorbable membranes used. The average healing period was seven months [9]. Bear in mind that most clinical trials have been performed by experienced specialists, with results that are unlikely to be achieved by less experienced dentists. Ridge expansion and ridge split can gain an average of 3mm width. The complication rate of up to 26% mainly involved a fracture of the buccal bone. Most papers on bone augmentation have not focussed on the clinical scenario obtained prior to augmentation but have simply reported the results [10].

For bone harvesting from other sites, CBCT is essential to determine the amount of bone available. Triangular or trapezoidal flap and releasing incision in the periosteum increased swelling is expected after surgery, so it is recommended that you administer Dexamethasone 8mg intramuscularly (if it is permitted in the country in which the dentist practices). Pressure immobilization will reduce dead space. Post-operative manual astriction and pressure immobilization using taping and/or a cold compress will reduce post-operative swelling.

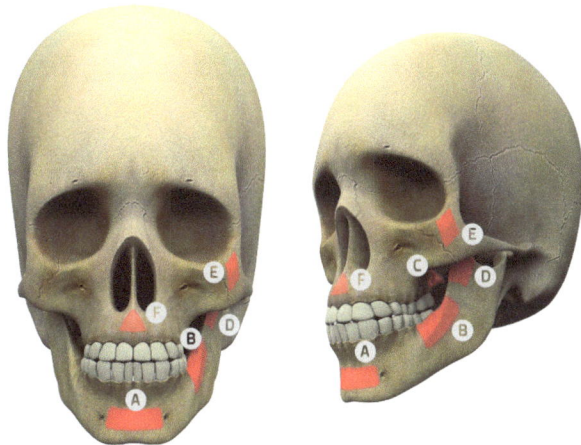

Figure 7.12 Left: Intra-oral harvesting bone from different areas and from the apical area of the implant if space is available. A) chin, B) anterior border of ramus/retromolar region, C) Maxillary tuberosity, D) Mandibular coronoid process, E) Zygoma, F) Anterior nasal spine and above the apex of a dental implant. Condition of available space.

The Apex of the Implant:

The apex of the implant is another source of the bone, the apex of the implant needs to be filled with a bone substitute, and a barrier membrane must be applied.

Maxillary Tuberosity:

When using bone from this source, the quality of the bone needs to be considered. The thin cortex and the soft quality of the cancellous bone not only make its use as a block questionable but can contraindicate the use of screw fixation for primary stability.

Retromolar Area:

Small cortico-cancellous bone blocks can be harvested from this area to augment an alveolar deficit in the posterior mandibular region under the same flap. The block can be stabilised using screws and protected with a membrane. Blocks can be used as the solid base at the centre of a defect, with bone chips in the surrounding areas. The only question to be answered when using two different kinds of bone (cortical and cancellous) simultaneously is how to decide the time interval needed for adequate graft healing prior to placement of the implant. Whilst there is a belief that a membrane can act to prevent bone resorption, its actual effect when used with a bone block and/or bone chips is uncertain.

Chin:

The quantity of bone available for harvesting from the chin can be assessed by studying an OPG, a True Lateral Cephalometric image, CBCT, or clinical observation.

A 5mm safety margin from the apices of the lower anterior teeth is necessary. The amount of bone that can be harvested depends on the patient's anatomy. It is highly recommended that the lingual cortex be kept intact.

The likelihood of post-operative pain and continued long-term discomfort is the downside of choosing this area. The symphysis provides a sufficient volume of cortico-cancellous bone, but its availability is accompanied by increased morbidity. In contrast, the mandibular ramus is mostly cortical bone and less likely to result in post-operative pain, but a higher frequency of post-operative bleeding has been reported. Soft laser is a good indication for incision in the lower labial sulcus to reduce bleeding and discomfort during and after surgery.

Anterior Nasal Spine:

When inserting dental implants in the upper anterior region, bone, if needed, may be harvested from the anterior nasal spine. This can be affected by a trephine drill, mono- or bi-cortical tablets, or rongeur. The quality of the bone is dense and has been shown to be easily and safely accessed. Its removal will not cause permanent changes to the overall nasal shape [11].

Basal Alveolar Bone:

This area of the mandible is an area from which bone can be harvested for grafting, but there seems to be no research to assess the efficacy of this technique. Harvesting bone using piezo surgery cutting tools is more straightforward than using standard rotary devices because piezo chips are thinner than fissure bur, which minimises bone loss. It is also easier to handle, but the disadvantage is that it takes time to set up the piezo surgery.

The advantages of harvesting bone from the oral cavity are:
• the operation has a shorter duration,
• there is reduced post-operative morbidity,
• there are no external scars.

The bacterial species isolated from different bone debris are common salivary flora related to all types of oral infections.

Since Streptococcus Viridans are implicated in bacterial endocarditis, an intra-oral graft may be hazardous for immunosuppressed or otherwise vulnerable patients [12-13].

Although a pre-operative chlorhexidine mouth rinse reduces oral bacterial levels, there is no evidence for its efficacy in bone or when applied to bone collected by the bone filter. The trephine drill showed the fewest bacterial colonies. Prophylactic antibiotic therapy is recommended because there is a risk of infection during intra-oral augmentation procedures.

The choice of intra-oral bone-harvesting device and the technique employed should be based on the requirements of each individual patient.

The use of intra-oral bone for bone augmentation may have favourable results and long-term predictability because of its intramembranous developmental origin. However, the limited availability of bone volume limits the intraoral donor sites to one or two dental implants. Bone blocks are associated with a low incidence of soft tissue complications even when bone chips and membranes are involved.

One of the difficulties of using autogenous bone chips without a membrane is maintaining the bone chips in position and supporting primary wound closure.

The author favours interposition graft due to its subsequent rapid vascularization and healing. Due to the need for a little envelop flap, the mobilized segment receives adequate circulation from the periosteum. The bone segment in between has maximum stability and vascularization, along with a pool of blood cells and bone cells.

Extra-Oral Bone Harvesting:

There are different areas in which bone is harvested for mandible or maxillae reconstruction; the common one is the iliac crest. Understanding iliac crest bone harvesting morphology can give the dentist an understanding of the limitations. Many disciplines do the surgery, primarily orthopaedic surgeons.

Iliac crest:

Iliac Crest Morphology:

On the base of the cross-sectional morphology of the iliac crest and the type of bone graft required, three types of bone blocks can be harvested:

Triangular: This type of acute undercut occurs above the iliac crest. Accordingly, an onlay block can be harvested without sectioning the lateral or medial cortex.

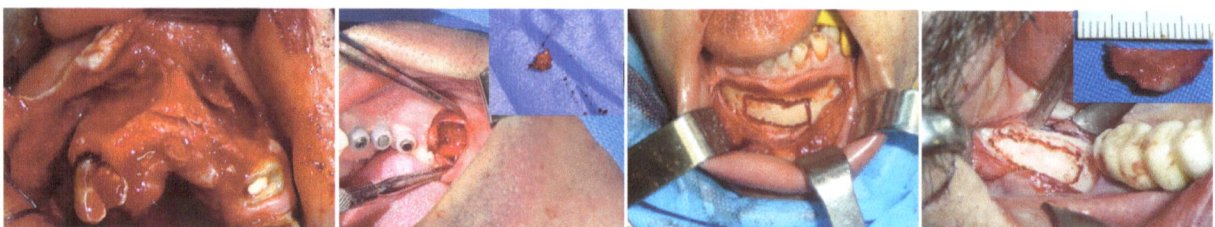

Figure 7.13 Intra-oral bone harvesting from left, maxillary nasal spine, maxillary tuberosity, chin and lower retromolar area.

Bullet-shaped: The lateral surface of the iliac crest is convex, as opposed to the concave medial surface. Depending on the type and volume of graft, bone may be harvested from the lateral or medial aspect of the crest. However, in this type, due to the conical cross-section of the crest, a more significant amount of bone needs to be removed.

Rectangular: This presents the most favourable morphology for bone-block removal, whether from the medial or lateral aspect.

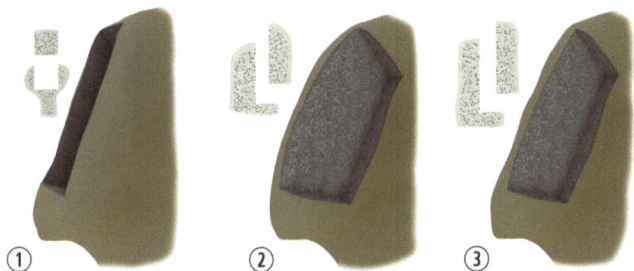

Figure 7.14 Cross section of the iliac crest: 1. triangular, 2. Bullet-shaped, 3. rectangular.

7.4. Bone Augmentation

In order to minimise post-operative morbidity in harvesting iliac crest grafts, it is essential to:

i) perform limited soft tissue surgery - the incision being placed between muscle attachments rather than through muscle tissue, ii) minimise manipulation of abdominal structures by gentle retraction of the reflected abdominal muscles, and ensure early post-operative patient mobilisation.

A prophylactic low-dose heparin against thromboembolism should not be required if the abdominal structures have minimal manipulation in conjunction with early postoperative mobilization.

Should there be a marked amount of bone loss occurring in the first year, this will have been due to an unacceptable degree of functional loading on a graft which, although united and vascularized, still has a large amount of dead, resorbing donor bone within the vital new bone at the grafted site.

The advantages of a staged approach compared with immediate implant placement are:

• As the graft has healed, a larger vital exposed surface contributes to new bone formation,

• Implant positioning can be preferable, allowing a better aesthetic result to be achieved,

• Better implant primary stability

The advantages of simultaneous grafting and immediate implant placement are:

• Less morbidity,

• Less operating time

• Lower cost

A removable prosthesis is more likely to be hazardous for all the above grafts, even though the buccal flanges are removed and relined with tissue conditioner.

There is controversy over the healing period necessary for iliac crest grafts, which is recommended to be between 4 and 6 months. The author's protocol, which is not scientifically based, is five months - unless the original bone is soft when it can be extended to 6 months.

Applying cancellous hip bone between the blocks and/or between the blocks and the alveolar bone of the jaw is a potential problem, as small cancellous fragments may become loose and perforate the mucosa. This can be prevented by applying a resorbable barrier membrane over such small fragments.

Major bone grafts have the potential for failure. Consequently, a 2-stage grafting technique, followed several months later by implant placement, is preferred, rather than one where both procedures are performed simultaneously.

In this way, implant positioning is more predictable because the quality and quantity of the healed graft can be observed visually during implant placement.

It is commonly believed that a keratinized gingival cuff around dental implants is highly desirable, though not essential - provided the patient maintains a high standard of oral hygiene. However, the author believes that a non-mobile soft tissue cuff (keratinized or non-keratinized) is necessary. The soft tissue cuff around the implant must be fixed to the adjacent periosteum, as there is a high risk of loss of soft tissue attachment from the implant if the peri-implant soft tissue is left mobile and susceptible to lip and cheek movements.

The treatment of a soft tissue breakdown over a bone graft during the healing period remains contentious. However, our experience is that it is preferable in such cases not to intervene surgically but rather simply to maintain an impeccable standard of oral hygiene. The exposed graft surface then acts as a dressing for the deeper bone, which is united with the graft bed and becomes re-vascularised. Eventually, a 1-2 mm thick

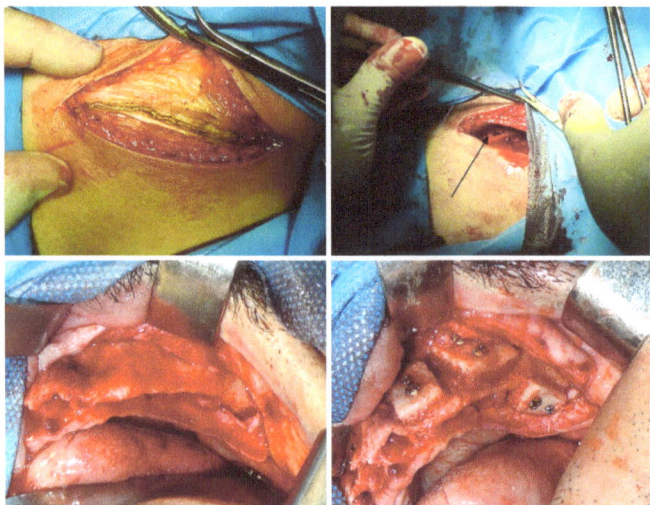

Figure 7.15 Harvesting bone from the iliac crest and screw to the maxillae.

sequestrum separates from the surface of the revascularised graft, and the soft tissues heal over the latter. Exceptions to this pattern are cases in which major soft tissue breakdown occurs, but these are rare.

Soft tissue flaps in bone grafting procedures may be designed so that they derive their blood supply from either the buccal or palatal mucosa.

During bone grafting, the advantage of a palatally-based partial thickness flap is simultaneous vestibuloplasty, which is usually in the anterior region. The advantages of the labially-based full-thickness flap are the cortico-cancellous block is covered by periosteum, minimises the ischaemic effect created by the vessels' traversing dense tissue at the crest, primary closure of the soft tissue (less discomfort for the patient) is possible. By contrast, a palatally-based flap creates a mucosal defect, which subsequently epithelialises in the lip.

Even though complications may occur (usually observed more in the mandible than maxillae), these are almost always minor and do not significantly affect the overall results.

One of the main issues of bone grafting is the degree to which soft tissue coverage provides an adequate width of keratinized soft tissues over bone blocks and around dental implants.

Full mouth flap, Maxillae:

Two approaches to the alveolar ridge are employed as required:

1. labia/buccal-based full-thickness flap: A palatal paracrestal incision (away from the crests, lingually or buccally) is performed between the first molar regions. The flap retracted to the labial\buccal surface of the alveolar cortex. Releasing incisions were made in the second molar region, approximately 10 mm distal to the proposed distal end of the graft. The nasopalatine neurovascular bundle is incised to free the palatal flap.

After cortico-cancellous block graft placement, relieving incisions are made parallel to the alveolar crest to release the flap without perforating it. This permitted the extension of the flap over the graft, facilitating wound closure without tension. Vicryl sutures were used to suture the edge of the keratinized labial/buccal flap to the palatal flap, utilising a horizontal mattress and running sutures.

2. Palatally based partial thickness flap: A labia/buccal parasulcular incision is made from the first molar to the other, and a mucosal flap is elevated to the mucogingival junction, where a full-thickness periosteal incision is made. A full-thickness mucoperiosteal flap is made, then retracted to the palatal side to expose the ridge crest. The mucosal flap is sutured to the palatal mucosa by mucoperiosteal elevators to reduce soft tissue trauma. A labio/buccal subperiosteal flap is reflected buccally from the periosteal incision line. Thus, the entire alveolar ridge, piriform fossa, and lateral wall of the maxilla to the zygomatic buttress are exposed.

The adaptation of the blocks consisted of removing some cancellous bone green stick fractures and splitting the block into smaller pieces. The graft was adjusted as necessary to adapt well to the residual alveolus. The three-dimensional size and contour of the graft are determined by the shape of the ridge required to support (i.e. labio-buccally) dental implants. The cortical surface is facing the soft tissue.

The last posterior block's distal margin is tapered and not placed beyond the second molar. The cortex of the alveolar ridge is perforated to increase angiogenic and osteogenic contact with the graft. The blocks are secured by the appropriate length of the bone screws, usually two per block or occasionally by titanium mini plates; the head of the screws is countersunk.

Miniplates can be used in those cases where hip block placement cannot be screwed for reasons of anatomy – proximity to the sinus in the posterior maxillae or inferior dental canal in the

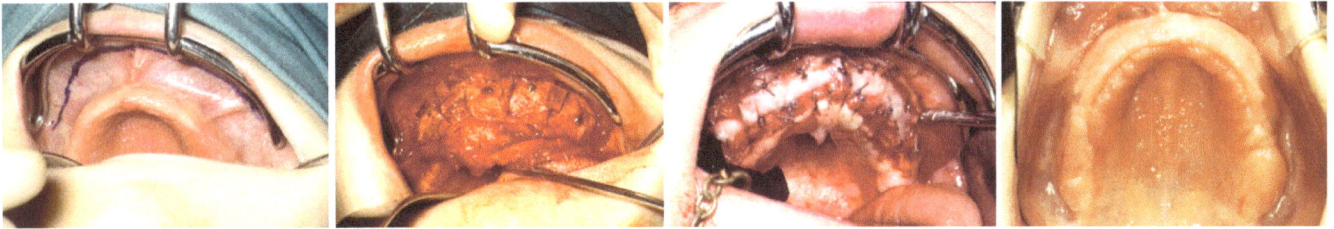

Figure 7.16 Full maxillae, iliac crest graft and free gingival graft.

mandible. Although a variety of complications have been reported at the hip donor site, strict attention to surgical technique is needed to prevent hip haematoma and hip wound dehiscence. If a gap exists beneath the blocks, it is filled with cancellous bone or a mixture of these autogenous bone and artificial bone substitute particles. If a dead space exists between the block and the labial/buccal cortex, the cancellous bone is pressed to fill the space.

The wound is sutured using Vicryl sutures. External pressure dressings are applied to the operated area.

Mandible:

A split-thickness incision inside the lip between the premolars is performed in full jaw reconstruction. A submucosal dissection is performed to a line 2 mm below the mucogingival junction. At this position, the periosteum is incised parallel to the mucogingival junction, and a full-thickness flap is reflected and exposed to the mandible's labial/buccal and lingual crestal cortex. The periosteum elevated down the labio-buccal aspect of the mandible. The mental nerve was identified, which delineated the posterior extent of the graft. Occasionally, if a distal extension is needed, the mental and inferior dental nerves are repositioned. The cortico-cancellous graft is placed and stabilised with the appropriate length of bone screws.

The head of the screws is countersunk to avoid trauma to the flap post-operatively.

A split-thickness incision inside the lip between the premolars is performed in full jaw reconstruction. A submucosal dissection is performed to a line 2 mm below the mucogingival junction. At this position, the periosteum is incised parallel to the mucogingival junction, and a full-thickness flap is reflected and exposed to the mandible's labial/buccal and lingual crestal cortex. The periosteum elevated down the labio-buccal aspect of the mandible. The mental nerve was identified, which delineated the posterior extent of the graft. Occasionally, if a distal extension is needed, the mental and inferior dental nerves are repositioned. The cortico-cancellous graft is placed and stabilised with the appropriate length of bone screws. The head of the screws is countersunk to avoid trauma to the flap post-operatively.

To provide a good soft tissue seal within the base of the newly created sulcus, a minimum clearance of three millimetres is needed from the edge of the block to the margin of the vestibuloplasty flap. The margin of the flap is sutured in two layers, 3 mm behind the margin with mattress sutures and at the flap edge with interrupted or continuous sutures. Once this technique is developed, marginal wound dehiscence does not occur (figure 4.9).

In order to provide keratinized soft tissue around dental implants

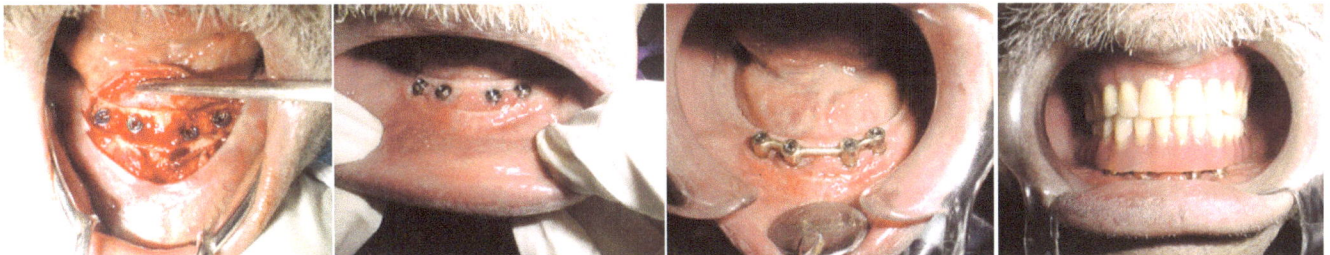

Figure 7.17 Secondary epithelialisation of the labial sulcus provides a stable, non-keratinized and non-mobile mucosa on the labial surfaces of the dental implants.

150

in bone-grafted cases, it is sometimes necessary to use keratinized palatal mucosa as the source of the free gingival graft. But sometimes, it is clear that the width of the available gingival graft will be inadequate. In these cases, a deliberate gap may be left between the margin of the otherwise inadequate graft and the crestal keratinized tissue.

The gap will still heal by secondary epithelialisation. The healed scar tissue will be non-mobile and non-keratinized (figure 7.17). Each type has potential complications and can treated as follows:

Cancellous bone loss: These are small fragments packed into the joints between cortico-cancellous blocks or between the cortico-cancellous blocks and the recipient maxillae. The fragments occasionally dehisced through the mucosa and need to be removed.

Screw dehiscence: Early removal of such screws can be carried out once the primary union of the graft has occurred. A bone block is always retained with two screws, and the removal of a screw after four weeks does not affect the stability of the graft.

Minor wound breakdown: Strict oral hygiene must be maintained until the wound has healed and/or the graft surface has been sequestrated. Once the site has healed, the dental implant can be placed. The main reason such dehiscence occurs is the presence of a sharp edge to the graft.

When a small sharp piece of bone is outside the soft tissue, the best thing is not to do anything; explain to the patient that it becomes necrotic and soft tissue will separate it and dislodge it, and the patient one day feels it and put it in the bin. Removing the sharp edge will promote more bone resorption.

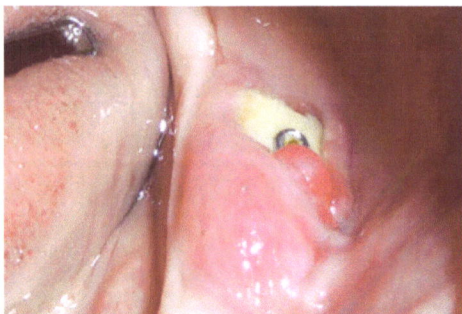

Figure 7.18 Screw and bone block dehiscence.

Membrane dehiscence: Strict oral hygiene must be maintained along with the excision of the exposed surface of the membrane. In the case of barrier membrane infection, immediate removal of the membrane is necessary.

Mental nerve paraesthesia: Review the position and provide assurance.

Forced deep placement of implants: This will occur where bone loss has rendered the planned position of the implant unfeasible. An implant, thus placed too deeply, will invite soft tissue problems. These will require the construction of a modified (extended) abutment to cope with increased soft tissue thickness.

Signs of infection of the grafts are Mild inflammation, wound breakdown, open drainage, and bitter taste.

When a bone graft complication arises, and dentures can bring or cause the complication, the dentist will request that the denture should not be used. Patients may wear dentures during sleep when the bone graft has not healed. Any case where denture function and/or aesthetics have been compromised can significantly affect the patient's quality of life, not least because of the psychological implications.

Although, in our experience, most of these patients may not be classified as psychologically ill, we feel, nevertheless, that it would be advantageous to have such patients screened by a clinical psychologist not only at the time of initial presentation but also during and after treatment to monitor the effect of prolonged, complicated treatment on these patients' well-being. Extensive bone grafting can be associated with limping for two weeks.

7.5. Non-autogenous bone substitute and membrane

There are several classifications for non-autogenous grafting bone substitutes and barrier membrane materials.

One of the simplest options is as follows: Allograft (derived from the same species) - freeze-dried bone allograft (FDBA) or demineralized freeze-dried bone (DFDBA).

Grafts or blocks can be cortical, cancellous, cortico-cancellous, or particulate. The disease-transmission risk is less than that of a blood transfusion. In Europe and the USA, tissue banks are monitored under strict guidelines to minimise the chances of HIV, Hepatitis B and C, and Treponema Pallidum cross-infection through infection tests. Patients with Creutzfeldt-Jakob and Human T-lymphotropic virus infections are excluded as donors.

Immunogenicity is reduced during processing by eliminating donor cells. Major Histocompatibility Complex (MHC) protein, a human leukocyte antigen, may initiate an immune reaction. However, the effect may be reduced by long-term freezing [14].

A xenograft is derived from demineralized bovine bone mineral (DBBM), algae-derived, and sea-derived (coral).

Alloplast: This is synthetically produced, hydroxyapatite [HA], β-tricalcium phosphate [TCP], Bioglass, and Calcium Sulphate. Jensen and co-workers studied more than 2000 papers regarding GBR and concluded that complete defect fill is not predictable. When augmentation procedures that deal with fenestration-type defects have been studied, the results show reduced membrane exposure and fewer complications from infection than those with dehiscence-type defects. This may be due to the greater distance between the membrane and the incision line. The conclusion was that there was a high level of evidence to support that the survival rates of implants between augmented bone and pristine bone are similar [15].

It is the author's experience that the most predictable horizontal ridge augmentation is the autogenous bone graft or a three-fold combination of autogenous bone particles and bone substitute materials with a low substitution rate when protected with a non-resorbable membrane for non-space making defect and resorbable membrane for space-making defect.

Vertical ridge augmentation has a high vertical bone loss, regardless of using different techniques and materials, including titanium mesh, titanium-reinforced membrane, and mini plates. In contrast, the block graft gains more height, but the rate of dehiscence increases. This is due to the stretching of the covering mucosa, which can compromise any tension-free primary closure. It can also be due to the reduced thickness of the mucosa. Establishing tension-free soft tissue closure that preserves proper vascularisation of the site is essential. That is fundamental to success.

Another more favourable technique due to providing a space-making defect is internal alveolar split bone and bone block graft between the osteotomized bony segments. A horizontal incision is made below the mucogingival line and raises the mucoperiosteal flap, one horizontal cut and two vertical bone cuts on the extremities of the horizontal cut using piezo surgery tips to complete the osteotomy. Two millimetres adjacent from the adjacent teeth. Raise upward the bone segment to leave a space for the bone block without disturbing the lingual periosteum. The autogenous bone block or allogenic bone block is inserted interpositionally and placed in the middle of the space, and the rest with bone graft particulate and fixation with miniplates between the basal and the cranial segment is unnecessary.

During pregnancy, soft tissue reacts to mechanical forces by cell proliferation, like abdominal skin, which has led to the development of soft tissue expanders. A soft tissue expander is a rubber balloon that expands soft tissue by expanding its volume without reducing its thickness, colour, or texture. More significant tissue gain has been achieved using rectangular or crescent-cross section form expanders rather than round expanders.

The original versions of expanders needed repetitive inflation, and this repetitive increase in pressure, even if intermittent, reduced tissue vascularity. Self-inflating osmotic soft tissue expanders have now been developed without repetitive inflation. The latest osmotic hydrogel expanders, with an impermeable silicon shell, have flat ends that do not expand. They also have screw fixation, which prevents their migration. The perforations in the impermeable silicon shell permit the influx of surrounding fluids for a slow, steep swelling curve. Hemispherical and cylindrical shapes are recommended for intra-oral use.

Placing the expanders too close to the incision line can lead to a minor perforation.

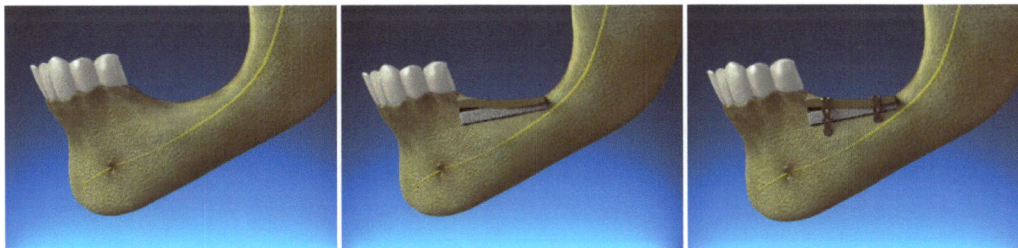

Figure 7.19 Segmental osteotomy and placing a bone block in the middle to increase the height of the alveolar bone.

The soft tissue profile gain at the attached gingival level is about 3mm. This will likely be reduced to about 2 mm at the time of implant placement. Less bone graft resorption is also expected compared with a conventional flap procedure.

Usually, expanders are placed subperiosteally, but also submucosal placement has been recommended, with the rationale that this avoids the replacement of the periosteum with collagen-rich connective tissue with no osteoblasts or precursor cells [16].

In vertical bone augmentation, soft tissue expansion carried out before augmentation significantly reduces the incidence of post-operative graft exposure. A scar at the surgical site indicates previous mucosal perforation by the tissue expander or limited expansion. However, the gain of keratinized mucosa is limited, mainly lining mucosa expansion, which is observed as all the expanders are placed in the vestibule.

Placing a soft tissue expander under the oral mucosa using the tunnel technique requires skill. The expanders start to swell on contact with fluid, so the moist environment demands rapid and dexterous surgery.

To prevent migration of the expander, screw fixation is essential, mainly due to the presence of a flat side on the expander that lacks sufficient expanding capacity. Also, it should be positioned away from the incision line.

Tissue expansion can be repeated in the same area. Both bone resorption and new bone formation beneath expanders have been reported. Connective tissue capsule formation requires a minimum of two weeks [17]. If subperiosteal expanders are left too long, the periosteum will become replaced by fibrous connective tissue [18].

Barrier Membranes:

• Regeneration of bone in small osseous defects may be achieved using barrier membranes. The membrane containing a blood clot or an augmentation material is laid over the defect. The main task of the barrier membrane is to prevent the migration of soft tissue cells across the membrane during the bone healing period, such as soft tissue cell occlusion. Mechanical separation of the soft tissue from the augmented area is sufficient to inhibit or delay the soft tissue invasion of the defect till the osteoblasts have enough time to migrate inside the cavity (figures 7.6, 7.21).

Regeneration of bone in minor osseous defects may be achieved using barrier membranes. The membrane containing a blood clot or an augmentation material is laid over the defect. Mechanical separation of the soft tissue from the augmented area is sufficient to inhibit or delay the soft tissue invasion of the defect till the osteoblasts have enough time to migrate inside the cavity (figures 7.6, 7.21).

Micropores are believed to permit fluid diffusion but prevent the access of soft tissue cells, such as fibroblasts, to the defect. However, the author believes that the defects are too minor and that the existence of pores is essential.

The membrane has been used to increase the width and height of the alveolus, cover denuded implant surfaces when the alveolus is narrow, treat peri-implantitis, and prevent recession adjacent to implant sites that will receive dental implants. In this book, we are not planning to discuss the increase in height using barrier membranes due to limited success and controversies.

Murray, in 1957, demonstrated that if a bone defect is protected with a plastic bag, the defect will be filled with bone. Lack of movement is a primary request for healing, including soft tissue and bone integration of the membrane.

A gore-tex membrane, an expanded polytetrafluoroethylene, is a non-resorbable material with a two-part design. The outer portion has internodal distances of 20-25 um, which encourages connective tissue attachment, but the central portion is relatively stiff and has smaller interstitial spaces.

One of the main complications of using e-PTFE is the membrane's premature exposure, which often necessitates premature membrane removal, jeopardising the treatment's effectiveness, which reduces the gain width by half to about two millimetres (figure 7.20).

In cases of extraction and immediate GBR, primary soft tissue closure is not easy, especially in the molar areas when the surface requiring coverage is not small and the crestal soft tissue defects at the opening of the tooth socket. Applying a membrane in this situation is impractical in that the membrane should have two millimetres of clearance from soft tissue wound margins, and in addition, it should also overlap on the bone beyond the margin of the defect so that it will not collapse into the cavity. In such cases, there are two options: first, to delay the augmentation procedure for eight weeks after extraction, by which time soft tissue healing over the socket will have occurred, or apply a rigid, non-resorbable membrane which can close the buccal opening of the defect and can remove after a minimum of four

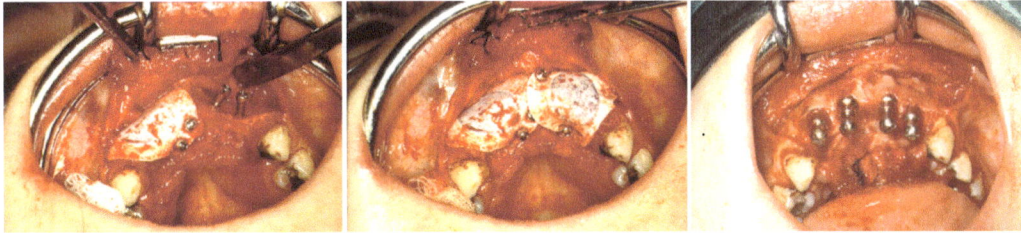

Figure 7.20 Gore-tex membrane fixation is a predictable technique to increase the ridge width.

An important and unresolved problem is the duration of required membrane protection. If 4-6 weeks is adequate, resorbable membranes may be appropriate, as their use does not involve further surgery to remove the membrane.

Dense e-PTFE or non-porous membranes are more infection-resistant than porous membranes, so closing and sealing the flap is not essential. In this case, compromising the flap's vitality due to releasing incisions will not occur.

Identifying the risk factors will increase the success rate.

Immediate implant insertion and membrane application have a higher complication rate of up to 50% than delayed replacement. Titanium-reinforced e-PTFE has been used to prevent the collapse of the membrane, and titanium membrane has been used. However, complications of premature exposure, infection and loss of the membranes occur.

For placing membrane fixation screws or tags, a favourable bone cortex is needed, and this can be problematic (figure 7.20). Also, the lack of direct attachment of the membrane to the tissue and air bubbles under the membrane prevent osteogenesis.

Soft tissue management and strict infection control are mandatory. Crestal incisions had a higher premature exposure rate compared with palatal incisions. Washing talcum-powdered gloves before touching the membrane during the trimming procedure is recommended. Different surgical instruments in a separate table, especially surgical suction tips, have been recommended.

RESORBABLE MEMBRANES:

A resorbable membrane is recommended as surgical trauma to the periosteum is expected to remove the membrane. A series of factors should be considered when choosing an ideal resorbable membrane: Calculable absorption time, stability during placement, prevention of invasion of fibrous tissue, resistance to collapse, resistance to infection, complete resorption with no residue in the tissues and elimination from the body. Clinically manageable pins or screw retention for primary stability of the membrane have been recommended. The screws or pins should be manufactured from the same material. Resorbable membranes have two groups: natural collagen polymers and synthetic polymers. Depending on the degradation mode, polymeric biomaterials can be classified into hydrolytically degradable polymers and enzymatically degradable polymers produced by macrophages and neutrophils. Most of the naturally occurring polymers undergo enzymatic degradation.

Natural collagen membranes

Type I collagen is one of the most common natural membranes provided by bovine or porcine tendons, pericardium, skin, or dermis of animals.

The natural collagen membranes have excellent cell affinity biocompatibility and bone regeneration capacity; they have limitations such as losing space-maintaining ability in humid conditions, inferior mechanical strength, and too rapid biodegradation [19].

Proteolytic bacterial enzymes may play a part in the degradation of collagen barrier membranes used for guided tissue regeneration [20].

As absorbable membranes are primarily metabolised through enzymatic degradation once exposed, they have a greater susceptibility to infection and a faster degradation rate. Membrane exposures compromise space maintenance and cell exclusion properties, leading to detrimental effects. During the first week of exposure, the outer surface of the barrier is colonised by bacteria, and by a couple of weeks, the bacteria have invaded the entire thickness of the membrane. Bacterial invasion results in membrane resorption, and even with the long-lasting crosslinked collagen barriers, bone regeneration outcomes are compromised once membranes are exposed.

Natural collagens have unpredicted resorption patterns,

possible inflammation due to the degradation process, and speedy degradation by the patient's saliva enzymes. Physical properties change when it is impregnated with blood, which is challenging to handle. Due to the lack of rigidity, space maintenance, and the thickness of the membrane, suturing without tension is more complicated, and difficulty in diagnosing the membrane exposure must be considered. Collagen membranes often collapse on the biomaterial granules; some studies have reported the superposition of two collagen membranes, making it more challenging to handle and suture.

In order to reinforce the mechanical and biodegradable stability, various chemical, physical and biological cross-linking methods have been introduced to cross-link collagen. Via cross-linking, the tensile strength of collagen was enhanced, and their degradation time was prolonged. However, the residual reagents or secondary products during collagen implant degradation may have toxic effects and thus limit their applications. Physical treatments, such as dehydrothermal (DHT) treatment, heat treatment, ultraviolet irradiation, gamma irradiation, microwave irradiation, and biological methods, are used as an alternative to introducing cross-link efficiently.

Exposed collagen membranes are difficult to manage because many enzymes present in oral fluids can rapidly degrade the collagen, leading to exposure of the biomaterial granules with bacterial contamination of site [21].

It has also raised certain ethical, religious and cultural issues. The limitations, such as poor mechanical properties and rapid degradation, are associated with the shortened functional period, greater susceptibility to infection, and the regeneration of new tissue, which makes the author think twice about applying this type of membrane unless to protect autogenous bone particles or a mixture of a bone substitute and autogenous bone particles in space-making defects.

The author opposes using animal or human bone for elective surgeries like guided bone regeneration (GBR). The memory of the UK infection crisis, where up to 30,000 people were affected by contaminated blood and thousands died, remains vivid in our considerations.

At that time, HIV had not been diagnosed, and hepatitis B was in the developing stage. There could be a risk of transmission to humans from animal or human-derived collagen. Prions could be a concern, but we were lucky that prions were diagnosed before marketing collagen-derived membrane or bone substi-

tutes. The prion paradigm has been expanded to misfold other diseases. What if tomorrow, the scientist discovers another disease? Furthermore, why have the concern when so many other options are available for elective surgery?

An adequate amount of keratinized tissue, a thick tissue biotype, a deep vestibular depth, and high flap flexibility with the use of absorbable membranes might minimise the incidence of wound opening. The primary closure is one of the impediments to resorbable membranes, especially natural collagen membranes. A periosteal releasing incision is needed for appropriate access to the augmented field. However, periosteal-releasing incisions might cause more swelling, bleeding, and patient discomfort. Importantly, they also may compromise blood circulation, and re-positioning the flap coronally may affect the gingivae aesthetic problems in the anterior regions. It is less needed with rigid, non-resorbable membranes, which may be placed by sliding over the needed area without any displacement.

Collagen membranes are completely degraded between 2 and 16 weeks, a period too short for a proper barrier function. Furthermore, their structures are variable by nature, leading to uncontrollable permeability of cells and tissues.

Resorbable synthetic barrier membranes

The resorbable synthetic barrier membranes have a predictable degradability and some mechanical resistance, and they degrade by hydrolysis in 4 to 6 months with limited signs of inflammation.

The main advantages of synthetic materials are reproducibility and unlimited quantities.

Membranes made of poly-lactic Acid (PLA) and poly-glycolic Acid (PGA) under different commercial names are available. The tensile strengths are based on the ratio of polymers PLA/PGA, which is a wide range. Cross-linking increases the tensile length, but the degradation timeline will subsequently increase. The membrane is broken down by proteolytic enzymes from polymorphonuclear cells into lactic acid or glycolic acid and exerted by the kidney or as pyruvate (figures 7.21,1.5).

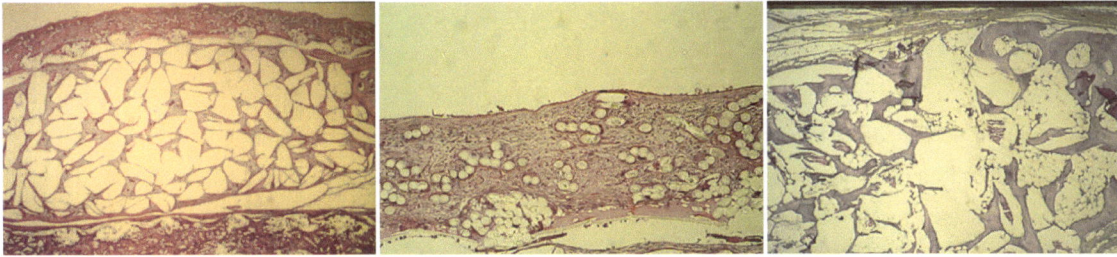

Figure 7.21 In space-making defects, rabbit parietal bone and 10 mm cavities were prepared and filled with bioglass particles protected by synthetic resorbable membranes. After eight weeks, the left demonstrates inflammation around the membranes and Bioglass particles. Middle: higher magnification demonstrates inflammation around the membrane. Right: after 16 weeks of membrane resorbing, most Bioglass particles were resorbed and replaced by bone tissue.

Augmentation without using a barrier membrane

The use of barrier membranes has its complications; there is a tendency for some clinicians to use allogenic materials and/or autogenous bone without membrane application in GBR cases. Based on the author's histology and clinical studies, only in the space-making defect is applicable when only autogenous bone particles or different types of bone substitute in the depth of the defect and 3 mm of the occlusal of the defect autogenous bone particles or chips are placed. The latter needs less autogenous bone particles and does not need a membrane.

Interposition grafting

This technique, which is invasive but has a low incidence of complications, has been introduced and applied by an oral surgeon. A linear incision is made above 3 mm of the mucogingival junction, and the mucoperiosteum is detached. Micro-saws make vertical and horizontal cuts, and the chisels finalise the osteotomy and mobilize the bony segments. The palatal soft tissue remains intact, and the bone block from the ramus of the mandible is provided; the cortical portion of the interposed bone faces buccal. The grafted block is fixed using Y-type microplates.

Distraction Osteogenesis

The author does not have clinical experience with this procedure, but that does not mean the technique is not applicable.

Ilizarov established the application of distraction osteogenesis through gradual traction of the pedicle bone fragment. This demonstrated the principles of tension stress and mechanical load accompanied by the development of local vascularization and simultaneous osteogenesis. But it does have limitations. There is a dispute over the minimum bone height necessary.

A vertical bone deficiency with a broad, round ridge is a good prospect for distraction osteogenesis. Posterior maxillae have not been used for this type of treatment. In deficient and/or scarred soft tissue cases, alveolar distraction osteogenesis is an option to prevent possible incision breakdown. It can be helpful in the anterior region, where aesthetics is very important. Usually, the fractured and mobilized segment is a pedicle attached to the lingual mucoperiosteum. The horizontal osteotomy must be a distance from the crestal bone but at least two millimetres above the inferior alveolar nerve. The mean latency period is one week to allow the mucoperiosteum to heal and reduce the risk of wound dehiscence. The mean distraction rate per day is 0.7mm, with a rhythm of 1-2 times daily. 5-6 mm of distraction length has been achieved at this rate. 1mm per day is acceptable for vertical movement, but 0.5 mm is needed for horizontal movement.

Too slow a distraction rate will result in premature bone union; too rapid can lead to non-union.

The complete healing period is about 12 weeks, and the implants can be placed four weeks after removing the distraction device.

The variables involved make distraction osteogenesis a complicated treatment technique for any patient: the rhythm required is empirically determined, the augmentation rate depends on the type of device employed, and the latter varies with the needs of the case, as does the distraction distance. All the patient needs is the added discomfort of turning the screw – daily [22].

While the author does not use this technique and does not presume to comment authoritatively upon it, he urges readers who find it attractive to investigate it.

For his part, the author uses and recommends a sandwich or interposition technique that he finds compelling. The method is intensive, and the patient needs to feel that they can bear the stress of the prospective surgery and the number of sessions that may be involved. Above all, their decision and tone should be taken only after a series of consultations during which each step is explained clearly. Make full use of audiovisual aids and brochures. However, what the patient has been told in writing will likely be forgotten once the patient is outside the door. At each stage of the programme, explain what is to be done at that visit, and afterwards, explain what may be experienced by the patient postoperatively. Explain that you will be available anytime the patient is concerned.

Fresh socket augmentation

Neither clinics nor dental hospitals produce either guidelines or recommendations on preserving the alveolar ridge of the fresh socket. Most change takes place in the first three months, and it has been estimated that there is a 50% reduction in the buccal-lingual width [23].

In the first six months, an average of 3.8mm of width is lost, while 1.24mm of height is lost. Resorption of mandibular bone is faster than that in the maxillae [24].

A Cochrane study evaluated the effectiveness of different grafting procedures and their ability to preserve ridge anatomy and prevent bone resorption. The study concluded that there is not enough evidence to recommend any particular ridge preservation technique over any other. No 'best procedure' could prove more beneficial for implant placement [25].

Different types of grafting materials have been used: autogenous, allograft, xenograft and alloplasts. Barrier membranes (resorbable or non-resorbable) have been used, with the latter having a better tissue response if they are not exposed. Resorbable membranes do not need to be removed, and it is claimed that they elicit minimal tissue reaction when exposed. Resorbable membranes have a distinct disadvantage since the minimal tissue reaction will not alert the dentist to early exposure. It has been claimed that grafting particles delay the healing process, but all had new bone formation. However, initiated, there are similar after three months; graft particles fill the ridge more than other methods [26].

Alveolar bone resorption can be detected after tooth extraction. It is usually first signalled by the lack of buccal bone. A clinician's main mistake is failure to scrutinise the alveolar bone walls. This is the best knowledge during curettage with a sharp curette. When the wall is thin and a dull curette is applied, it may induce too much force and fracture the thin but stable alveolar bone. Usually, the dentist does not detect either dehiscence or the fenestration.

A failure to carry out a proper socket examination can lead to a wrong diagnosis, which may be used as a basis for a faulty treatment plan. This will have a roll-on effect on implant placement decisions, so both implant placement and subsequent aesthetics may be compromised.

An intrasulcular circumferential incision is made to the coronal level of the alveolar bone around the tooth.

7.6. Prevention and Preservation of Alveolar Bone loss (socket preservation)

Minimally Invasive Dentistry is the application of "a systematic respect for the original tissue."

Even though some patients seem to be convinced that the only things that count are replacements and are prepared to pay for a filling but not for a procedure that can help avoid having one.

The concept of preventive dentistry has been taught in undergraduate courses in cariology and periodontology. Preventive treatment, diagnostic tools, and new techniques for cutting teeth and removing decays have evolved in cariology. In periodontology, there is a preference for non-surgical therapy; when periodontal surgery is required, it should be minimally invasive with periodontal regeneration. However, the oral surgery department is less taught, and the dentist becomes a spendthrift in the alveolar bone in extraction.

The replacement of enamel, dentin and tooth has been improved in the last decades; however, the replacement of the alveolar bone is traumatic for patients and dentists, costly, and less predictable.

This subject has been the author's interest for the last 25 years, as he has seen complicated cases that may have been avoided if the school of thought had changed, and this needs to start at the undergraduate level.

This subject will be discussed in three time zones: before and immediately after tooth extraction.

a) Before Extraction:

Decision tree for indication of extraction:

Indications for tooth extractions are caries, periodontitis, periapical disease, trauma, orthodontics, and others such as tumours. The main blurred subject of the indication is periodontitis. The main question would be when to extract a tooth. Was the patient informed that delaying extraction may jeopardise future dental implant placement or that a major bone graft will be needed due to delay?

Diagnosing and informing the patient is mandatory, and trying to eliminate the general risk factors like alcohol, obesity, diabetes, smoking, stress and replacing Statin with another drug.

Before starting any periodontal treatment, the dentist needs to investigate if the patient suffers from any systemic disease, takes medicine affecting periodontal status or has a poor diet. It has proven the associations between lack of fatty acids, vitamin C, vitamin E, beta-carotene, fibre, calcium, dairy, fruits, and vegetables with periodontal disease [27].

In Relapsing periodontitis in supportive periodontal care, which needs to repeat subgingival instrumentation of the residual pockets, the antiseptics do not provide significant benefits; one study on probiotics and one on the use of vitamin D and calcium supplementation showed significant improvements in periodontal parameters [28].

Many factors will affect the dentist's judgment to recommend extraction, from the degree of bone loss, attachment loss, furcation lesions, mobility, and crown-root relationship to financial aspects, patients' expectations, and motivations.

Oral hygiene and the level of the remaining alveolar bone need to be registered. Periodontists more often prefer to maintain the teeth with follow-ups, and dentists with more years of experience opt for more extractions. Grade 3 tooth mobility, exposure to root bifurcation, smoking and drinking habits played a significant role in the tooth's poor prognosis, and the dentist may prefer extraction [29].

Reasons to indicate the extraction of teeth with periodontitis are the presence of mobility, severity of attachment loss and radiographic bone loss greater than 50%. Mobility can be reduced by treatment of the inflammation, and the severity of attachment loss does not indicate the disease status; only oedema, erythema, bleeding, and suppuration indicate the inflammation [30].

Radiographs are the primary determinants that can affect the treatment plan, demonstrating the bone crestal level, inter-radicular bone resorption, and crown-root ratio [31].

To put it in simple terms, the author recommends, first, the dentist start non-surgical periodontal treatment and if the bone loss of 50% continues to worsen or in bifurcation grade 3 when the bone loss height between the roots is more than 2 millimetres, then extraction should be recommended to the patient. Extraction is recommended for mobility grade 2 with other above risks or grade 3 with or without above general and local risk factors.

Commercialising dental implants has made extractions more common, and patients always have the right to receive all information on the therapeutic options and decide on treatment plans.

b) At the clinical session of extraction

Atraumatic extraction means less gingival laceration, crushing the crest of the socket, buccal cortical plate fracture, postoperative pain, and bleeding. Bear in mind that the pressure and compression by instruments may induce bone necrosis.

The knowledge of instruments for extractions is necessary to prevent crushing the bone.

The author's concept is that forceps should be used only as an instrument to lift out the tooth without force, except for using upper or lower cow horn forceps (but not eagle beak forceps) for extracting molars. Cow horn forceps work below the socket crest, reaching deep in furcation and initiating occlusal movement by wedging and sliding the tooth out of the socket. If it is not moving or stopped in the middle, a barrier impedes the movement, and if force is applied, the root or bone may fracture. Instead, the dentist can study the scenario and find the impediment.

Before using any instrument, the first extraction step is to sever the soft tissue attachment surrounding the root. A straight elevator can be used, but the author prefers rigid, flat plastic.

The next step is to penetrate the PDL space, about 0.15-0.21 mm wide, using different instruments. There are generally two types of tips: spoon shape or flat. They have different names, but the concept is the same. Generally, the straight elevator tips are spoon-shaped and cut or detach the gingiva, then the periodontal ligament and expand the space, which increases the degree of freedom of the root inside the alveolar socket.

The tip of the elevator, which is the active part called the blade, looks more like the bowl of the spoon. The blade has two surfaces, convex and concave; concave is in contact with the root surface with different lengths (3-4mm). The bowl's design is different in size, shape, depth of depression, and thickness.

There are no guidelines or ISO regarding its design; the front edge, The radius of the curvature, the Side edge, and the front edge converge, and the length of the bowl have not been standardized.

Usually, the elevator is slowly rotated and moves toward the least significant resistance areas, occlusal and labial/buccal, as the bone cortex is thinner labial/buccal. Maximum width (the amount it can rotate and dislodge the root) is different, graded 1,2 and 3 without any standards. The width of the bowl decreases from the maximum to the back edge of the bowl. The maximum edge is nearer to the front. Lengthwise, the maximum concavity is toward the back edge.

Mechanical principles of elevators:

1. Lever: the long lever arm and the short effort arm make small movements against great resistance. Depending on the location of the fulcrum concerning the object raised, a push or pull force will dislodge the object upward. The author recommends not using lever type 1, as it will crush the crest of the socket. Only apply leverage type 2 or use the wedge technique.

By lodging the straight elevator #1 against the tooth root and rotating the instrument on its long axis, a large rotational leverage force can be applied in a very controlled manner over a short distance. As the tooth and bone are forced apart, the un-cut periodontal ligament is stretched and torn beyond the instrument's tip if tension is long enough. By working systematically around the root's circumference, it will be loosened to the point where it can simply be lifted from its socket or, if not, placing a wider straight elevator with the same manoeuvre and rarely is needed to use #3.

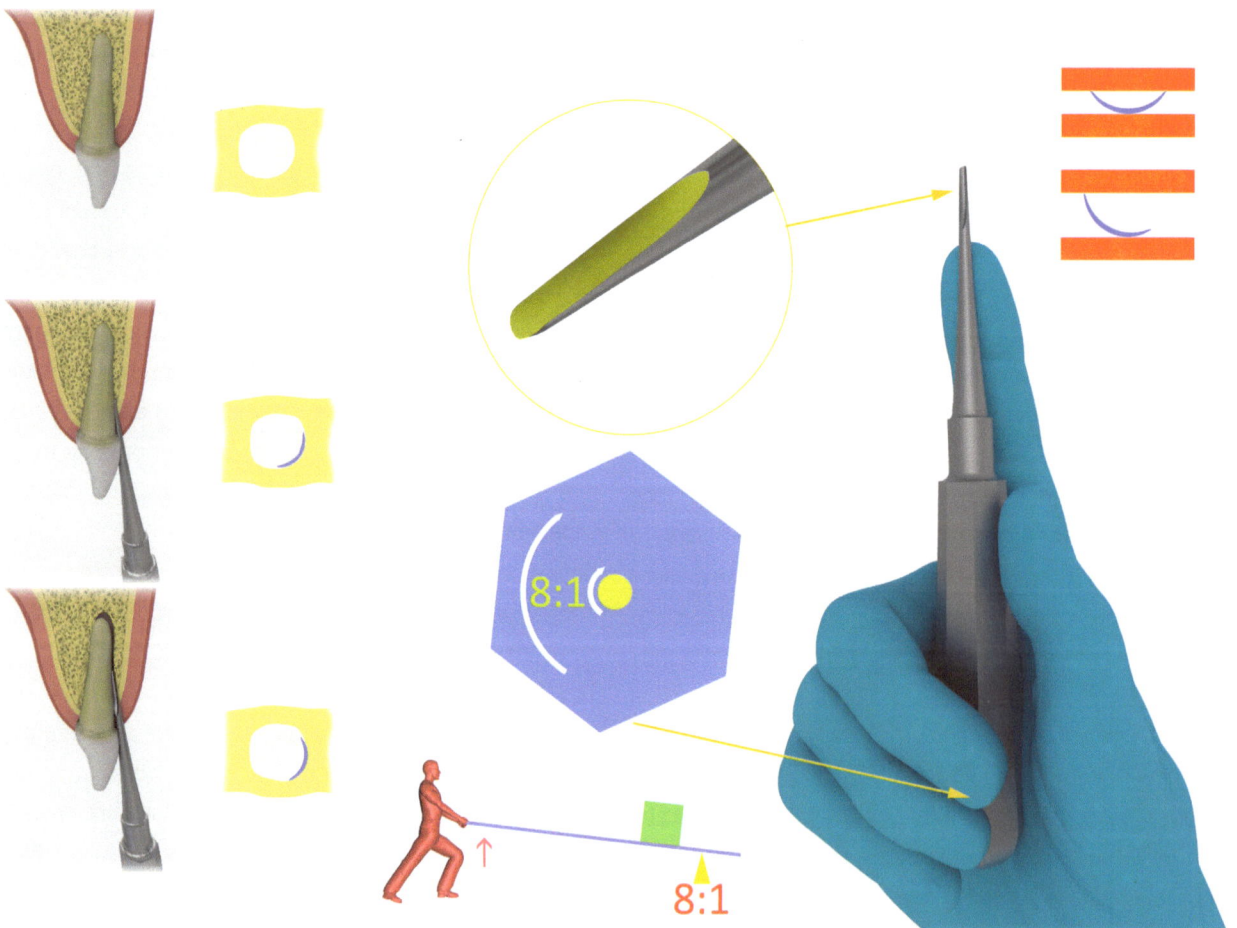

Figure 7.22 The spoon-shaped blade of the straight elevator and the tangential concave surface are placed toward the root. A more considerable leverage is placed by rotating the instrument along its axis, which expands the socket and loosens the root. Only the type 2 lever is recommended because lever 1 crushes the crest of the plate of the alveolar bone.

159

2. Wedge principle:

The wedge principle is when a wedge instrument is used to displace the root of the socket by expanding the socket and displacing the root—reminder: the root gets smaller toward the apex.

Different approaches can use this principle. The blade can be flat (Periotome) or spoon-shaped (straight elevator). For a straight elevator, rotate slightly to wiggle the blade and work it towards the apex. It is placed parallel to the long axis of the root between the socket wall and the root, and when purchased is obtained, the strongest portion of the alveolar socket is used for the fulcrum of the leverage. Usually, this manoeuvre is not recommended on the buccal surface as it is too thin.

The family of flat blades includes the Coupland chisel, Luxator, Periotome, and pre-elevator.

Coupland and luxator are single bevels (like chisel), and Periotome and pre-elevator are bi-bevelled. In engineering, single bevels are designed for peeling and shaving, and double bevels are for cutting, chopping, and pushing away from both sides. As the root is more resistant to the bone, the push is more toward the bone, expanding the socket.

The principles of safe use of elevators:

In the palm grip, the handle rests against the palm heel for heavy forces and the finger grip for delicate pressure (figure 7.22). The elevator or luxator must be supported by placing the finger of the holding hand down the long axis of the elevator, in which the tip of the finger is leaned on something firm, like a tooth, to control and prevent slipping when pressure is applied. When the elevator is in position, it is rotated with the force by the thumb and forefingers.

Never use it as a class one lever, as it will fracture the crest of the alveolar socket or even the alveolar bone. During wiggling to penetrate, there is a chance of fracturing the crest of the socket. Elevators can be used to displace roots out of the socket, but if the apex is close to the maxillary sinus or Inferior Dental Nerve, the force should be applied with total control, and if it doubts, do not do it. However, when the tooth is loose, a forceps can be used to pull out the tooth without any force.

There are different types of extraction elevators like Warwick James (right, left, and straight), Coupland (sets of three each of increasing size), Straight elevator (are thicker with a slightly bowed shoulder on the back side and are less sharp), the Straight elevators have two general designed tips winged and non-winged. The wings help to hug the root, so there is less chance of slipping, but they have the tendency to dig and crush the alveolar bone ridge, and the author does not recommend them. Never use force; as a rule of thumb, only use fingers or wrist, not the arm.

Coupland elevators are in three sizes and use pulley levers; as the author recommends the wedge technique, he does not recommend Couplands.

Luxation elevators are straight (have thin, sharp blades to cut PDL about 3 mm). When applying apical pressure, cut in circular cutting motions, not prying motion, and use a deep-wedged luxator to push against the root. The shape of the handles of luxators is the same as a straight elevator, and young dentists may use too much force or wiggle movements, which are prohibited, which may be why it is not taught at the undergraduate level. The problem is that when young dentists go to practice, many luxators are available, and it is better to be taught in dental school under supervision. The blade is thin and must not be used to lift the tooth out as the tip may fracture (figure 7.23).

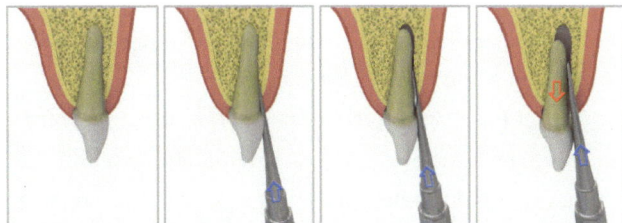

Figure 7.23 Using the wedge technique, the straight elevator, luxator, or Periotome is pushed in the PDL space (blue arrow), and the root is luxated or pushed outside (red arrow).

The luxating elevators have different types of curves and bends. Inwards give better access to the mesial and distal root surface outwards.

There are different types of Periotome flat tips: Rigid (soft or hard), flexible, which do not resist bending and act like a spring, bent freely and ensures the approach to the tooth root to find its path in the narrow PDL space (0.15-0.21 mm). Gently but firmly push the blade of the Periotome deep into the periodontal space of the tooth to be extracted, and do not lift or twist with excessive force as straight elevators do (figure 7.24).

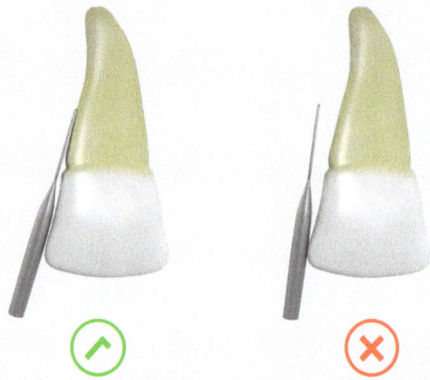

Figure 7.24 Periotome blade with tangential attachment to the root surface (left Periotome's blade). If not, as the cancellous bone is soft, the Periotome may penetrate the cancellous bone and not cut the PDL and provide the space between the bone and the root (right Periotome's blade)

The pre-elevator or Periotome are inserted at an angle of 10-20 degrees as a wedge against the tooth and then pushed deep into the PDL space to break down the periodontal ligaments.

It is rocked back and forth to gently advance in PDL space with the metronome motion, the tip is fixed, and the arm is moved right and left along the axis of the root.

The grip of Periotomes/pre-elevator is like holding a fountain pen: keep the handle in your palm with a firm grip and rest it between your thumb and index finger. The ring, little finger, and palm are pressed against the tip of the blade to provide stability. Some of the handles have been designed to use a mallet with short and gentle strokes.

A gentle mallet can push the tip toward the apex if the handle is designed for it. Usually, the mallet is unnecessary unless the root is ankylosed, and this technique is the most conservative technique to remove an ankylosed tooth or dental implant. It is recommended to tell the patient that tapping like a woodpecker you will feel.

When the tooth is loose, a straight #1 elevator is used and may continue to #3, and whenever it is loose, the dentist can use a forceps with gentle reciprocal 45 degrees and gentle pull (like a tweezer) to extract the tooth. If there is resistance, do not use force; go back and find where the resistance is and use the Periotome and or straight elevator.

Piezotome, which is a bone-cutting tool that transmits ultrasonic high-frequency vibrations through a metallic tip to cut bone while sparing the surrounding soft tissues, has also been on the market [32].

Pre-elevator technique:

The lack of a 1 mm width can change the treatment plan, and bone preservation is necessary. The author recommends the pre-elevator technique. The limited PDL space does not allow a spoon-shaped design of an elevator tip to penetrate without crushing the crest. In the first stage, using a flat-end shape instrument is safer. It is better to use a fine flat end after providing a pocket along the root; then, if it is needed, a straight elevator tip penetrates the prepared pocket safely. On this concept, the author designed an instrument called a pre-elevator.

The Author designed the Pre-elevator, a type of Periotome with a rigid tip made of titanium grade 5 (figure 11.2). The tip is wedge-shaped, and the handle is designed to accept the surgical mallet's light force. As it is wedge-shaped, after the final push, the opening of the bone pocket is wider than the Periotome.

Because of the thin tip, rigid and wedge silhouette, and sharp profile, the pre-elevator can fit better into tight apical spaces than the Periotome. It should be used with a metronome movement with the tip as the pivot point. The back-and-forth with metronome motion, in which the fixed point is at the apical end, will expand the socket smarter than Periotome. If the root is ankylotic, the ankylose section will be dislodged using a short, light mallet stroke without damaging the external cortical plate.

The cross-section of the external cortical plate is that it is thin in the bone crest and usually thickened toward the apex but not in the labial surfaces of the upper anterior teeth. Working in the upper anterior region requires more meticulousness due to the thin labial alveolar plate and the aesthetic region. The sagittal root position in relation to the anterior maxillary alveolar process has three types. In type 1, the long axis of the tooth is parallel or lingually inclined; in type 2, the root is slightly inclined toward the buccal bone; and in type 3, the root is inclined toward the buccal bone [33] (figure 7.25).

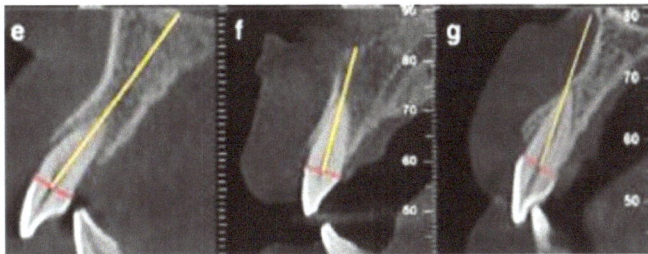

Figure 7.25 The maxillary alveolar process sagittal position is type 1-3 from left to right. The surgeon needs to know and react accordingly during extraction and immediate implant replacement.

In the upper anterior region, the proximal and buccal approach is a default approach; however, if the remaining solid root is on the half palatal surface, the palatal approach parallel to the long axis of the root is recommended.

In extraction and in remaining root removal, adequate vision is essential; use surgical suction (small tip) or pressure for a few minutes on a gauze.

The molars are recommended to be separated, and separation can be achieved by bur, chisel or elevator; the upper molar can be sectioned in two as the buccal roots are short and can purchased together with ease. The fulcrum is placed on the interdental area, and the root is by the heel of elevators; this is the only area using fulcrum type 1 that can be applied. If the purchase is unsuccessful, the elevation is done through an adjacent empty socket with a Cryer, in which the interseptal bone is removed together or at a separate stage.

If the alveolar plate is fractured and attached to the periosteum, it should be retained to preserve the alveolar bone's shape and prevent collapse.

Retained root or ankylosis:

As default, the dentist aims to expose the point of the application for elevators by providing a gutter of bone around the tooth but leaving the buccal and lingual plate intact using surgical micromotor with irrigation and a fine fissure bur vertically with its point apically, but do not pressure the bur as it may fracture.

As alveolar bone resorption after extraction is inevitable, the dentist must maximise his effort to minimise it [34].

c) Immediately post-extraction

Immediately after extraction, a medium-sized curette is placed inside the socket and gently scrapping the socket to remove the PDL and debridement and, at the same time, examine the integrity of the socket, primarily external buccal and lingual external plates.

Considerations for Irrigation After Tooth Extraction

There is a debate regarding the irrigation of the socket post-extraction. Advocates for irrigation argue that it aids in removing debris, improves the visualisation of the socket, and prevents dry-socket occurrence by eliminating foreign materials. On the other hand, opponents of this practice contend that irrigation can dislodge the blood clot, which is crucial for the initial healing phase and the prevention of dry-socket. Furthermore, there is a concern that irrigation might introduce bacteria into the socket, increasing the risk of infection and potentially disturbing the natural healing process.

The author recommends a balanced approach to irrigation following curettage. Specifically, the socket should be gently irrigated with isotonic saline, which does not disrupt the osmotic balance. This should be performed using a Frazer surgical tip number 12, applied with low pressure by removing the hand from the thumb control hole. After irrigating, the socket should be thoroughly examined, and the saline should be removed. It is important to assess whether the socket is bleeding; if it is not, it is rare; further curettage may be necessary to promote bleeding and ensure proper healing.

This method aims to maximise the benefits of irrigation while minimising potential risks, thus supporting optimal post-extraction care.

If a bony wall is missing, a flap is raised with a rigid flat plastic, extended to the socket's mesial and distal line angles, and then extended down to the mucogingival junction of the mucoperiosteum. A subperiosteal pocket (for example, the lingual surface) is created with the metronome movement to provide a trapezoidal flap without releasing incisions; thus, the dentist can feel and study the surface anatomy of the buccal surface. Studying surface anatomy will visualize undercuts, dehiscence, or fenestration without releasing incisions. After irrigation, a rigid, non-resorbable membrane is slid inside the pocket, and 2mm should be counter-sunk off the alveolar ridge and on the mesial and distal of the defect (figure 7.26).

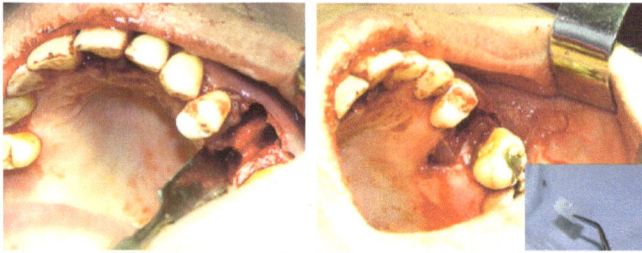

Figure 7.26 When a wall of alveolar bone is detected, a non-resorbable membrane should be placed to prevent soft tissue invasion in the socket. It is recommended to be placed 2 mm below the alveolar ridge.

The membrane should be placed without any tension or folded angles. The proximal papillae are sutured, with one sutured in the middle to stabilise the soft tissue and bring the soft tissue's margins as close together as possible. Placing any type of bone substitute in the socket is not recommended, and the socket only needs to be protected from soft tissue (epithelial and connective tissue) invasion in the socket. Whenever the membrane is exposed, or signs or symptoms are observed, using a tweezer, it can pull out without any surgeries and let nature take its course, which usually takes 2.5-3 months.

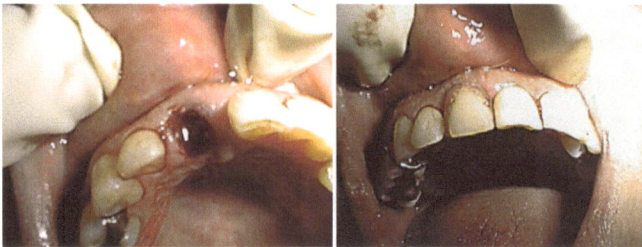

Figure 7.27 the buccal flange of the 11 is removed, and the denture is relined with tissue conditioner.

With this method, vertical incisions are not made, and the buccal vestibule will not be compromised.

Digital pressure with or without sterile gauze is forbidden. The patient may be prescribed antibiotics and analgesics for seven days, but their influence on success is uncertain.

Suppose a removable provisional prosthesis is placed. It is essential to remove the buccal flange (figure 7.27).

7.7. Sinus Lift Augmentation

The sinus mucosa is delicate and attaches to the periosteum on its osseous surface. A thin layer of respiratory epithelium lines the Schneiderian membrane. It cannot be differentiated as a separate layer from the periosteum of the bone to which it is tightly adherent. Blood supply to the antrum comes from branches of the internal maxillary artery, the alveolar artery, suborbital, ethmoidal, facial, palatal and ostial branches. Venous drainage is by the sphenopalatine vein and pterygomaxillary venous plexus.

After extraction of maxillary teeth, inadequate alveolar bone and pneumatization of the maxillary sinus are frequent findings. The following classification has been mentioned in chapter two and can be used as a guideline for treatment planning.

Closed sinus lift:

It is recommended that the minimum height implant placed in this region should be 11 mm. However, sometimes, the dentist has to make a choice - should he apply the closed sinus lift in a less invasive manner and place an 8mm implant, or perform an open sinus lift and place an 11 mm implant?

In clinical cases where the height of the alveolar bone below the maxillary sinus is class II, then a single osteotome intra-socket sinus lift is recommended. However, if the quality of the bone is not soft, then class III only with the 4mm of bone height would be enough to push the sinus floor with the remaining bone at the lateral aspect of the cavity and apical region (figure 4.19, 7.28).

Bone Width	Mm	Bone Height		Implant Angle		Crown Height	
A	6.5mm <	I	8mm <	A	0-15 °	1	Equal
B	3-6.5mm	II	4-8mm	B	15-40 °	2	+ 3mm
C	3mm >	III	4mm>	Γ	40 ° <	3	3mm<

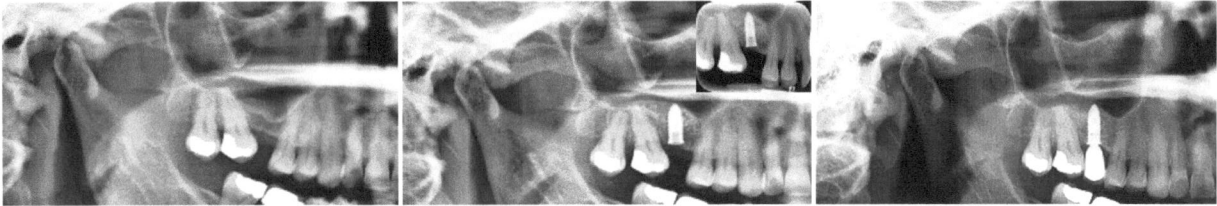
Figure 7.28 Intra-socket sinus lift is predictable and has minimal side effects.

Under local anaesthesia, a palatal para-crestal incision is made, and a full-thickness flap is elevated. Usually, a releasing incision is not required.

The following issues need to be considered.

The thickness of the cortex, The quality of the cancellous bone, The amount of bone height remaining, The amount of bone height which needs to be increased, The patient's psychological state (e.g. anxiety),

The need for sedation?

After the round drill penetrates the cortex, the pilot drill (diameter 2 - 2.2mm) prepares to three mm short of the sinus floor. This point can be detected by suddenly increased resistance to drilling. An osteotome with the same diameter, or one size smaller than the diameter of the dental implant, is used to fracture the sinus floor, and the membrane is raised by tapping the implant to its final length. When the bone quality is medium or hard, consecutive drills are used to prepare the site, but if the quality of the bone is soft. The preference is to continue using the serial osteotomes, and then the implant is inserted.

A collagen sponge may be used as a plunger to assist in hemostasis. It will also serve as a shock absorbent and a space-maker for bone formation. On average, some 2-4 mm of height can be gained. The prerequisite for this technique is a minimum presence of 4 mm of good-quality bone. When the bone quality is soft, it has been recommended that implants with micro threads and a tapered design be used. The claim is that this form will prevent the implant from sinking into the maxillary sinus under occlusal load, but the reference is unreliable 35.

The quality of the bone dictates the choice of surgical technique. This area usually has Type A bone width, Type II bone height, and poor bone quality. It can be treated by a closed (one-stage) osteotomy or "no waste bone technique" (full push forward technique) in these cases. In one stage, osteotomy, after making a dig in the cortical bone. The following instrument is an osteotome, which is one size smaller than the final diameter of the implant. The cortico-cancellous bone particles push more apically, gaining bone height in the approach.

Type III bone height can be treated only by an open sinus lift.

The worst scenario is BIII or CIII. In these instances, we cannot simultaneously expand the ridge and perform an open or closed sinus lift. Nor is there enough bone mass to be pushed toward the sinus floor.

When Types II and III bone height are found, and if the patient is lucky enough to have 3mm of bone width posterior to the sinus, it is more logical to place an implant in the palatal surface of the sinus. An acceptable angle will likely be available, but the maximum angle should be type beta.

Hazards are Screw implants, sealing screws, and soft bone. The dentist bears in mind that the apex of the implant will not have solid support; the bone is soft, and during the implant placement or sealing screw placement, the implant can fall into the sinus cavity. Thus, implants with a diameter at the crest larger than the apex can help prevent the scenario.

Poor height diagnosis from OPG; perhaps one of the sides of the prepared cavity has less bone, and the implant will not have contact with bone at the apical area of the dental implant.

Open sinus lift

No significant study has determined which graft material is superior, although it is usually accepted that autogenous bone is superior to an allogenic substitute.

In 1986, Tatum introduced a modified Caldwell-Luc procedure and lateral osteotomy, which fractured inward of the anterolateral wall and elevated sinus membrane and produced a cavity to insert graft particles.

The osteotomy approach uses a round head bur and elliptic window with a longer diameter mesiodistally, and no sharp edges exist to perforate the Schneiderian membrane. The sinus lift procedure is more reliable using specially designed mucosal elevators with long shanks. One stage and two stages of augmented sinus have been recommended if the primary stability of the implant immediately after the graft placement is predictable. In the two stages, augmenting in one stage of surgery and placing the implants after a few months, biopsy core samples of the augmented sinus are the ideal method to study the quality of the new bone formation during implant placement, which can reflect the length of the healing period.

Autogenous specimens demonstrate new bone formation with increased quantity and improved quality when compared to the specimens obtained from the sites grafted with allogenic bone. The author prefers a mixture of 50% allogenic and 50% autogenous bone to augment the sinus.

Due to the low bone density at the time of implant exposure, an instrument should be used to resist the torsional force during the removal of healing abutments. Gradual implant loading and control of occlusion to avoid overloading the implants is recommended.

Realising that the sinus floor is flat is essential in one-stage sinus lift surgery using a block graft. Underwood's septa increase the risk of sinus mucosa rupture, prevent stabilisation of a bone block, and impede the view of the sinus floor. The septa can be a complicated factor that the surgeon must bear in mind: a chisel and hemostat remove such septa.

The implant-bone interface was studied from a deceased patient who had had simultaneous bilateral maxillary sinus augmentation and implant placement after eight months. Two implants were observed: One implant was totally submerged in bone and graft material, and the other was devoid of bone at the apex. They concluded that eight months would not have been enough healing time before loading [36].

There is a debate on the merits of using a barrier membrane to cover the defect in the lateral wall of the sinus. Following sinus augmentation surgery, some reports of graft migration in the sinus and migration of connective tissue into the maxillary sinus can be observed [37,38].

Some implantologists prefer to use a barrier membrane that is better stabilised using pins to cover the window. However, a laborious second surgical procedure and possible site contamination are the downside of this procedure.

In order to determine the appropriate augmentation material, it is crucial first to understand the nature of the cavity that needs to be filled (figure 7.29).

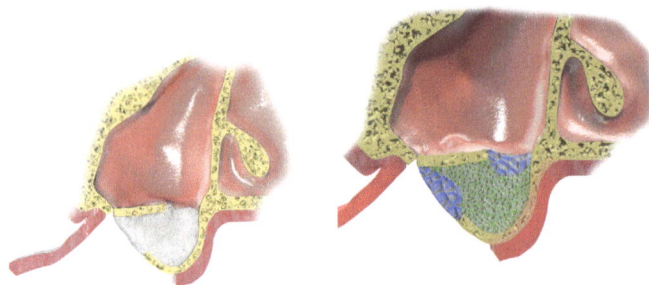

Figure 7.29 Coronal section of the maxillary sinus after reflecting the sinus membrane. Green sticks are fractured, pushing the cortex like opening the car's hood. The grafted area is green, and in the area without cortical bone support, the soft tissue (blue) may invade the grafted area.

There is an incomplete superior wall; the medial bony wall is covered by mucosa, so it does not have osteogenic potential; the inferior wall is bone, but in advanced cases, dehiscence can be observed, the inferior lateral wall is bone, but the rest of the lateral wall has been displaced as part of the preparation of the surgical site. Cortical bone does exist, but it is fragile (figure 7.30).

The main vulnerable area will be the superior area, which is better filled with predictable osteoinductive material.

It is recommended to use a trephine drill (less than the diameter of the implant) to remove the bone core and study the quality of the bone. The bone quality can be studied using histology sections; if the means are unavailable, a simple X-ray can show the bone quality (figure 7.31). That can affect the length of the healing period. If the quality is poor, a minimum of six months is recommended.

Other alternatives could be mentioned in a severe atrophic edentulous jaw where the patient is a poor candidate for major augmentation.

Digital technology enables the fabrication of custom-made subperiosteal implants (Mal Implants) using 3D printing, with data acquisition facilitated by CBCT (Cone Beam Computed Tomography) [40].

Quad zygoma implants have a high success rate in the maxillae, which can be immediately loaded with cross-arch stabilisation [41].

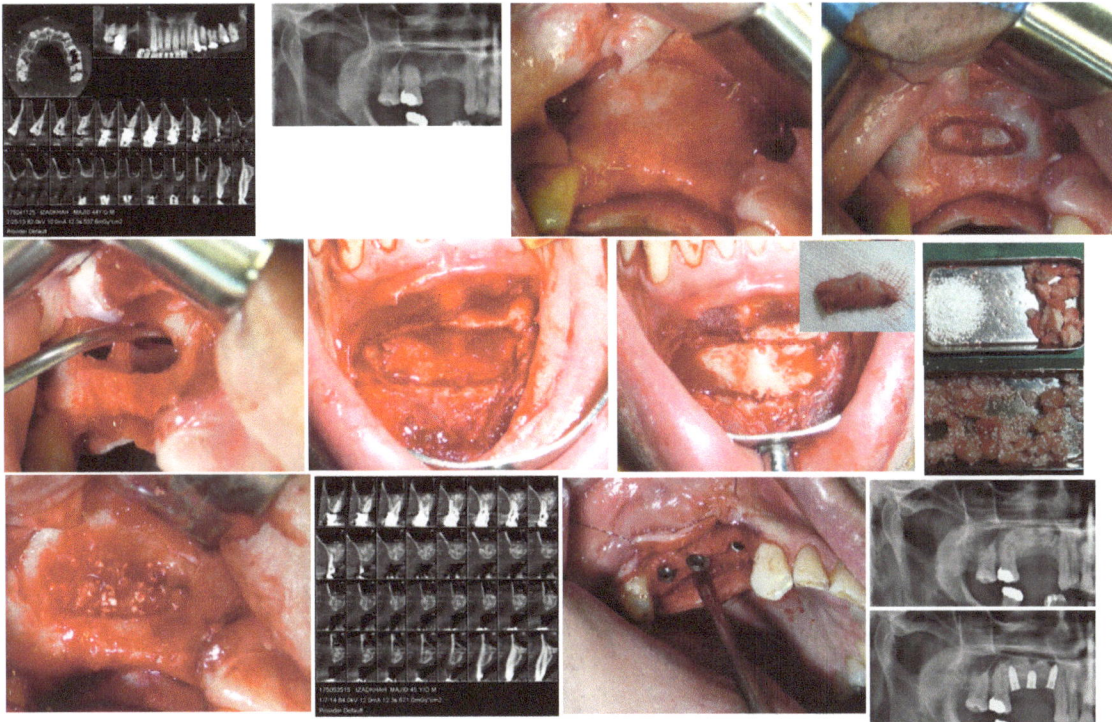

Figure 7.30 An open sinus lifts access through the anterolateral wall; sometimes, Underwood septa are observed at the sinus floor. Bone harvested from the chin, crushed and mixed with the bone substitute, will increase the volume and the radiopacity, making a better radiographic measurement. The final placement of the implants.

It is suggested that patients with sinus inflammation or infection and upper airway hypersensitivity should not be treated. Also, caution should be exercised with patients with compromised soft tissue (injury, post-radiation).

Aspergillosis and Escherichia coli infection, neurogenic pain, resorption of the graft, migration of the implant to an undesirable angulation in one-stage sinus lift, implant placement into the maxillary sinus during abutment connection, recurrent sinus infection are the main complications of the sinus lift augmentation and implant placement.

Smoking and raised intranasal pressure (e.g. nose-blowing, sneezing) are prohibited for several weeks following sinus surgery. Broad-spectrum antibiotics and nasal decongestants are prescribed. The graft should be placed below the level of the ostium.

If the Schneiderian membrane is perforated and is more than 1 mm, it needs to be sutured using 7/0 sutures or protected with membrane. One of the options is magnesium membrane [39].

Complications of sinus lift include sinusitis, malposition of dental implant, infection and prosthetic complications [42].

Zygomatic implants have been proposed to eliminate the need for major bone grafts to reconstruct atrophied maxillae. The literature has reported a high success rate but needs general anaesthesia.

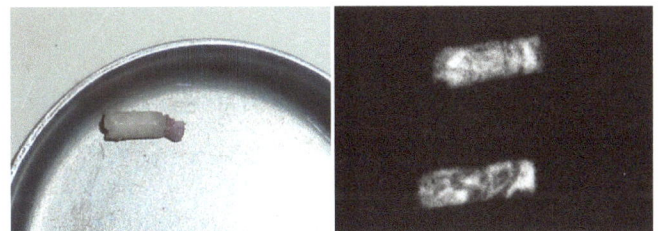

Figure 7.31 A biopsy of the grafted area and a micrograph were used to study the quality of the healed bone.

166

However, a host of complications have been reported. These include nasal or antral cavity penetration, loss of zygomatic implants due to overloading, speech alteration, difficulties in maintaining oral hygiene, invasion of the infratemporal fossa, chronic gingivitis, and intracerebral penetration. Thus, well-experienced dentists with a good background in oral surgery or ENT surgeons should apply the technique. If the angle is mesially inclined, the implant will end up in the nasopharynxor sphenoid sinus; if laterally-inclined - the infratemporal fossa; if cranially-inclined - the pterygopalatine fossae or temporal fossae will be invaded. The application of computed tomography cannot provide the necessary accuracy (figure 7.32).

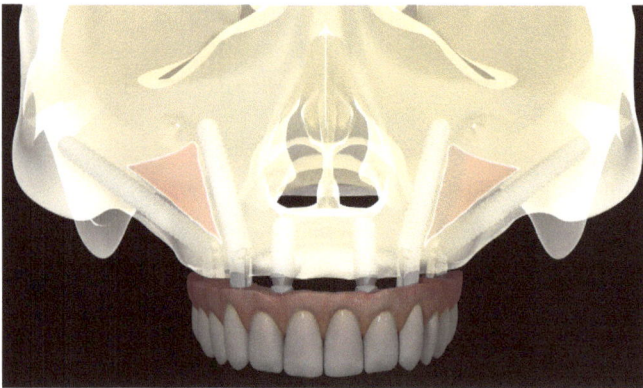

Figure 7.32 Zygomatic implants can be placed in different positions: intra-sinus, in the wall of maxillae and extra-sinus. The author prefers the wall of the maxillae technique.

References:

1. Schropp L, Wenzel A, Kostopoulos L, Karring T: Bone headlining and soft tissue contour changes following single-tooth extraction: a clinical and radiographic 12-month prospective study. Int j Periodontics Restorative Dent 2003;313-323.

2. Jensen SS, Terheyden H. Bone augmentation procedures in implant dentistry. Int J Oral Maxillofac Implants 2009;24(suppl):218-36.

3. Chipasco M, Casentini P, Zaniboni M. Bone augmentation procedures in implant dentistry. Int J Oral Maxillofac Implants 2009;24(Suppl): 237-59.

4. Aghaloo TL, Moy PK. Which hard tissue augmentation techniques are the most successful in furnishing bony support for implant placement. Int J Oral Maxillofacial Implant 2007;22(Suppl):49-70

5. Milinkovic I, Cordaro L. Are there specific indications for the different alveolar bone augmentation procedures for implant placement? A systemic review. Int J Oral Maxillofac Surg 2014;43:606-625.

6. von Arx T, Kurt B. Implant placement and simultaneous ridge augmentation using autogenous bone and a micro titanium mesh: a prospective clinical study with 20 implants. Clin Oral Implants Res 1;10:24–33.

7. Elangovan S. Implants Placed In Bone Augmented With Intra-Oral Grafts, Compared To Iliac Crest Grafts, May Have Better Survival Rates. J Evid Based Dent Pract. 2023 Dec;23(4):101927.

8. Al Haydar B, Kang P, Momen-Heravi F. Efficacy of Horizontal Alveolar Ridge Expansion Through the Alveolar Ridge Split Procedure: A Systematic Review and Meta-Analysis. Int J Oral Maxillofac Implants, . 2023 Dec 12;38(6):1083-1096.

9. Zitzmann NU, Naef R, Scharer P. Resorbable versus nonresorbable membranes in combi-nation with Bio-Oss for guided bone regen- eration. Int J Oral Maxillofac Implants 1997;12:844–52.

10. Milinkovic I, Cordaro L: Are there specific indications for the different alveolar bone augmentation procedures for implant placement? A systematic review. Int J Oral Maxillofac Surg. 2014 May;43(5):606-25. doi: 10.1016/j.ijom.2013.12.004. Epub 2014 Jan 19. Review.

11. Cho Y-S, Hwang K-G, Park -J. Postoperative effects of anterior nasal spine bone harvesting on overall nasal shape. Clin. Oral Impl. Res. 24, 2013, 618–622.

12. Kürkçü M, Oz IA, Köksal F, Benlidayi ME, Güneşli A: Microbial analysis of the autogenous bone collected by bone filter during oral surgery: a clinical study. J Oral Maxillofac Surg 2005, 63:1593–1598.

13. Takamoto M1, Takechi M, Ohta K, Ninomiya Y, Ono S, Shigeishi H, Tada M, Kamata N. Risk of bacterial contamination of bone harvesting devices used for autogenous bone graft in implant surgery. Head Face Med. 2013 Jan 11;9:3.

14. Gad LM, Wein M, Schmal H. Evaluation of MHC 1 and MHC 2 in alloge-neic bone blocks used for alveolar ridge reconstruction. J Biomed Mater Res B Appl Biomater 2015.

15. Jensen SS, Terheyden H. Bone augmentation procedures in localized defects in the alveolar ridge: clinical results with different bone grafts and bone-substitute materials. Int J Oral Maxillofac Implants. 2009;24 Suppl:218-36.

16. Kaner D, Friedmann A. Soft tissue expansion with self-filling osmotic tissue expanders before vertical ridge augmentation: a proof of principle study. Journal of Clinical Periodontology 2011, 38: 95–101.

17. Mertens C, Thiele O, Engel M, Seeberger R., Hoffmann J, Freier K. The use of self-inflating soft tissue expanders prior to bone augmentation of atrophied alveolar ridges. Clinic Implant Dent Relat Res 2017, 17(1): 44–51.

18. Abrahamsson P, Walivaara DA, Isaksson S, Andersson G. Periosteal expansion before local bone reconstruction using a new technique for measuring soft tissue profile stability: a clinical study. J Oral Maxillofac Surg 2012; 70(10): e521–e530.

19. Hoogeveen E.J, Gielkens, PFM, Schortinghuis, J, Ruben JL, Huysmans M, Stegenga B. Vivosorb as a barrier membrane in rat mandibular defects. An evaluation with transversal microradiography. Int J Oral Maxillofac Surg 2009, 38, 870–875.

20. Sela MN, Kohavi D, Krausz E, Steinberg D, Rosen G. Enzymatic degradation of collagen-guided tissue regeneration membranes by periodontal bacteria. Clin Oral Implants Res 14(3):263-8.

21. Hürzeler MB, Quiñones CR, Schüpbach P. Guided bone regeneration around dental implants in the atrophic alveolar ridge using a bioresorbable barrier. An experimental study in the monkey. Clin Oral Impl Res. 1997;8:323–331.

22. Saulacic N, Lizuka T, Martin S, Garcia G. Alveolar distraction osteogenesis: a systemic review. Int J Oral Maxillofac Surg 2008;37:1-7.

23. Schropp L, Wenzel A, Kostopoulos L, Karring T. Bone healing and soft tissue contour changes following single tooth extraction: a clinical and radiographic 12-month prospective study. Int J Periodontics Restorative Dent 2003;23(4):313–23.

24. Tan WL, Wong TL, Wong MC, Lang NP. A systematic review of post-extractional alveolar hard and soft tissue dimensional changes in humans. Clin Oral Implants Res 2012;23 Suppl 5:1–21.

25. Atieh MA, Alsabeeha NH, Payne AG, Duncan W, Faggion CM, Esposito M: Interventions for replacing missing teeth: alveolar ridge preservation techniques for dental implant site development. Cochrane Database Syst Rev. 2015 May 28;(5).

26. Araujo MG, Linder E, Lindhe J. Effect of a xenograft on early bone formation in extraction sockets: an experimental study in dog. Clin Oral Implants Res 2009;20(1):1–6.

27. O'Connor JLP, Milledge KL, O'Leary F, Cumming R, Eberhard J, Hirani V. Poor dietary intake of nutrients and food groups are associated with increased risk of periodontal disease among community-dwelling older adults: a systematic literature review. Nutr Rev 2020 Feb 1; 78 (2) : 175-188.

28. Calciolari E, Ercal P, Dourou M, Akcali A, Tagliaferri S, Donos N. The efficacy of adjunctive periodontal therapies during supportive periodontal care in patients with residual pockets. A systematic review and meta-analysis. J Periodontal Res 2022 Aug;57(4):671-689.

29. Tolentino PHMP, Rodrigues LG, de Torres EM, Franco A, Silva RF. Extractions in Patients with Periodontal Diseases and Clinical Decision-Making Process. Acta Stomatol Croat 2019 Jun;53(2):141-149.

30. Armitage GC. Periodontal diseases: diagnosis. Ann Periodontol 1996;1(1):37-215.

31. Moreira CHC, Zanatta FB, Antoniazzi R, Meneguetti PC, Rösing CK. Criteria adopted by dentists to indicate the extraction of periodontally involved teeth. J Appl Oral Sci 2007 Oct;15(5):437-41.

32. Alraqibah MA, Dayashankara Rao JK, Alharbi BM. Periotome versus piezotome as an aid for atraumatic extraction: a randomized controlled trial. J Korean Assoc Oral Maxillofac Surg. 2022 Dec 31; 48(6): 356–362.

33. Zhang X, Li Y, Ge Z, Zhao H, Miao L, Pan Y. The dimension and morphology of alveolar bone at maxillary anterior teeth in periodontitis: a retrospective analysis-using CBCT. Int J Oral Sci. 2020 Jan 14;12(1):4.

34. Couso-Queiruga E, Stuhr S, Tattan M, Chambrone L, Avila-Ortiz G. Post-extraction dimensional changes: A systematic review and meta-analysis. J Clin Periodontol 2021 Jan;48(1):126-144.

35. Kim HY, Yang JY, Chung BY, Kim JC, Yeo IS. Peri-implant bone length changes and survival rates of implants penetrating the sinus membrane at the posterior maxilla in patients with limited vertical bone height. J Periodontal Implant Sci 2013;43(2):58-63.

36. GaRey DJ; Whittaker JM; James RA; Lozada JL: The histologic evaluation of the implant interface with heterograft and allograft materials ;an eight-month autopsy report, Part II. J Oral Implantol 1991, 17 (4) :404-8.

37. Misch CM, Misch CE, Resnik RP, Ismail YH, Appel B: Post-operative maxillary cyst associated with a maxillary sinus elevation procedure. A case report. J Oral Implantol 1991;17:432-7.

38. Avera AP, Stampley WA, McAllister BS: Histologic and clinical observations of resorbable and nonresorbable barrier membranes usued in maxillary sinus graft containment. Int J Oral Maxillofac Implants 1997;12:88-94.

39. Elad A, Pul L, Rider P, Rogge S, Witte F, Tadić D, Mijiritsky E, Kačarević ZP, Steigmann L. Resorbable magnesium metal membrane for sinus lift procedures: a case series. BMC Oral Health, 2023 Dec 14;23(1):1006.

40. Zielinski R, Sowinski J, Piechaczek M, Okulski J, Kozakiewicz M. Finite Element Analysis of Subperiosteal Implants in Edentulism-On the Basis of the Mal Implant® by Integra Implants®. Materials (Basel), 2023 Nov 30;16(23):7466.

41. Davó R, Fan S, Wang F, Wu Y. Long-term survival and complications of Quad Zygoma Protocol with Anatomy-Guided Approach in severely atrophic maxilla: A retrospective follow-up analysis of up to 17 years. Clin Implant Dent Relat Res 2023 Dec 12. doi: 10.1111/cid.13296. Online ahead of print.

42. Lan K, Wang F, Huang W, Davó R, Wu Y. Quad Zygomatic Implants: A Systematic Review and Meta-analysis on Survival and Complications. Int J Oral Maxillofac Implants. 2021 Jan-Feb;36(1):21-29.

CHAPTER EIGHT:

INTERDISCIPLINARY CARE: COLLABORATIVE COMMUNICATIONS WITH SPECIALITIES

8. INTERDISCIPLINARY CARE: COLLABORATIVE COMMUNICATIONS WITH SPECIALITIES

Aim:

To emphasise the significance of interdisciplinary collaboration between young dentists and medical specialities, illustrating how such partnerships can elevate patient care. Special attention is given to the intersection of dental implantology with diverse fields of medicine, demonstrating the collective impact on overall patient health and treatment outcomes.

Necessary Knowledge base:

It is assumed at this stage that you have a general knowledge of basic science related to dental implantology, documentation and record keeping, patient assessment and treatment planning, dental implant and augmentation surgical techniques.

Learning Outcome:

• Understand the key aspects of interdisciplinary communication with ENT surgeons, oral surgeons, general anaesthetists, and other dental surgery disciplines.
• Appreciate the impact of effective collaboration on patient care and treatment outcomes in the context of complex dental surgeries and procedures.

> Dental implant and bone graft surgery can be treated under local anaesthetic , IV sedation or general anaesthesia. Management of the airway will be more difficult as the Mallampati score increases.
>
> When I.V. sedation is not recommended or even unsuccessful, then day surgery under general anaesthesia will be the next option.

Dental implant treatment planning involves orthodontics, periodontics, and restorative prosthetics. Conscious sedation or general anaesthesia may be considered based on the type of surgery proposed and the patient's tolerance. The dentist must have a general knowledge of the other disciplines to communicate with other physicians and dentists, especially general anaesthetics, ENT surgeons, and different dental specialists.

8.1.   General anaesthesia and sedation

Dental implant surgery could be associated with patient anxiety, which may increase symptomatic activity. Mindfulness meditation can be used as a sedation technique. It decreases the bispectral index (quantifies the level of hypnosis by the algorithm of electroencephalographic signals, which 71-90 indicates sedation), heart rate, and blood pressure, and increases SpO2 and decreases cortisol level [1].

Dental implant and bone graft surgery can be treated under local anaesthetic, IV sedation or general anaesthesia (as a day case). The use of IV sedation in dentistry has gained popularity, and we now have 25 years of experience using Midazolam without any complications.

Each country has its regulations or guidelines which need to be respected, but generally, in a dental office or surgery, the patient must be ASA I, a non-smoker, and under 70 to be treated by I.V. sedation with Midazolam. In elderly patients, the reduced total body water content and cardiac output require a reduced initial dose, and we recommend that it not be performed in a dental clinic [2].

The patient's medical status and airway need to be studied.

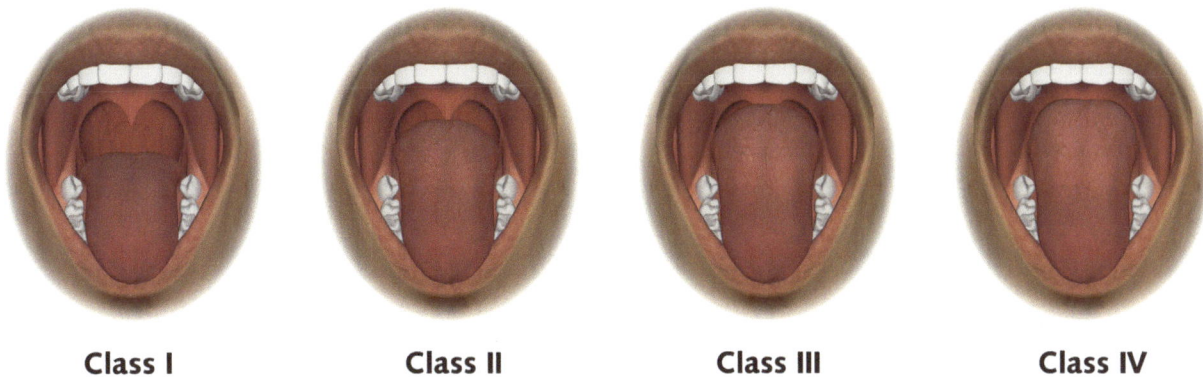

Figure 8.1 Positions of the tongue classified by Mallampati.

Mallampati classified the position of the tongue to:

Class I Complete visualisation of the uvula, tonsillar pillars, and soft palate

Class II Partial visibility of the uvula and complete soft palate

Class III Only the soft palate is visible

Class IV Only the hard palate is visible

Management of the airway will be more difficult as the score increases.

It is recommended that at the initial appointment, the patient's blood pressure, pulse, and ECG are recorded using one hand-held lead and oxygen concentration using a pulse oximeter. The same procedure is repeated on the day of surgery, and if there are any significant differences, then any elective surgery under sedation must be reconsidered and very likely not performed.

I.V. conscious sedation is defined as a drug-induced depression of consciousness during which patients respond purposefully to verbal commands alone or when commands are accompanied by light tactile stimulation. No interventions are required to maintain a patent airway, the patient maintains normal breathing, and cardiovascular function is normal.

Administration of incremental drug doses is given until a desired effect is reached. Knowledge of each drug's time of onset, peak response and duration of action is essential to avoid overdose.

Assessment categories				
Responsiveness	Speech	Facial Expression	Eyes	Score
Responds to name	Normal	Normal	Clear, no ptosis	5 (alert)
Lethargic response to name	Mild slow	Mild relaxation	Mild ptosis	4
Respond to loud voice to name	Slurring	Marked relaxation (slack jaw)	Marked ptosis (half the eye or more)	3
Respond to mild shaking.	Few recognisable voices	-	-	2
Does not respond to shaking	-	-	-	1 (deep sleep)

Table 8.1 Sedation assessment by scores 1-5.

If movements, hyperactivity, and combativeness have been observed during the surgery under I.V. sedation, it is recommended not to continue the surgery and the sedation. This scenario should be predicted/anticipated and mentioned to the patient during treatment planning.

Post-operative instructions should be handed to the patient before the surgery, and a letter should be sent to the patient afterwards.

Printed instructions given to the patient before the operation might include:

"When you are home:

Printed instructions given to the patient before the operation might include:

• Eat a healthy meal to restore your energy.

• You should be able to return to your everyday activities the next day.

• Avoid driving, operating machinery, drinking alcohol, and making legal decisions for at least 24 hours.

• Check with your doctor before taking any medicines or herbal supplements.

• If you had surgery, follow your doctor's instructions for recovery and wound care".

When I.V. sedation is not recommended or even unsuccessful, then day surgery under general anaesthesia will be the next option. The definition of day surgery in the UK and Ireland is clear: the patient must be admitted and discharged on the same day, with day surgery as the intended management programme. It is still counted as in-patient treatment in the UK but not in the US. Shortened hospital stays and earlier mobilisation also reduce the risk of hospital-acquired infections and venous thromboembolism (VTE).

General anaesthesia is ideal for phobic patients, for whom conscious sedation may not be enough to deal with their anxiety, for cases when oral surgery or complicated dental procedures are needed, and when the patient wants the experience to be completely pain-free. When the dentist and the patient agree that the surgery will be done under general anaesthesia, the dentist must request a blood test, chest X-ray (if indicated), and a letter to the anaesthetist to visit the patient at least 24 hours prior to the surgery.

One of the complications of general anaesthesia is vomiting or nausea. Even though the surgical staff is not important, for the patient and their families beside him, it is a traumatic experience. It undermines the psychological relationship between the patient and the medical staff and undermines all the hard work done by the dentist and the medical staff.

Nausea is a subjective and unpleasant awareness of the presence of vomit. Vomiting is a forceful expulsion of stomach contents via the mouth by powerful contractions of the abdominal muscles. This is caused by anxiety and the swallowing of blood. The stimuli of nausea and vomiting are psychogenic, olfactory, visual, and vestibular. These affect the higher brain centres, although the mechanism is not clear. The associated signs and symptoms are increased salivation, pallor, tachycardia, hot and cold sensations, sweating, gastrointestinal motility and relaxation, duodenal retro peristalsis, and decreased gastric acid secretion.

Severe nausea and vomiting are complications of GA, which patients themselves rate as worse than post-operative pain. The incidence rate is 25-30% in hospitals, is lower in outpatient clinics, and can lead to delayed discharge.

Benzamides are the least expensive and safest agents for preventing and treating nausea and vomiting. If the patient has been identified as high-risk, they should be treated prophylactically. The use of a Scopolamine patch has been shown to be effective, but it does enhance sedation [3]. Some patches are placed in the back of the ear before the general anaesthesia.

Anticipating problems around general anaesthesia:

The placement of a breathing tube may leave the patient with a sore throat for a couple of days; injury to the lips, tongue, or teeth may happen when the breathing tube is inserted. The risk of dental damage increases, if the teeth are already loose or cracked or vulnerable crowns or bridgework are not noted. There is always the risk of postoperative nausea with most types of anaesthesia, especially if the patient is predisposed to motion sickness or has difficulty with narcotic pain medications. Anaesthetists prefer to establish an airway via the mouth. Placing a tracheal tube for a period of time runs the risk of drying the laryngeal and tracheal mucosa, impairing their ciliary activity. For oral surgery and dental implant surgery, nasal intubation is necessary, and a north-polar tube, formerly known as a maxillofacial tube, should be used, attached to the forehead (figure 8.2). During intubation, the anaesthetist must be careful not to damage the surgical area, especially if one-piece implants have been placed. It is recommended that the one-piece implants be splinted prior to removal of the tube.

Steps to prepare the patient for general anaesthesia:

In some countries, dentists can request routine laboratory and urine tests, white and red blood cell counts, coagulation studies, and kidney function tests like Blood Urea Nitrogen (BUN), Creatinine, blood glucose, and electrolyte levels. The urine test is used to reveal any urinary tract infection or diabetes or to diagnose dehydrated patients. Usually, hospitals do not accept the tests after six weeks.

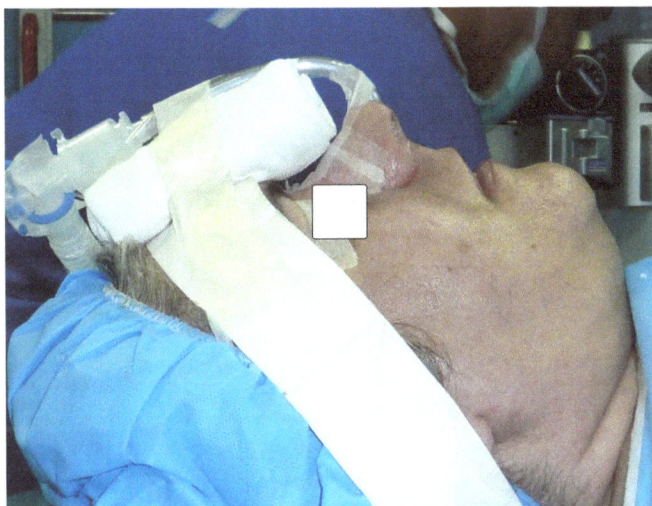

Figure 8.2 Nasal intubation using the north polar tube.

In other countries, they refer the patient to the hospital, and the hospital management takes over.

Clinicians may predict most abnormal preoperative and chest radiographs based on the history and physical examination, and chest radiography only rarely provides unexpected information that influences preoperative management.

The patient should clearly understand the instructions regarding medication they should or should not be taking and when precisely before surgery. They must be instructed, verbally and in writing, when to stop eating and drinking prior to surgery. They must stop eating and drinking before surgery to prevent impairment of the normal reflexes that close the vocal cords, thus preventing inhalation of partially digested food stomach acids. This

is despite the use of endotracheal tubes during general anaesthesia to prevent this complication. The dentist should explain the procedure, stating that a tube is placed in the patient's throat to protect the airway and ensure the passage of oxygen (and anaesthetic gases like nitrous oxide) [4].

In 2001, the American Society of Anaesthesiologists (ASA) recommendations on pre-operative Chest X-rays stated, "Clinical characteristics to consider: include smoking, recent upper respiratory infection, COPD, and cardiac disease, asthma, age more than 55'.

The anaesthetist must conduct the pre-anaesthetic visit a minimum of 24 hours before the surgery. In meeting the patient, the anaesthetist can identify potential complications and alleviate the patient's anxiety.

Elective surgery, like dental implant surgery, is not recommended for patients with the following conditions or habits:

• diabetes, seizures, asthma, respiratory and cardiovascular problems, tuberculosis, smoking

• excessive alcohol intake

• drug abuse

• previous adverse reactions to anaesthetics

• pregnancy

• taking medications that can reduce the effect of the anaesthetics or may interact adversely with the anaesthesia.

8.2.　ENT Surgeon
Benign　Paroxysmal　Positional　Vertigo (BPPV)

A maxillary sinus lift is a safe and predictable procedure for increasing alveolar bone height in the postero-superior alveolar region. It enables both effective oral rehabilitation and the restoration of full masticatory function, even in the case of a previously atrophic maxilla.

Two types of sinus lift procedures have been documented: closed (direct) sinus lift and open (indirect) sinus lift.

The open sinus lift begins by creating a window through the anterolateral wall of the sinus and then pushing up the sinus membrane.

The closed sinus lift is the lifting of the floor of the sinus, with its membrane, through the implant placement osteotomy, but without gaining access through the anterolateral wall of the sinus. This procedure involves the use of the mallet, and one of

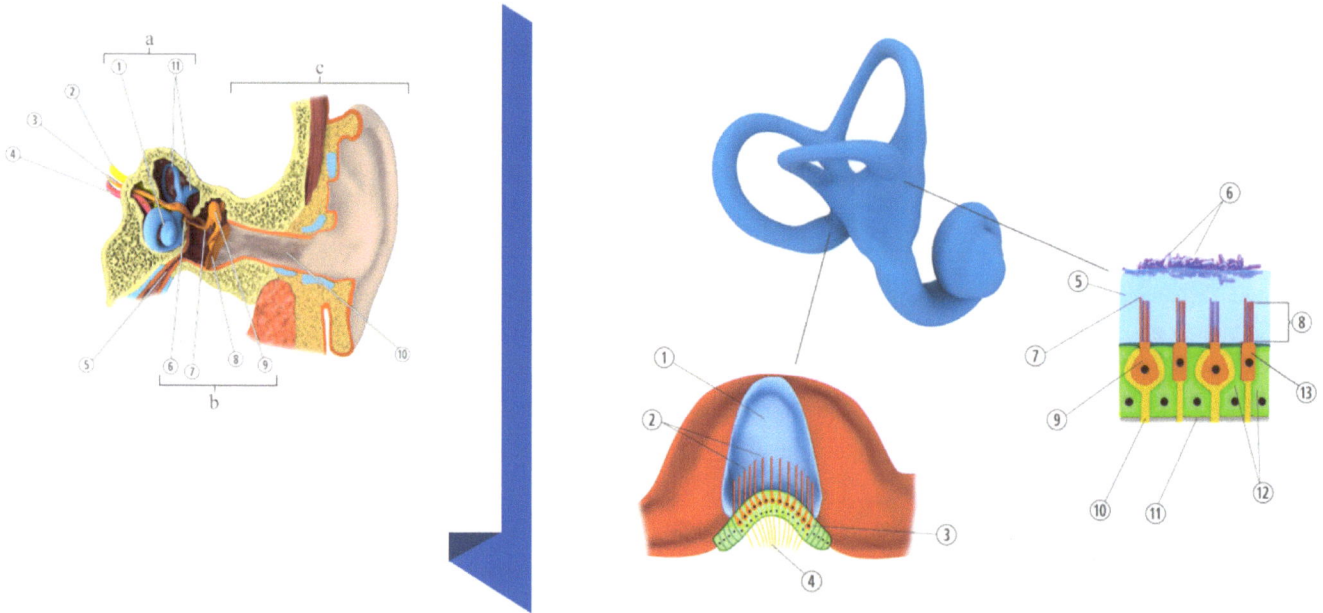

Figure 8.4 The internal anatomy of the ear demonstrates the position of otoconia and its relationship with the vestibular system.

Left: a (inner ear), b (middle ear), c (outer ear). 1-Cochlea, 2-Facial nerve, 3-Vestibular nerve, 4-Auditory nerve, 5-Eustachean tube, 6-Stapes, 7-Incus, 8-Ear drum, 9-Malleus, 10-Ear canal, 11-Semicircular canals. Right: Vestibular system, lower left; enlargement of Crista; 1) cupula, 2) hair bundles, 3) hair cells, 4) nerve fibre. Right: enlargement of the macula; 5) otolithic membrane, 6) otoconia, 7) kinocilium, 8) stereocilia, 9) type I hair cells, 10) nerve fibre, 11) basement membrane, 12) supporting cells, 13) type II hair cell.

possible (if rare) complications is Benign Paroxysmal Positional Vertigo (BPPV). Only one case of BPPV during an open sinus lift has been reported.

The mallet causes tiny crystals of the calcium carbonate called Otoconia, a normal part of the inner ear's anatomy, to detach the from the otolithic membrane in the utricle and collect in one of the semi-circular canals. The fibrous otolithic membrane is in the inner ear's vestibular system and plays a central role in the brain's equilibrium interpretation.

While the head remains still, these crystals will settle through gravity. As soon as the head moves, the crystals shift and stimulate the cupula, sending false signals to the brain. The cupula is a jellylike cap that is displaced by water movement, and the hair beneath it is bent, activating the nerve.

This produces vertigo, nystagmus (involuntary eye movements), nausea, and vomiting. These signs will typically arise immediately after the surgery or the following day.

The symptoms of BPPV may recede without treatment. The em-

ployment of Epley or Semont manoeuvres will usually reduce the symptoms or even eliminate them. Antihistamines, sedatives, or scopolamine can be used, but the patient needs to be referred to an ENT surgeon for examination. Gentle malleting or the avoidance of hyper-extension of the neck may prevent the unwanted event in the first place [5].

The symptoms are dizziness or vertigo, lightheadedness, a feeling of imbalance and nausea. Changing the head position, getting out of bed, or rolling over in bed brings on the symptoms. The leading cause is degeneration of the inner ear's vestibular system, which is worn or torn by otoliths. Ear rock or Otoconia are calcium carbonate, and they are not able to migrate into the canal system unless predisposing factors are present. Precipitating factors can be head injury, prolonged supine positioning during dental treatment, or vibration from drilling. There is a relationship between BPPV and migraine. Viruses or medications like Gentamicin can also cause BPPV [6].

The diagnosis is based on history, physical examination, and

175

the result of vestibular and auditory tests, which are not usually necessary.

The Dix Hallpike manoeuvre involves moving the head of the patient 45° to one sight, moving the patient from sitting to the supine position, and, after 30 seconds, moving the patient back to the sitting position.

If no nystagmus is observed as a diagnostic marker, the procedure is then repeated on the left side.

Nystagmus is a vision condition in which the eyes make repetitive, uncontrolled movements. These movements often result in reduced vision and depth perception, affecting balance and coordination. These involuntary eye movements can occur from side to side, up and down, or in a circular pattern. https://www.youtube.com/watch?v=wgWOmuB1VFY is an excellent animation to observe.

If further investigations are needed, the patient should be referred to an ENT specialist to organize/perform Electronystagmography (ENG) or MRI tests.

The treatment is usually to wait 12 months and see if most symptoms disappear by then. If patients accept this, they must avoid sleeping on the wrong side. When they wish to rise from the bed, they need to get up slowly, sit on the edge of the bed for a minute, and avoid extending their head or picking something up from the floor. Usually, the patient opts for treatment instead of waiting too long. There are different diagnostic and treatment approaches, of which the most common is the Epley manoeuvre, which is as follows:

After diagnosis of the affected side, the patient sits on the bed's edge and turns his head to the affected side. The patient lies down, but a pillow is placed under the shoulder (not under the head). The head position should not change, and wait for 30 seconds till the vertigo stops. Then, turn the head 90 degrees to the other side and wait 30 seconds. Finally, slowly sits up but stays on the bed for a few minutes. The movements should be applied three times before going to bed at night, and after the dizziness stops, continue for 24 hours.

Sometimes, a second treatment is needed. If neurological symptoms like weakness or numbness are elicited, then this means that vertebral arteries are under compression, and if this is allowed to persist, a stroke could occur.

To reduce the chances of recurrence, the patient must sleep semi-recumbent (45 degrees) for the next night. During the following day, the patient must keep their head vertical, and any dental treatment or hair appointment should be cancelled. For one week following this diagnosis, the patient must use two pillows to sleep on and avoid extending the head. After one week, the patient can cautiously adopt the position that made them dizzy. Surgery is the last option that the ENT surgeon will have in mind.

Sinusitis:

The sinus lift procedure has a well-recognised impact on the delicate homeostasis of the maxillary sinus.

The presence of persistent nasosinusal or maxillary sinus disease may encourage the development of postoperative complications (particularly maxillary rhinosinusitis), which can compromise an otherwise good surgical outcome.

Because of these considerations, the management of sinus lift candidates should include the identification of any situations which may contraindicate the procedure. If naso-sinusal disease is suspected, a clinical assessment by an ear, nose and throat specialist is essential. This should include nasal endoscopy and, if necessary, a computed tomography scan of the maxillo-facial region, particularly the osteomeatal complex.

This first stage in the clinical assessment is preventive and diagnostic and should be dedicated to detecting potentially irreversible contraindications to a sinus lift.

The second stage is preventive and therapeutic. It is aimed at correcting (mainly with the aid of endoscopic surgery) such potentially reversible ear, nose and throat contraindications as middle-meatal anatomical structural impairments, phlogistic-infective diseases and benign naso-sinusal neoplasms, the removal of which allows the recovery of naso-sinusal homeostasis. This can restore the physiological drainage and ventilation of the maxillary sinus.

The third stage is post-operative and is diagnostic and therapeutic. It is only required if mainly infective and sinus complications arise after sinus lift surgery. It aims to ensure early diagnosis and prompt treatment of maxillary rhinosinusitis to avoid implant loss and related adverse sequelae.

Thus, before undertaking a sinus lift, the surgeon must consider its impact on sinus physiology to avoid unwelcome complications. An ENT surgeon should be asked to provide the primary specialist opinion. This should hold for any approach to a sinus lift procedure, as the ENT surgeon's help will be a vital aspect of the procedure if surgical success is to be assured.

There have been attempts at experimental surgical strategies, such as the combined two-step procedure, in which the ENT surgeon first restores maxillary sinus ventilation endoscopically by resolving the pathological process or the anatomical alteration which initially contraindicated implant surgery. Then, after a period of at least 3-4 weeks, the oral surgeon performs the sinus lift and places the implants.

As an expert in nasosinusal physiology, the ENT surgeon should also play a helpful role in defining, with the implantologist, a prophylactic regimen for the candidate for sinus lift to reduce the risk of complications.

These would include instructions to:

- Stop smoking
- Avoid dehydration,
- Avoid pollutant inhalation,
- Avoid exposure to low temperatures or dry air,
- Avoid consumption of atropine-like drugs.

These are only a few examples of the hygiene rules indicated for the patient.

8.3. Dental Specialist

Implant treatment is a prosthetic-driven surgical speciality. Placing a dental implant in a surgically formed bony space immediately calls for the cooperation of associated specialities for future crowns, and the artificial root called dental implant or fixture must be provided. That is why other disciplines in dentistry could be involved.

The loss of teeth over a long period of time can lead to the extrusion of opposing teeth, which their surrounding bone and gums may accompany. Correcting occlusal discrepancies may or may not involve orthodontics.

Occlusal reduction with or without endodontic treatment is clearly an option, but the financial and time concerns must be considered.

In severe cases, or when the patient does not wish to have endodontic or orthodontic treatment to intrude on the teeth, partial segment osteotomy offers an option.

Incomplete or unsuccessful orthodontic treatment and lack of space apically to place a dental implant is one of the complications that may arise when there is no communication between an orthodontist and the dentist responsible for implant placement.

8.4. Communication with other specialists:

This section covers the patient's general health, especially the presence of any systemic disease which may impact any proposed implant treatment. This requires communication with the patient's doctor and any appropriate medical specialist.

Although dentists are generally aware of the need for such communication, doctors are less so.

This demands a sound understanding of systemic disease and how this applies to the patient. Some countries like the UK have strict guidelines regarding dental management of medically compromised patients, and many do not and are left to the dentist's judgment and school of taught. The guidelines between countries differ. It is recommended that the dentist be aware that in this book, we are just giving general knowledge, and the dentist needs to adjust him/herself to the country's regulations.

ENDOCRINE DISEASE

Diabetes

Diabetes is a risk factor for periodontitis. Periodontal infection can affect glycaemic control in diabetic patients, leading to tooth attachment to alveolar bone loss. This is known as the "sixth complication" of diabetes. Unfortunately, GMPs are sadly unfamiliar with dental pathology and, therefore, less concerned with preventing or curing periodontal disease and its attendant complications. Diabetes can cause delayed healing, unstable fibrointegration, and infection. The quality of glycaemic control is essential for successful dental implant treatment.

Diabetes Type 2 - Patients with HbA1c values of 0-8% have a higher success rate, but any delay in healing should be checked for before the final impression is taken.

Dental implant surgery is feasible in selected diabetic patients with the employment of careful patient preparation and follow-up. These conditions reinforce the need for a dialogue between dentists and diabetologists in order to offer patients the best chances of success.

Thyroid and Parathyroid

Both the thyroid and parathyroid glands influence the level of blood Ca2+. The thyroid reduces the level of blood Ca through the effect of calcitonin, which inhibits osteoclastic activity, while the parathyroid raises blood Ca through the effect of PTH hormone, which inhibits osteoblastic activity,

Anaemia

There are different types of anaemia, but all may induce ulceration, glossitis and angular cheilitis. People who bruise or bleed easily and develop anaemia may have problems with their blood's ability to clot.

Afro-Caribbeans especially, along with Mediterraneans, Middle Easterners and Indians, have a tendency towards sickle cell anaemia. In these cases, the need for haemoglobin electrophoresis needs to be emphasised.

Bleeding disorders

Platelet disorders and coagulation defects may impede implant treatment. The patient should be managed at a special centre or through direct liaison with the patient's doctor.

Aspirin is the most common cause of bleeding; the effect may last up to one week.

As dental implant surgery is elective surgery, it should be embarked upon only when platelet levels are at least 50*109 /L. Ideally, it should be above 75*109/L.

If active bleeding is noted, tranexamic acid, preferably as a mouthwash, should be used. If necessary, platelet transfusion should be given immediately before or during the surgery.

Coagulation defects may arise in haemophiliacs, patients on anticoagulants or those with liver disease. These cases must be managed through liaison with the relevant specialist or the patient's GP.

Patients using anticoagulants like Heparin (IV or subcutaneous) may find that the effect wears off in about 8 hours, and only in an emergency should protamine sulfate be used. The activated partial thromboplastin time (APTT) needs to be measured.

Low-molecular-weight heparin (subcutaneous) has little effect on APTT and is usually used for short-term deep-vein thrombosis. Its use for the reversal of protamine sulphate is partially effective.

The effects of oral Warfarin last up to 48 hours. The INR should be 2-4; Vitamin K1 and/or fresh frozen plasma are needed in an emergency.

Metronidazole is used a lot in dental implant surgery, and the dentist needs to remember that the patient taking Warfarin and given a concurrent prescription for Metronidazole has an increased anticoagulant effect. Metronidazole inhibits CYP2C9, the enzyme responsible for S-warfarin metabolism. The delayed metabolism of Warfarin enhances the anticoagulant effect and increases the likelihood of bleeding complications. There are reports of ototoxicity after using Metronidazole, which, after four to 6 weeks following withdrawal, gradually recovered.

Vitamins E and C can also have slight blood-thinning effects.

The Scottish Dental Clinical Effectiveness Programme (SDCEP) has provided guidelines which the author advises even non-UK-based dentists to study. If the treatment may cause bleeding, it is advised to plan treatment early in the day and week, provide pre-treatment instructions, treat atraumatic as possible and only discharge the patient once haemostasis has been achieved. Provide post-treatment advice and emergency contact details.

Do not interrupt anticoagulant or antiplatelet therapy for patients with prosthetic metal heart valves or coronary stents. History of pulmonary embolism or deep vein thrombosis in the last three months of the patient for cardioversion, it is better for non-urgent treatments to be delayed till after three months.

For high bleeding risk of dental procedures with low certainty evidence, treat in the morning and first do limited initial treatment area before complex procedures.

There are four categories of drugs which will increase bleeding in invasive dental procedures:

1. Direct Oral Anticoagulant (DOAC) drugs, which are scheduled twice a day (Apixaban, Dabigatran), miss the morning dose and are taken at the usual time in the evening. Drugs taken once a day (Rivaroxaban, Edoxaban) delay the morning dose till 4 hours after haemostasis, and if taken in the evening, take it at the usual time in the evening.

2. Vitamin K antagonist (Warfarin, Acenocoumarol): The last 24 hours of INR should be between 2 and 4.

3. Injectable Anticoagulant (Dalteparin, Enoxaparin, Tinzaparin): Consult with the clinician as the implant is a selective surgery.

4. Antiplatelet drugs (Aspirin, Clopidogrel, Dipyridamole): the medication should not interrupted even in invasive dental surgeries.

Few dentists believe that stopping aspirin for a couple of days will reduce the tendency to bleed. Bear in mind that the half-life of aspirin is about 20 minutes; however, after a single dose of aspirin, platelet COX activity recovers after about ten days.

It is advised to discuss the issue with the patient as having more swelling or bruise after implant placement is safer than stopping anticoagulant therapy.

Stages of Hypertension	Systolic Blood Pressure (mm Hg)	Diastolic Blood Pressure
Normal	<120	<80
Prehypertension	120–139	80–89
Stage 1 hypertension	140–159	90–99
Stage 2 hypertension	≥160	≥100
Hypertensive urgency	Severe hypertension	>120, no end-organ damage
Hypertensive emergency	Severe hypertension	>120, end-organ damage
d ptosis	d ptosis	d ptosis

Cardiovascular diseases

Blood pressure (BP) above 140 systolic and 90 diastolic for more than three months is considered hypertension. About 95% of cases are classed as essential hypertension, and the rest are considered to be due to renal dysfunction or endocrine disorder[7]. Having the pulse rate and blood pressure taken at the consultation appointment is essential. The patient's baseline BP is recorded in the reception room, where their stress level is likely lower than in the surgery itself. On the day of the surgery, the pulse and BP need to be re-checked at reception. If it is high, the author recommends that the surgery be cancelled and the

patient referred back to his GP. If a BP of 160/10 is observed (Stage II hypertension), some believe that surgery can still be carried out. The author disagrees and believes that no surgery should be undertaken when a patient has developed Stage II hypertension. He believes surgery should be cancelled and the patient referred to the GP or specialist.

Patients with a PMH of rheumatic fever with a damaged heart valve do not require prophylaxis. It is recommended that a minimum of 3 months elapse after an MI before surgery can again be undertaken, subject to specialist approval. For surgery, it is imperative to use adequate local anaesthesia, which may still be better with sedation. The best choice of local anaesthetic is plain Mepivacaine 3%.

Respiratory diseases

General anaesthetics and sedatives which reduce the respiratory drive should be avoided. It is not a bad idea for simple spirometers to be used during the recent virus pandemic, but they are not recommended in dental surgeries for cross-infection control reasons. NSAIDs may exacerbate asthma.

Patients suffering from COPD may prefer to be treated sitting upright; always ask the patient.

Dry mouth due to mouth breathing needs to be considered. If the patient is using a corticosteroid inhaler, there is a chance of oral candidiasis and rinsing the mouth after inhaler application should be recommended.

Gastro-intestinal diseases

Patients with GI tract conditions may be on medication, and the contra-indications relevant to those drugs need to be considered. Bear in mind that the patient may be under steroids or immunosuppressants. The dentist might be tempted to prescribe NSAIDs, but the patient's GI condition could preclude their use. Small and large bowel disorders may reflect anaemia and chronic deficiencies.

Hepatic diseases

The increased likelihood of bleeding should be expected. Anaemia and hepatitis B, C, and D must be considered, and the relevant cross-infection guidelines for prevention and against transmission are strictly applied. Metabolism and excretion of drugs may be affected. It may be better to arrange for a general blood and coagulation screen. Vitamin K and/or fresh frozen plasma should be available.

Excess alcohol reduces platelet numbers and function. History can help as bleeding or bruising easily if there is doubt, FBC and liver function tests (Albumin, Alanine aminotransferase or ALT, Alkaline phosphatase as ALP, serum bilirubin, Gamma-glutamyl transferase or GGT, Aspartate aminotransferase or AST) recommended. Also, prothrombin time (PT) and international normalised ratio (INR) are used to study clotting.

Renal disorders

Patients with renal disease carry a heightened risk of infection, which may be exacerbated by any immunosuppressive drugs which may be prescribed. Renal patients have a bleeding tendency. They may also fail to excrete some drugs fully, and this can induce toxicity.

Renal disease can also lead to renal osteodystrophy and osteoporosis. Renal osteodystrophy itself can result in secondary hyperparathyroidism, and both can, in turn, produce bone lesions in the jaws. DPT and CBCT features will show bone demineralisation by decreased trabeculation and decreased thickness of cortical bone. There will be the typical ground glass appearance (a hazy opacity) of bone and metastatic soft tissue calcification and radiolucency consisting of giant cell lesions and generally lytic areas in the bone.

There is a possibility that the renal patient may be a carrier of HepB and/or HIV. If the patient is under dialysis and due for surgery, the best day is the day after dialysis when the INR result is available.

The author recommends being more considerate of the bone around dental implants in these cases.

An extension to the healing period and the use of a provisional crown with lowered occlusal force before the final restoration, which is called progressive loading, in which the bone gradually matures under tension, is recommended. In a partial long-span bridge, incrementally increase the occlusal table's height from infra occlusion of more than 0.16 mm (16 um), which is controlled by double layers of shim stock passing freely through the occlusal contact to complete occlusion. In single tooth replacement, the author recommends that 0.12 mm (12 um) be off occlusion using black/red Arti-Fol metallic (Bausch) [8].

Immunocompromised patients

Of those patients who are immunocompromised, the group of individuals who face the worst scenario are those with AIDS. There is a high tendency towards infection, so cross-infection control needs to be strict. CD4 T-lymphocyte defect or reduction of numbers can start with a simple flu-like illness.

Osteoporosis

Osteoporosis is a lack of bone matrix with inadequate bone mineralisation. The patient may be under steroid therapy with its attendant precautions.

There are three families of drugs which are used,

1. Bisphosphonates (e.g. Alendronic acid),

2. Rank L inhibitors (e.g. Denosumab),

3. Anti-angiogenic (e.g. Sunitinib)

As there are different guidelines in extractions, patients are under these groups of drugs. In the UK, the drug should not be stopped in primary care, and antibiotic coverage is not recommended. Informing the patient that if the extraction site has not been healed after eight weeks, the dentist will refer the patient to secondary care (specialist).

If the patient took bisphosphonate for less than five years or Rank L inhibitor for the last nine months, the patient is classified as low risk.

Suppose the patient has been taking bisphosphonate for more than five years or simultaneously under cortico-therapy or Rank L inhibitor for the last nine months with simultaneous cortico-therapy or anti-angiogenic for cancer treatment, and a history of MRONJ is classified as high-risk. In that case, however, the protocol does not change.

It is limited to no antibiotics, oral hygiene instruction, and reduced sugar, alcohol and smoking.

It is essential that dentists follow the guidelines of each country in which they practice.

However, the hypothesis that increasing bone mineral density (BMD) by drug therapy and the main approach is prevention had debates. After decades of use, the effectiveness is uncertain, and the adverse effects are certain. There is not enough evidence to demonstrate the effect of bisphosphonate and other groups on short and long-term effects on dental implants [9].

Like many other subjects, this subject needs randomised and multicentric studies with longer follow-ups to ensure we are guiding our patients [11].

There is a lack of communication between medical professionals and dentists, and the patient needs to be warned against the potential adverse effects on the alveolar bone, with or without dental implants.

The author recommends that dentists with prospective implant patients on bisphosphonates should contact the relevant physicians to ask them to change the treatment and use this as a last resort. Inform the patients to continue to be exposed to the effects of the drug long after they have stopped taking it.

The author's experience was that although the implants were stable in five years, there was unusual significant bone loss around the implants.

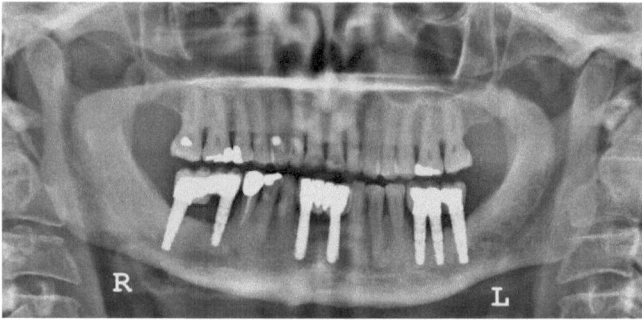

Figure 8.3 Sudden bone loss around dental implant after three years of low-dose Bisphosphonate treatment.

Whether or not it is appropriate to use dental surgery to screen for common systemic diseases is a cultural, personal and pragmatic decision for the dentist. However, the dentist must be adequately trained not to stress the patient unnecessarily.

Treat the patient, not the tooth, and always start with the most straightforward surgery and the one with the most prolonged treatment period, bone graft, or upper jaw. Bone grafts and easiest contradict each other; the potential benefits must counter-balance the risks.

Mental illnesses, such as depressive disorders or anxiety disorders, exert a significant impact on a substantial portion of the adult population. Among the prominent pharmacological interventions for these conditions is the administration of Selective Serotonin Reuptake Inhibitors (SSRIs), which have been demonstrated to correlate with diminished bone mineral content and density [11]. Notably, empirical evidence indicates a three-fold escalation in early implant failure rates, with a compounded effect observed when two or more SSRIs are concurrently utilized. Furthermore, there exists an association between the administration of SSRIs and heightened marginal bone loss surrounding osseointegrated dental implants [12].

Forensic dentistry

Forensic identification of the deceased involves various methods, among which radiographic recognition of dental implants is one of the methods used to identify the individual.

Implant recognition software, radiographic recognition of dental implants and assessment of batch numbers help forensic odontologists identify the victims by comparing them with the antemortem records of the affected victims.

Radiographic recognition of dental implants is one of the methods used to identify the individual.

The implant batch numbers can be identified using a microscope. The fire and oxidation layer depends on the thickness of the oxidation layer.

Imaged using a WILD Heerbrugg microscope attached to a digital camera. The batch number is clearly visible within the implant before firing. Following the firing, the number is still visible where there is an oxidation layer. The survival of the identifying batch number will depend on the etched number's depth and the oxidation layer's thickness. Companies need to be convinced to insert serial numbers on each implant to establish a new approach to identifying deceased persons.

Forensic identification by determining the restorative material radiodensity that is used for implant restoration adds additional evidence to dental identification. Also, the failed dental implant has helped to identify the deceased [13,14].

181

References:

1. Turer OU, Ozcan M, Alkaya B, Demirbilek F, Alpay N, Daglioglu G, Seydaoglu G, Haytac MC. The effect of mindfulness meditation on dental anxiety during implant surgery: a randomized controlled clinical trial. Sci Rep, 2023 Dec 7;13(1):21686.

2. Mallampati SR. Clinical signs to predict difficult tracheal intubation (hypothesis). Can Anaesth Soc J 1983;30:316–7.

3. Cruthirds D, Sims PJ, Louis PJ: Review and recommendations for the prevention, management, and treatment of postoperative and postdischarge nausea and vomiting. Oral Surg Oral Med Oral Pathol Oral Radiol. 2013 May;115(5):601-11.

4. Smetana GW, Lawrence VA, Cornell JE. Preoperative pulmonary risk stratification for noncardiothoracic surgery: systematic review for the American College of Physicians. Annals of Internal Medicine 2006;144:581-95.

5. Reddy K S, Shivu ME, Billimaga A. Benign paroxysmal positional vertigo during lateral window sinus lift procedure: a case report and review. Implant Dent. 2015 Feb;24(1):106-9.

6. Ishiyama A, Jacobson KM, Baloh RW: Migraine and benign positional vertigo: Annals of Otology, Rhinology and laryngology 2000, 109 (4):377-80.

7. Southerland JH, Gill DJ, Gangula PR, Halpern LR, Cardona CY and Mouton CP: Dental management in patients with hypertension: challenges and solutions Clin Cosmet Investig Dent. 2016; 8: 111–120.

8. Esposito M, Grusovin MG, Achille H, Coulthard P, Worthington HV. Interventions for replacing missing teeth: different times for loading dental implants. Cochrane Database Syst Rev. 2009 Jan 21;(1):CD003878.

9. Erviti J, Perry T: Rethinking the Appraisal and Approval of Drugs for Fracture Prevention, Front Pharmacol, 15 May 2017;1-6.

10. Fiorillo L, Cicciù M, Tözüm TF, D'Amico C, Oteri G, Cervino G: Impact of bisphosphonate drugs on dental implant healing and peri-implant hard and soft tissues: a systematic review. BMC Oral Health. 2022 Jul 17;22(1):291.

11. Feuer AJ, Demmer RT, Thai A, Vogiatzi MG. Use of selective serotonin reuptake inhibitors and bone mass in adolescents: an NHANES study. Bone. 2015;78:28-33.

12. Kotsailidi EA, Gagnon C, Johnson L , Basir AB, Tsigarida A: Association of selective serotonin reuptake inhibitor use with marginal bone level changes around osseointegrated dental implants: A retrospective study. J Periodontol 2023 Aug;94(8):1008-1017.

13. Deepalakshmi TK, Prabhakar M: Role of dental implants in forensic identification. J Forensic Dent Sci, 2014 6(2): 145–147.

14. Byraki A, Costea AV, Curca GC, Hostiuc S: Radiographic recognition of dental implants as an aid to identifying the deceased. J Forensic Dent Sci. 2014 May-Aug; 6(2): 145–147

CHAPTER NINE:

RESTORATIONS

9. RESTORATIONS

Aim:

This chapter examines the advantages and disadvantages of provisional restorations utilized during different stages of implant therapy, including an analysis of current provisional treatments, their indications, and contraindications for removable and fixed provisional prostheses in implant dentistry.

Necessary Knowledge:

It is assumed at this stage that you have a general knowledge of basic science related to dental implantology, documentation and record keeping, patient assessment and treatment planning, and dental implant surgical techniques.

Learning Outcome:

The advantages and disadvantages of different provisional restorations constructed for patients at various stages of implant therapy, currently used provisional treatments – indications and reasons for their use, and Contraindications for removable and fixed provisional prostheses/implants.

> No matter what type of provisional prosthesis is provided for the patient
> CHEWING HARD FOOD SHOULD BE AVOIDED.
> providing a stable rigid bite is essential and Duralay (Inlay pattern resin) is a material of choice, resin frame with wax is tested in the patient first and then is fabricated in the laboratory.
> Digital intra-oral impression can be used when the finish line is clearly visible, and it is possible to keep it dry.

Provisional and interim prosthesis terms have been used to provide a fixed or removable prosthesis to create or improve stabilisation, aesthetics, and function during dental implant healing. The author described provisional prosthesis as delivery of the prosthesis immediately after dental implant placement; moreover, if it is delivered after one week of dental implant placement, it is an interim prosthesis.

Ideally, the laboratory should be close to the clinic, so if needed, the laboratory technician can come to practice for shade confirmation, or if there is a misunderstanding of the clinical issue, it could be straightforward.

9.1. Provisional Restorations

Aesthetics and function need to be planned and incorporated into the provisional prosthesis during the healing period. The patient usually needs a little chair time and the reassurance of an immediate improvement in their appearance and function. Rigid and semi-rigid splinting can be used successfully, and a provisional restoration can be selected as a semi-rigid splint [1].

The best patient-dentist relationship is based on mutual trust. It depends initially on each liking the other, on the dentist demonstrating an understanding of the patient's needs and wants, and on the dentist's ability to devise a treatment plan that is understandable, practical, logical, and seen to be such by the patient. Above all, the dentist must offer a treatment plan at a level that he knows he can achieve, and the patient should understand that the dentist has the necessary skills. Mutual respect, mutual trust, and proper skills are essential for success.

When 3-piece dental implants have been placed, the provisional restorations can be removable, soft tissue-borne, tooth-supported, and implant-retained, using provisional narrow dental implants.

In cases where 3-piece dental implants are placed, a fixed partial denture or resin-bonded prosthesis is recommended. A removable denture may exert undesirable pressure on the healing implant, and it will be detrimental to the implant's survival.

Placing only one stage of a 3-piece implant will increase the harm.

Sealing screw loosening and continuous repeatable trauma on the soft tissue from the periosteum may provoke fistulae and bone loss, it may be with discomfort, which is usually negligible by the patient, and that means the patient will come to the dentist too late.

Removal of the buccal flange with relief of the fit surface will leave a gap between the alveolar ridge and the neck of the denture teeth, and this can be relined with tissue conditioner, which is soft and can last for a few weeks but can still put the dental implant under unwanted pressure, leading to harmful consequences. Using other more challenging soft liners can magnify the pressure and is likewise not recommended. Removable dentures are also less popular, are bulky, and can compromise speech. They can provoke the gag reflex, and some patients cannot tolerate them.

One millimetre countersinks the three/two pieces of dental implants can prevent the side effect; however, if possible, not by invading the I.D. canal or maxillary sinus.

Most changes in gingival height occur in the initial three months. Narrow implants with a diameter of 3.5 mm suffer less gingival recession. Also, the implant platform is positioned buccal-lingually, buccal bone thickness, gingival biotype (thin or thick), flapless or minimal soft tissue reflection, and horizontal defect dimension affect the gingival contour and height.

When the implant platform is placed more buccally than palatal, the resulting gingival recession is greater, especially in the implant placement with immediate restoration [2].

The Essix provisional occlusal appliance (supported by occlusal coverage of the adjacent teeth) has been recommended. It is simple and affordable, but patients are not fond of it.

The appliance is made from transparent thermoplastic sheets, either in the surgery or in the laboratory. The technique is easy to follow. In the model, the missing teeth are replaced by denture teeth. A sheet of thermoplastic baseplate is heated and vacuum-formed over the "restored" model. Because the occlusal surfaces bear the occlusal pressure, the gingival surfaces around the implant and the dental implant itself are protected. As aesthetics are usually not acceptable for the patient, and mastication is difficult, it can only be used for a few days.

An alternative to the Essix-type appliance is a fixed provisional prosthesis. The pontic areas can be provided by any tooth - natural, denture tooth, or handmade composite tooth - bonded to the neighbouring teeth. A cast metal or Maryland bridge can also be used if appropriate.

If you use natural teeth, these can be sectioned, the pulp removed, the tooth cleaned and autoclaved and filled with composite from the apical end. The enamel surface is etched and bonded. Bulk composite on the proximal sides, placed to retain the pontic, will have little effect on the aesthetics. Overall, the addition of composite to the enamel will hardly be noticed.

If you use reinforced cast metal, tooth preparation may be needed; it is expensive, and sometimes, the grey colour of the metal retainer cannot be masked. It debonds frequently. Adding a clasp can be helpful as the provisional restoration may be used for a long time. The occlusion may prevent the addition of composite to the palatal surface.

Dislodgement or fracture can occur, but that demonstrates that the patient is chewing hard food.

Placing a one-piece thin provisional dental implant between the implants is another option for immediate provisional restorations, usually applied in full mouth rehabilitation.

There is a need for a transitional thin implant in full jaw rehabilitation or where a long-span edentulous area is involved. The implants are immediately loaded, and the prosthesis needs to be fixed.

Neither prosthesis nor implant can tolerate heavy mastication and may fracture if this limitation is not respected. A minimum space of 2 mm is mandatory between the provisional and definitive dental implants.

When one-piece dental implants are inserted, there are other options to provide provisional immediate restoration so that the patient can benefit from fixed prosthesis 3. Different scenarios are discussed below:

1: immediately after extraction, the extracted tooth is sectioned at the gingival level, pulp removed, cleaned autoclaved and filled with composite from the apical end (figure 9.1).

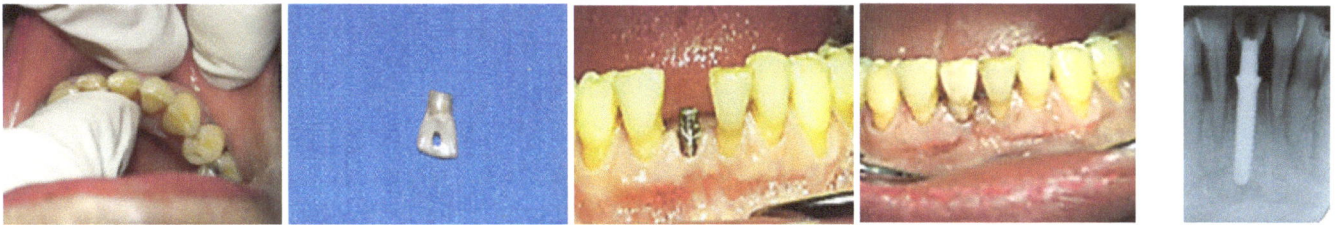

Figure 9.. Left to right, central incisor mobility, tooth sectioned after extraction, filled with composite, and cemented using adhesive cement.

2: Immediately after extraction and dental implant placement. The implant was placed more in the palatal position, and a small space-making defect was observed in the buccal surface. Using a rigid, Flat plastic instrument, push the buccal bone to have a green stick fractured towards the implant.

In a hand-mix formula, a polycarbonate provisional crown was selected, disinfected, and relined with the bis-acrylic composite. The crown can be cemented with any type of cement. The author prefers zinc oxide cement as the colour is yellowish and does not affect the colour after cementation, and moisture does not affect its settings. After removal of the excess and heavy irrigation under the flap, the flap is sutured.

A lower denture can be adjusted to a provisional acrylic bridge (figure 9.3).

If three-piece implants are placed and a screw-retained bridge is used, there is a need to place impression posts, scan or take an impression, and by different techniques, the provisional prosthesis can be screwed into the dental implant. With the author's experience, it is more time-consuming (takes about 4 hours), and during impression post placement and removal and screwing of the temporary abutments, the implant's stability may be jeopardized.

The technique of choice would be based on the school of thought, experience, and available laboratory experience.

The placement of the provisional restoration allows the patient to evaluate their initial appearance following tooth loss immediately after the extraction procedure.

It should reproduce the appearance, speech, and occlusal function and preserve or even enhance the peri-implant soft tissue anatomy. It allows one to evaluate and even alter the immediate result and help determine the contours of the final prosthesis.

The occlusion surface of a single tooth replacement should be completely shy of the occlusion in both centric relation and eccentric excursion. The occlusal parameters of the single tooth provisional or partial bridge are not the same as that of the full-arch prosthesis. The full arch prosthesis benefits from cross-arch stabilisation in eccentric excursions, but partial edentulous restorations should have light-centric contacts and be free of eccentric contacts during temporisation.

Provisional (Interim) prosthesis:

Due to many factors, such as bleeding and limited time, a provisional prosthesis is not good enough to achieve the goal of managing tissue with minimal gingiva inflammation. The stable occlusion, appropriate aesthetics, phonetics, and if there are doubts, another provisional prosthesis that is more accurate

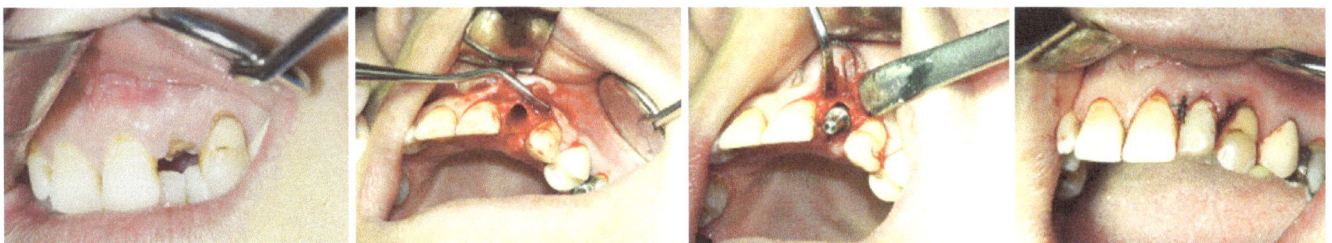

Figure 9.2 Left to right: upper left lateral Incisor root extracted, the buccal bone intact, and a one-piece dental implant inserted. The buccal defect is closed with a green-stick fracture of the buccal bone towards the implant, a provisional polycarbonate crown is selected and relined with bis-acrylic composite, after removal of the excess, it is cemented, and then the flap is sutured around the provisional crown.

186

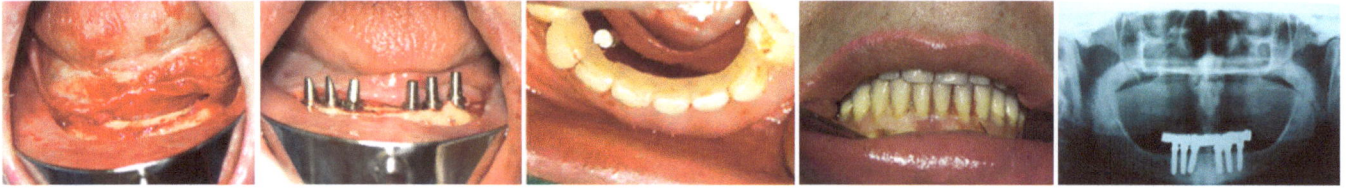

Figure 9.3 Left to right; after exposing the alveolar bone and placing the dental implant. Major discrepancies in the angle of the abutment are corrected. The lingual flange is removed, and bis-acrylic composite fills the empty spaces using the standard procedures. Make sure it is removed a couple of times on the moist preparation to prevent it from setting into the undercuts so the bridge can be removed easily later for final adjustments and polish. The bridge can be cemented with any type of cement. The right photo is the final DPT with the lower hybrid bridge.

can be provided, which we call provisional or interim prosthesis. This type of prosthesis aims to be used as an index for final restorations.

When the finishing margin of the abutment is a shoulder, then provisional protective caps can be used.

If the finishing margins do not need preparation, placing a fixed provisional restoration using a prefabricated impression cap is recommended, making the soft tissue around the dental implant easier to protect.

The downside is that the optimal natural soft tissue contour cannot be provided as the abutment cross-section at the gingival opening level will be round.

In the case of full mouth rehabilitation, or where a large span bridge is involved, which crosses the midline, or a fixed curved denture, make use of a hard(viscous) soft liner as a temporary cement for temporary fixation between weekly sessions. It reduces both the chairside time and the potential discomfort for the patient when the bridge is removed. It also reduces the chances of fracturing it during its removal and encourages sound, clean, soft tissue around the abutment.

Intra-oral fabrication of the provisional restoration may have poor marginal adaptation, especially when the finishing margin of the abutment is subgingival. Some believe removing any excess cement is difficult and can produce scratches on the restoration or the abutment.

The scratch resistance of a titanium dental implant abutment was studied using 14 N force.

The depth of the scratch produced was 0.34 um, which is less scratch damage than would be created in cementum, so according to some authors, metal curettes may be used on titanium abutments [4].

Fabrication of the provisional (interim) fixed bridge on the abut-

ment of the dental implants can be done directly, in the mouth or indirectly, through the laboratory.

The direct approach still requires initial input from the laboratory. An intra-oral impression allows the laboratory to construct a diagnostic wax-up from which a clear matrix is fabricated. The latter is used to generate the provisional bridge. The disadvantage of this method lies in the possibility that acrylic resin, applied at the chairside, may flow into abutment undercuts or available channels, like screw-access channels, and be difficult to remove. Nonetheless, the dentist has complete control of the procedure.

The indirect approach allows the laboratory to construct the provisional prosthesis. This may well be heat-polymerized, ensuring a good fit, good function, and better aesthetics and durability. The alternative would be employing a pressure pot, reducing porosity and increasing durability.

Denture teeth laminates may be used to improve long-term stability and aesthetics.

If the patient is partially dentate, teeth adjacent to the saddle areas will allow the correct positioning of the clear matrix.

If the patient is edentulous, the clear matrix will be seated on soft tissue, and the potential for inaccuracies will increase.

Here we present a step-by-step procedure for single tooth replacement:

Dental impressions are taken, and casts are made.

A provisional polycarbonate crown is selected based on size, form, and shade. Apply Vaseline or coconut butter on the abutment using an earbud or cotton roll.

Add resin to the provisional crown matrix and position it over the dental implant abutment.

Remove the excess, loosen the crown during the initial set,

187

adapt and repeat the procedure. When the resin starts to become warm, control the position of the crown on the abutment. If the finishing margin of the abutment has not been modified, check the finishing margin of the crown and make the final adjustment by removing the excess or adding to the finishing margin using flow composite. Adjust the occlusion according to the treatment plan - shy of occlusal contacts, progressive loading, or full occlusal contact.

Polish with a wet muslin wheel and fine pumice.

Several types of acrylic resin materials are used to fabricate interim restorations. These may be self-cured or light-cured resins such as polyvinyl methacrylate, polymethyl methacrylate (PMMA), bis-acryl composite, and visible light-cured urethane dimethacrylates.

The use of resin materials for computer-aided design/computer-aided manufacturing (CAD/CAM) has increased recently. Even permanent dental restorations can be milled from polymeric materials such as polymethyl methacrylate (PMMA)-based or poly-oxymethylene (POM) CAD/CAM blocks.

This approach provides more precise margins, better colour stability, and better physical and mechanical stability.

The conventional technique for fabricating fixed, provisional (interim) implant-supported prostheses for edentulous patients involves converting a transitional complete denture into a fixed interim prosthesis in order to provide aesthetics and enable the OVD record to be transferred.

The shape of the acrylic teeth can be modified to the patient's needs.

Making a duplicate prosthesis in case the initial one is damaged or breaks would be prudent. Cold-cure resin is porous and can become stained over time. It can also encourage soft tissue (mucosal) inflammation. Heat-cured resin is more colour-stable and has less porosity [5].

Many methods have been described, and the dentist must realize which one it suits it best. One of the methods is that a prosthesis can be duplicated at the chairside by impressing putty on a cast. Tooth-coloured resin is poured into the index, and after this has been set, a self-cure denture base resin is poured into a Lang duplicator to reproduce the remaining anatomical features [6-8].

9.2. Definitive restorations

The final station of the patient's treatment journey should be delivering a definitive restoration retained by a securely placed dental implant. Meeting the patient's expectations is the primary determinant of success. High expectations on the patient's part are all good, but failing to meet them can be a bad experience for both the patient and the dental team. It is essential to identify high expectations at the outset. Preparation is key.

Remember, the failure to give the patient sufficient information on other treatment options, the number of sessions, their risks, their costs, and maintenance requirements are the main reasons behind any failure to satisfy a patient's expectations.

In the final analysis, the patient and the implant team must agree on whether the final prosthesis is to be fixed or removed. This means a full discussion of each alternative prosthesis's pros and cons.

Two types of definitive restoration can be provided for the patient: fixed or removable. The removable restoration must be removed before the patient goes to bed, and it can be left out until the patient wakes in the morning.

The advantages of the fixed prosthesis are its improved ability to masticate, the feeling of a natural dentition, a reduced intrusion into the natural occlusal space, and the confidence imparted by a fixed prosthesis.

The disadvantages are the need for more precise surgery, more bone and soft tissue grafting to provide an aesthetic emergence profile, reduced access to hygiene maintenance, the difficulty or sometimes the impossibility of repair, and the higher cost.

The advantages of removable dentures, by contrast, are that they are easier to clean, provide lip support, so there is less need for soft tissue and bone grafting, are relatively easy to repair, and are relatively affordable.

The disadvantages of the removable denture are that it is less efficient for mastication, needs more maintenance as parts may need to be replaced, lacks the feel of natural teeth, has a greater chance of needing an early remake, and may be less comfortable - especially when the patient has a large tongue.

Also, the alveolar bone resorption speed will remain in the areas where dental implants have not been placed.

Oral hygiene is an essential factor in the continuing health of the final restoration, as fixed restorations need more care than implants next to removable prostheses. This is especially so where there has been vertical bone loss and/or accompanied by poor-quality soft tissue around the dental implant.

A number of materials can be used for the fixed restoration retained by dental implants, while that used for the removable prosthesis is usually plastic.

Most people show their incisors and gingival papillae when they smile, and while reproducing a natural tooth appearance is essential, if complex, reproducing soft tissue with multiple teeth is even more so. The inter-arch distance may influence the final restoration. As a rule of thumb, where the distance is less than 10 mm, a fixed prosthesis is recommended; where it is greater than 15 mm, a removable prosthesis will have fewer complications.

If it is decided to delay the placement of the definitive restoration after surgical exposure of the dental implant, it is crucial to protect the site, especially the surgical flap, to prevent displacement.

This means that the patient should not use a provisional removable prosthesis for two weeks post-operatively. This will significantly affect the patient's lifestyle if the aesthetic zone is in the process of being rehabilitated. If a provisional prosthesis cannot be avoided, then care must be taken not to put pressure on the transmucosal healing abutment.

Patients naturally prefer a comfortable experience, minimum sessions, and short chair times. They also want their appearance not to be compromised over the treatment period. Despite the development of techniques for immediate implant placement with immediate restoration, many dentists prefer two-stage surgeries. These will continue to challenge the dentist's ability to satisfy the patient's demand for aesthetics.

During dental implant treatment planning, the dentist needs to study the patient's lip line, the dental arch's shape, and the bone's morphology. Also needed will be a note of the interdental space, potential positions for the implant(s), the preferred characteristics of the prosthetic crown, and how the soft tissue can best be handled (figure 9.4).

The interdental space should be 5.5 mm mesio-distally, with an additional 1.5mm in the proximal regions to allow the formation of the gingival papillae. Allow for 5mm bucco-lingually to provide space for the future crown.

If the implant axis is the same as the crown axis, the crown height will be similar to that of the natural crown. When the crown height is increased from 10 mm to 20 mm, the lingual and

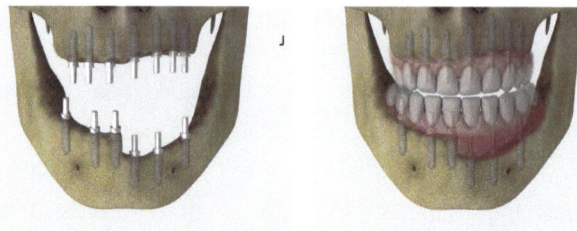

Figure 9.4 Interdental space needs to be noted. Compare the right and left sides of the patient; when the crown height is increased, the moments will increase significantly.

apical moments increase by 200%. When the crown height increases, the cantilever length should be reduced, and the number of implants should be increased (figure 9.4). Short implants are not well-defined but are usually less than 8 mm tall.

In the case of short implants, it has been reported that the failure rate of 5mm diameter implants is 25% in the maxillae and 33% in the mandible, but in the case of longer implants of 10 and 12 mm lengths, but with the same diameter, the failure rate in the maxillae was 10% and in the mandible was zero [9].

If the implant axis is lingually inclined, the compensating buccal overextension of the prosthetic crown will hamper proper hygiene control and adversely affect aesthetics.

Several procedural options that can affect the peri-implant gingivae:

1. Application of the template and to determine the optimal implant position,

2. Application of the implant-supported provisional prosthesis,

3. The size and form of the restorative platform,

4. The abutment material,

5. The final prosthetic material,

6. The mode of retention of the final prosthesis.

An assessment of the efficacy of the surgical guide or template has not been published. The facial positioning of an implant can be associated with gingival recession.

No studies have also focused on the aesthetic outcome of the provisional prosthesis. Papillae regeneration has apparently been seen in most cases, even though the lack of data has allowed no firm conclusion to be drawn. Horizontal offset designs have been reported, resulting in stable or a slight gain in the midfacial mucosal height.

The timing of the abutment/crown placement depends on the condition of the gingiva surrounding the implant and whether the cover screw is exposed or submerged. Most practitioners prefer mature tissue to be present before impressing; hence, a healing cap or an abutment with a provisional crown can be placed for 10-14 days before final crown placement.

The final abutment and crown can be placed simultaneously; I recommend a custom abutment. The dentist can take the impression and send it to the lab to fabricate the custom abutment and crown.

If the implant needs exposure followed by the placement of a temporary abutment, then it should be allowed to heal for six weeks to allow full maturation before the final impression is taken.

Abutments can be prefabricated to several different shapes, angles and sizes, allowing the clinician to select the best available fit. The clinician who adopts an 'average' approach to an 'average' population cannot provide optimum features for each scenario. Custom-made abutments which are screw-retained to the provisional or definitive crown can also be applied.

Abutment preparation

Abutment preparation is necessary for cement-retained restorations.

Retention forms are the features (surfaces) that prevent crown removal along the long axis of tooth preparation (like sticky foods). Factors which influence the retention are:

Total surface area: The dimensions of the dental implant cement-retained abutments are less than those of natural teeth unless the abutment is customised. Even though the stability or fracture of the customised abutments was not affected in the literature, the author's experience in the single tooth molar replacement is otherwise [10].

Resistance Forms are the features that prevent the removal of the crown by apical, horizontal or oblique forces (occlusal forces). Parallel walls, steps and grooves with a depth of 1 mm in the axial walls increase resistance.

Anti-rotation increases resistance but is only necessary for single-tooth prostheses. The bridges are not recommended unless the abutment's height is less than 5 mm.

The Taper of each axial wall is between 6°-16°, which, as it increases, the retention drops significantly. And changing the surface roughness from 10 um to 40 um doubles the retention. The submarginal contour shapes the surrounding supporting tissue or transitions from the round interface of a dental implant to the proper contour of a tooth at the gingival tissue. The emer-

gence profile should be smoothly contoured without any sharp undercuts, which make it difficult to clean the patient and facilitate the removal of excess cement.

The recommendation for the PEEK fixed cement-retained prosthesis abutment preparation is that the relationship between height and diameter is a minimum of 2:1. The height of the clinical crown to the height of the abutment is 3:1, and the occlusal distance between the abutment and the occlusal surface of the opposing teeth is 3 mm but less than 2 mm will not be acceptable.

For a PFM crown, the minimum thickness of layers needed on the buccal surface from the abutment to the external surface is as follows: spacer (0.3mm), Frame (0.4mm), opaque (0.3mm), dentin (0.5mm), the enamel translucent (0.2mm) which the result of the total would be 2.2. mm. The glaze reduces the thickness by about 10 um. For BIOHPP, the minimum thickness of the PEEK (frame) is 0.3mm, but 0.5 mm is advisable. The composite for the full anatomy by High Impact Polymer Composite (HIPC) is 1.5 mm, but 2.0 mm is advised.

Finishing margin

There is no doubt that the best surface for the gingival to be in contact with is titanium. However, for aesthetics and prevention of food entrapment, the crown's margin should be 0.5-1 mm in the crevicular sulcus and not encroach the biologic width. The choice of restoration material is crucial for compatibility and minimising inflammation risk.

There is no doubt that the marginal fit should be optimal, and the control method will be discussed later.

No finish line design has yet proven to be superior with regard to the marginal accuracy of the subsequent restoration. Instead, good detectability of the margin for the dental technician or intraoral

Scanning devices appear to be of primary importance.

The knife (featheredge) margin makes the best marginal seal but is difficult to visualise. You may need to contour the finishing margin of the crown. The crown thickness would be thin, which is no advantage for the implant, as the diameter of the abutments is usually thinner than the average prepared tooth.

For light chamfers, the thickness is between 0.3 and 0.5 mm, which is a better definition than the featheredge indicated for full metal crowns or PFM but with metal collars.

Heavy chamfers have a well-defined finishing margin of 1.0-1.5

mm, as indicated in the PFM and all ceramic crowns.

Shoulder with 1.0-1.5 mm thick indicated in PFM and all-ceramic restorations; however, for PEEK restorations, the shoulder is preferred.

Chamfer and feather-edge may be recommended as acceptable crown-abutment geometries for screw-retained implant-supported single-crown restorations because they offer a combination of good mechanical behaviour and marginal fit [11]. Insufficient evidence demonstrates the efficacy of finishing the margins with fine-grit diamond burs or tungsten carbide burs.

Materials for crown-retained dental implants

1. Gold: This is the oldest material that has been used. The main reasons are its durability and low reactivity compared with all other metals used in the mouth. Gold's hardness is close to that of tooth enamel, and it is well-suited for molars in patients suffering from bruxism. Gold, even when it's thin, is durable. It triggers the least sensitivity. It is an alloy and contains other low-reactive metals. It does, however, conduct hot and cold quickly, and it can wear, especially if opposing porcelain crowns. The weight of the upper long bridge is a negative factor in addition to the cost.

2. Full Porcelain to Emax.

3. Porcelain fused to metal (gold)

4. Porcelain fused to zirconia

5. Full zirconia

6. Dental composite (PEEK)

Gold alloys and palladium-silver alloys have passed the test of time. In the late 1980s, chrome cobalt - was available for accurate metal-ceramic construction. While it also suffered high shrinkage, this can be remedied. Deformation of the framework during the high-temperature ceramic fusion stage is lower than that which occurs with high noble alloys. One of the most widely used is high-strength lithium disilicate ceramics, but they require time-consuming crystallisation after milling, polishing, or glazing. The resin nano-ceramic hybrid material has sufficient strength, pleasing aesthetics and marginal adaptation, which is polished using abrasive discs and is a good alternative [12].

Titanium combined with low-fusing ceramics has also been marketed. CAD-CAM technologies for milling pre-processed metal and high-strength ceramics show promise, but a 10-year follow-up and comparison with a conventionally cast framework is needed.

The clinical requirements of the case determine the basis for the selection of dental materials. Would it provide a better environment and have more suitable physical characteristics if it is based on metal, ceramic or polymer? The materials with the closest match to the wear characteristics of enamel are gold and amalgam. The emphasis on the aesthetics of polymer composite has led to the evolution of lower and crystalline ceramics, such as zirconia, ceramics with higher elastic properties, such as alumina, heavy particle-filled resin cured at high temperature with pressure, like Lava Ultimat (3M) and Cerasmart (GC). Ceramic-based resin has an interpenetrating network (IPN), which can change its physical properties, such as fracture toughness, fracture strength, contact stability, and grinding damage tolerance. In its resistance to crack propagation, it behaves like bone. Examples are Vita Zahnfabrik's Enamic and the In-Ceram Alumina group.

Non-precious gold-colour (NPG+2) alloy is a copper-based dental casting alloy with 2% gold formulated for constructing fixed crown and bridge restorations. The main disadvantage is that it can only be applied as a full metal prosthesis. The author has over ten years of experience before other materials come to market. It was indicated in patients suffering from bruxism and used in the premolar and molar regions. Designing a shelf in the buccal surface to provide space for laboratory composite. It was one of the safest and most affordable designs. The margin of the crown contacting the soft tissue is NPG (figure 9.5).

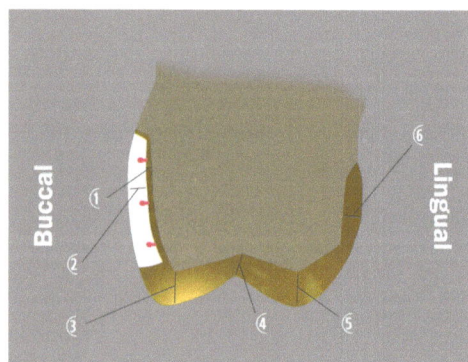

Figure 9.5 The upper first molar cross-section is covered with an NPG crown and the buccal surface of the laboratory composite. The minimum thickness is 6 (0.6 mm), 5 (1.3 mm), 4 (0.8mm), 3 (0.8 mm),2 (1.2 mm and 1 (0.3 mm). The white area demonstrates the area filled with composite, and the reds are the mushroom's projection for the retention of the composite.

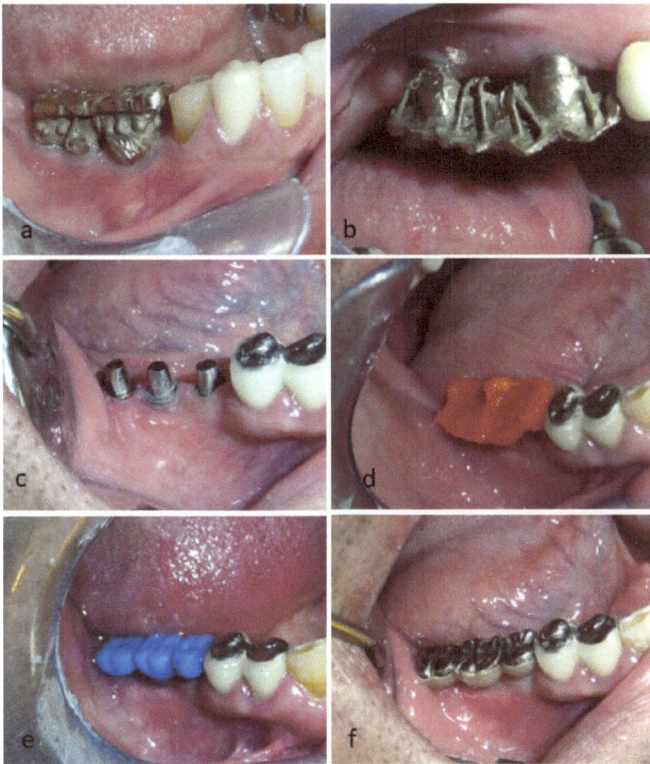

Figure 9.6 a,b; different mechanical retention types are recommended for the composite's retention, c-f: Providing a stable, rigid bite is essential, and Duralay (Inlay pattern resin) is a material of choice. A resin frame with wax is tested in the patient first and then fabricated in the laboratory.

Other types of retention have been suggested depending on the available space (figure 9.6).

When the patient has a dental implant and suffers from bruxism, the patient must understand that he must come for a dental checkup every six months. The BEWE score is recorded in each session, and photos of the occlusal surface are provided. Treatments or referrals are recommended if profound changes occur (Figure 7.9).

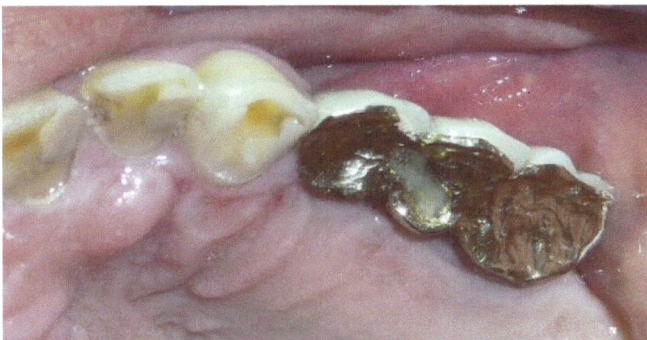

Figure 9.7. The attrition and breakdown of the composite filling in the anterior teeth are evident; also, abrasion of NPG is significant, and the perforation is temporarily closed with composite. This scenario should be diagnosed before this stage. However, the NPG abrasion saved the dental implant's integrity and prevented abutment fracture or bone loss.

In patients with heavy bruxism, the crown is abraded, and if the composite from the buccal surface falls off, it is replaced again in a dental chair without the need to remove the crown from the dental implant abutment. Nevertheless, when PEEK was introduced to the market, it was a blessing.

Poly-ether-ether-ketone (PEEK) has been introduced into the orthopaedic and dental fields. Modified PEEK containing 20% ceramic fillers is a high-performance polymer (BIOHPP, Bredent GmbH, Senden, Germany) that is biocompatible and has good mechanical properties, high-temperature resistance, and chemical stability. It is as elastic as bone (4GPa modulus of elasticity) and reduces stresses transferred to the abutments. The framework provides a better construction basis than conventional metal frameworks. Allergic reactions have not been reported, and the material has no metallic taste. It is highly polishable, has low plaque affinity, and has good wear resistance 13-17. Author indications are:

• Dentin exposed (total surface) due to abrasion/attrition

• The height of the crown (from the margin of the implant) is more than 150% of the natural clinical crown

• Cantilever and heavyweight (measure the difference)

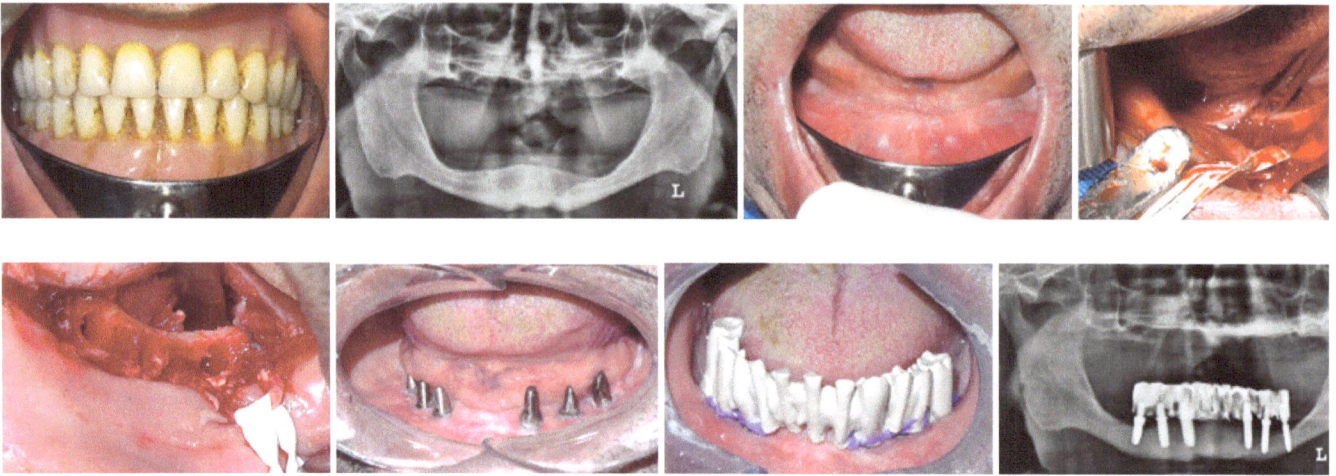

Figure 9.8 The patient is 62 years old and a heavy smoker; the upper left is the patient upper and lower dentures with stains. The patient warned that smoking would change the colour of the PEEK. The upper right and lower left demonstrate nerve positioning and then healed implants and abutments. The BIOHPP (PEEK) framework is checked using low-viscosity polyvinylsiloxane to check the finishing margins without any gaps. The lower right demonstrated the DPT and the radiopacity of the PEEK.

The PEEK fixed prosthesis does not make artefacts in future CBCTs as all metals do.

It has also been used successfully for mandibular RPDs when combined with acrylic denture material, but the loss after one year of the initial high-gloss surface has been reported as indirect contact with oral mucosa [18] (figure 9.8).

TYPES OF CEMENT:

There are screw-retained and cement-retained dental implant prostheses. A screw retains a screw-retained prosthesis, and the cement-retained prosthesis requires cement. Cement-retained restorations were introduced as having better aesthetics, simpler fabrications, lower cost, and improved passivity than screw-retained restorations.

Different types of definitive dental cement are in the market: glass ionomer, zinc phosphate, polycarboxylate and resin cement. The dentist selection is based on convenience, familiarity, and cost; the only trend that may be seen is that resin cement is used for either zirconium- or aluminium-based abutment.

Cement attaches the prosthesis by friction as zinc phosphate, and some are adhesives by a chemical bond, such as etch resin with enamel and dentin, which does not correlate to dental implant abutments.

The type of cement the dentist uses is based on the school of thought and type of material used.

There is not enough evidence the efficacy of the retentiveness of a particular cement for natural dentition may not correlate with dental implant abutment.

Issues are important, such as controlling the cement flow and diagnosing and removing excess cement immediately after cementation or after long-term follow-up. Dentists use different technique applications, such as loading only the margin of the crown, using a brush to place the cement inside the crown and loading inside the crown. Even though many dentists load about a quarter of the crown with cement, the author recommends that when the silicone dental impression material is used to demonstrate the leakage of the crown, it can removed and used as an index to brush the required amount of cement in each crown instead of doing blindly and putting too much or too little. Detection of excess cement is mandatory for the success of dental implant treatment.

The difference ISO 4049/2000 establishes that the radiopacity of the luting cement should be equal to or greater than that of the same thickness of aluminium 19; however, not all have the condition 20. The radiopacity of dental cement seems to depend more on the presence of elements with high atomic numbers than on the type of material like Zinc.

Another problem is that the resin cements are highly adhesive to titanium surfaces, even when machined smoothly, and removal may be tricky.

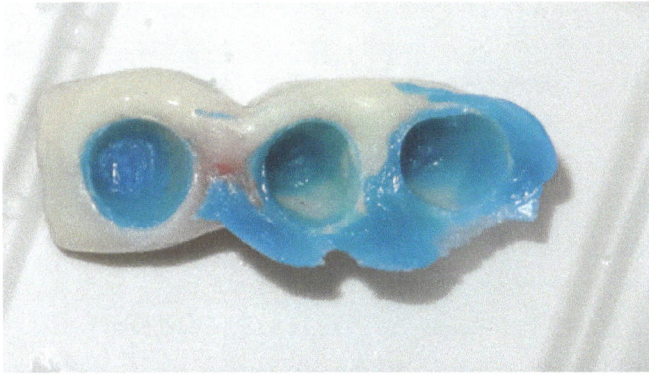

Figure 9.9 The silicone wash inside the crown/bridge can point to the leakage of the finishing line and the amount of cement needed for each crown's internal surface.

Cement detection is clinically affected by the implant diameter, undercut, and implant site. Deep subgingival cementation makes it more complex; thus, ideally, cementation margins should equal or exceed the free gingival margin level. However, a maximum of 1 mm is applied in the aesthetic region. In contrast to teeth, the peri-implant soft tissue lacks resistance because soft tissue does not attach to the implant surface, and connective tissue fibres align parallel along the abutment surface and do not provide a barrier and less resistance to the pressure of the cement.

The potential of maintaining the Standard abutment is more difficult than that of the platform switch with the larger abutment, even with the shallow cementation margin (figure 9.10). Logically, as the diameter of the implant increases, there would be less cement retention.

The author prefers zinc phosphate, which is radiopaque, less adhesive and has superior cleaning properties and resin cement (Panavia) only on single tooth replacement where the abutment height is short (less than 6 mm).

Temporary cements:
The author believes the need for a final prosthesis retained by a dental implant is rare.

Some dentists prefer to use temporary cement, as it may need to remove the fixed prosthesis due to colour correction, repair of ceramic fracture, occlusal correction, in the case of abutment loosening, treatment of peri-implantitis or implant failure.

Accidental detachment or multiple abutment prosthesis, the scenario of a couple of abutments having leakage and the other being well cemented. In this scenario, the prosthesis needs to be removed with potential damage to the prosthesis, abutment and/or dental implant, which is not a good experience.

Accidental detachment occurs more frequently with Zinc oxide than with acrylic/urethane cement 21.

The author recommends that after finalizing the bridge, if there are doubts and need a week for temporisation, use a self-curing temporary soft denture liner consisting of the resilient methacrylate formulation. Zinc phosphate is 50% for single tooth replacement, and coconut oil or Vaseline is 50% even though a single crown should not need temporisation.

The author advises against using zinc oxide temporary cement to attach crowns to dentin or enamel without coconut oil due to potential attachment issues. However, this cement is suitable for metal abutments in the hand and may be susceptible to removal by saliva. The author encountered situations where one of the retainer cements of a bridge washed away while the others remained intact, rendering the bridge immovable and unable to be removed.

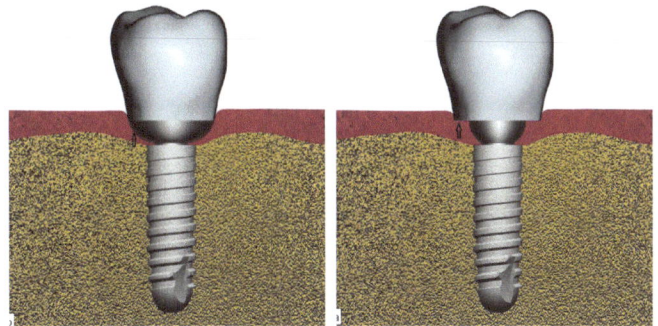

Figure 9.10 (Left implant), when there is a significant difference between the diameter of the abutment at the cement margin level and the crown, more space is available for cement retention compared to the platform switch (right implant) in which the abutment's diameter at the cement margin is close to the crown.

9.3. Dental Implant Prosthesis

In this chapter, we discuss the types of implants- abutment connections, abutment materials, abutment prosthesis connections - removable and fixed prosthesis and screw-retained (horizontal and vertical screw-retained) and cement-retained fixed prosthesis and cementation technique. Abutment preparation - extra-oral (lab or clinic) and intra-oral preparation will be discussed.

9-3-a: Implant-abutment connections:

a. External connection

b. Internal connection

While placing a one-piece implant will mean that the micro gap will be eliminated, there are still circumstances in which a conventional three-piece dental implant is preferable.

External connections were used for many years before the Branemark era, and a stable implant-abutment connection is a prerequisite for successful osseointegration[22].

The serendipity of Brandmark, using titanium and the external hexagon design to facilitate implant insertion, first was not used as an anti-rotational feature. The hexagon is a six-sided shape for the abutment implant interface that extends above the coronal portion of a dental implant. Other types with more sides have evolved, but the hex is the most commonly used.

The issues which need to address are soft tissue closure, the concentration of stress, the needed preload, stability of the joint and degrees of rotational freedom between abutment and implant, short crown height, aesthetics, screw loosening, misfit and microbial seal.

The external connection is easier to use when the implant is placed in an angulated position and if the height of the crown is less than 7 mm. However, the external cover, with a height of at least 1 mm, may make the soft tissue closure challenging.

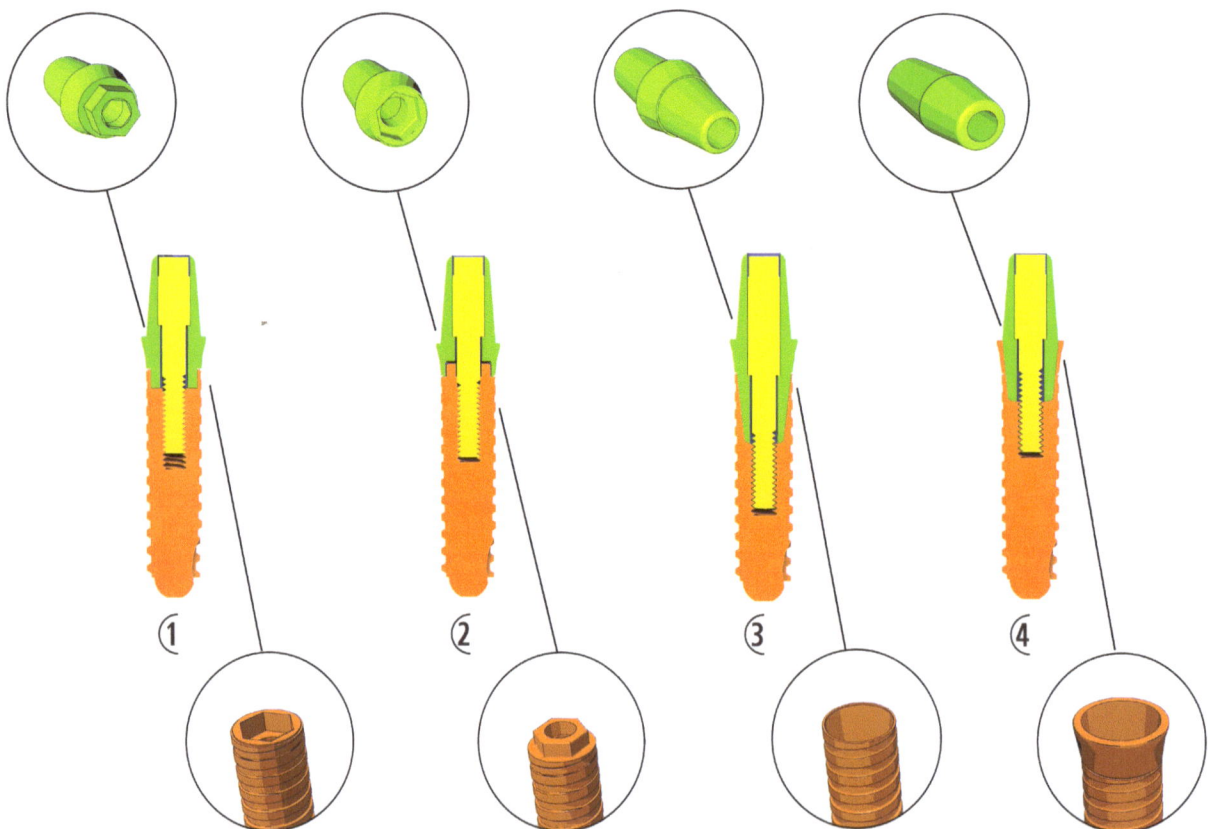

Figure 9.9 The silicone wash inside the crown/bridge can point to the leakage of the finishing line and the amount of cement needed for each crown's internal surface.

Some dentists believe that an external hex provides more positions for the abutment; however, tilting the external hex implant in 10 degrees can be detrimental [23].

The immediate solution was to increase the height from 0.7 to 1.2 height and the width from 2.0 to 3.4 mm, which extended abutment screw engagement and increased the fulcrum arm, reducing the tipping force and screw loosening, however increasing the height will bring other disadvantages during soft tissue closure.

The increased strain at the cervical area in the external hex design has been documented, and the internal hex strain is at the apex of the implant [24].

In the short dental implants, the stress is concentrated under axial loading at the crest in the external hex; however, it showed less stress at the crestal level under oblique loading.

Morse taper design, under oblique loading, showed a higher area with a tendency to direct stress toward the implant's apex and could be recommended for morse internal connection, especially in single tooth replacement with adverse crown-implant ratio [25].

The amount of bone loss affects stress distributions differently with the type of connection. After even 2 mm bone loss, the connection type affects the stress distribution in single tooth replacement. Within the internal connection, more stress is generated; however, greater stress was in the abutment screw restoration of the external connection [26].

Degrees rotational of freedom between the abutment and the implant cannot be ignored; most stable is less than 2° as less than 5° Significantly reduced the number of loading cycles to loosen the implant-abutment joint and as the degrees increases, the probability of screw loosening increases [27].

After the abutment screw loosening, increasing the torque from 30 to 35 Ncm, screw joint stability was improved without changing the geometry of the implant-abutment interface [28]. The result can be debated as it was demonstrated that the amount of the insertion torque may deform the implant-abutment connection, in which the internal connection is 36 Ncm and the external connection is 27 Ncm [29]. These studies have different dental implant systems, meaning different Titanium and geometry, so they cannot be related to all cases. The dentist needs to understand if the torque of the abutment screw is increased to prevent reoccurring abutment screws from loosening and what would be the consequences.

Metanalysis by Goiato found that, when considered from a mechanical, biological and aesthetic point of view, internal connections present better results than external connections and that conical connections have both the best sealing ability and greater stability [30].

There are different types of internal connections; one of the types is conical attachment. Due to friction between the external wall of the abutment and the internal wall of the implants, it locks. The lock or intimate contact provides a series of advantages as fewer micromovements that reduce screw loosening or fracture [31].

This unique contact even reduces bacterial colonization between the implant, abutment and the screw [32].

The conical connection is classified into two designs, no interface and platform switch, the latter having the most favourable stress transmission during nonaxial loading. For the platform switch, the diameter of the abutment is smaller than the implant platform [33].

The bone crest level is more protected by lack of movement than the micro-gap between the abutment and the implant [34].

Micro-gap:

A micro-gap will be present between the individual parts of a three-piece dental implant. This micro-gap will inevitably allow bacterial leakage between the parts, thus colonising the inner portion of the connections. This bacterial reservoir will induce local tissue inflammation and localised bone loss. It has been suggested that this is one of the causes of early crestal bone loss around dental implants. The inside of the connection is low in oxygen concentration and distant from any tissue, which can provide an inflammatory defensive response; therefore, it is a suitable environment for developing anaerobic bacteria that will produce peri-implant pathology (figure 1.12).

The precision fit between the components, the repeated screw loosening and re-tightening, and the loading force that the complex bears affect the size of the gap between the components. The loading force increases the micro-gap and the consequent pump effect between the inside of the dental implant and the peri-implant tissues.

Conical connections produce a superior seal with a micro-gap formation, accompanied by torque maintenance and abutment stability.

Using a mounter, which does not affect the prosthetic connection or minimise insertion torque, has been recommended since this can reduce microbial contamination [34].

Abutment materials:

Many different materials have been advocated for the construction of dental implant abutments. Commercially pure titanium and various titanium alloys have all been and still are used. Alumina, with its tooth-like colour, was tried until it was found to be susceptible to fracture during both laboratory and clinical procedures. Yttrium oxide-stabilised zirconia, with its improved mechanical strength, was introduced. Its mechanical properties, histological evaluation, plaque evaluation or bacterial adhesion and clinical survival rate have all been studied; however, limited review articles have been published. Although its mechanical strength is initially twice that of Alumina, it decreases after cyclic loading due to its ageing process. The method of its fabrication also affects its strength. Chair-side adjustment using a high-speed handpiece and diamond bur can also affect its clinical strength.

There is no difference in the peri-implant soft tissues around Zirconia or Titanium, but the tissue around zirconia may heal faster, with less plaque accumulation but no other clinical effect. While the colour of Zirconia is not Gray, it is still too white compared to that of natural teeth at the coronal cervix [35,36].

A better colour match is found when the mean buccal mucosal thickness exceeds 3 mm.

Regarding the shade of the soft tissue adjacent to the implant, It has also been concluded that no matter which type of restorative material is used, the soft tissue shade is different compared to that around neighbouring natural teeth. When the soft tissue thickness is less than 2 mm, gold zirconia or titanium nitride abutments provide a shade much closer to the neighbouring teeth [37, 38].

Gold-palladium and zirconia abutments with universal shade cement can be used, but the titanium abutment to support all-ceramic crowns can be masked by white opaque cement [39].

Soft tissue surgery or graft (sub-epithelial connective tissue graft or collagen matrix) may need to be advocated when using titanium abutments.

A single-component zirconia implant superstructure has been recommended. This consists of the zirconia abutment and framework in one component. The handling is easier, and the insertion procedure is friendly. Adequate support beneath the veneer ceramic is a necessity.

Abutments made from castable materials have been marketed. With these, the technician uses resin or wax to build the external implant surface of the one-piece crown abutment. The casting of the surfaces that enter the interior of the dental implant has not been validated, and this technique is questionable.

Gold hue titanium abutments can also help. These can be produced commercially or by a laboratory. Nano-silver coating prevents biofilm formation as the colour is pinkish [40].

High voltage anodisation by an electrochemical process has been used. This uses dilute phosphoric acid, and silver ion exchange from the solution forms a layer with a thickness of 5 um. This has a violet appearance, increased durability and an enhanced antimicrobial effect. It looks promising.

The anodic oxidation of titanium produces a superficially dark pink colour in abutments and does not influence the biocompatibility of the titanium surface [41].

Consideration of aesthetics should not be limited to that of the crown – that of the soft tissue should be considered, too. That soft tissue is more translucent because of the reduced vascularisation of the soft tissue around dental implants. We can use titanium nitride with a gold hue to eliminate the soft tissue's potentially grey cast. As mentioned previously, Zirconia abutments with their white appearance can have their appearance masked as long as there is soft tissue of a minimum of 2 mm thickness surrounding the zirconia [42].

Narrowing the abutment emergence profile increases the connective tissue's thickness and reduces the titanium's grey effect. However, discolouration has been reported despite using a zirconia abutment and an all-ceramic crown [43].

Material	Advantages	Disadvantages
Zirconia	Aesthetics similar to that of natural crown No alloy allergy CAD/CAM customised	More potential fracture Metal Ti base can debond Over-preparation weakens its strength Technique sensitive Colour shows through thin, soft tissue
Titanium	Strongest Not technique sensitive CAD/CAM milling potential	The grey colour shows through thin, soft tissue
Gold-Hue	Strongest Good aesthetics in thin, soft tissue CAD/CAM milling	Abutment preparation eliminates the aesthetic gold appearance

Table 9.1 A summary of the abutment materials and their advantages and disadvantages.

Polyetheretherketone (PEEK), to be used as an abutment, has an elastic modulus closer to that of bone and can be modified by reinforcing it with carbon fibres to achieve a modulus close to that of cortical bone. It was introduced to the market in 1998 (Invibio Ltd, Thornton-Cleveleys). The PEEK abutment has a higher stress concentration in the cervical region compared to that of Titanium. The CFR (carbon fibre-reinforced)-PEEK is black due to the carbon fibres and, therefore, unsuitable in the aesthetic area [43,44].

Abutment screw:

Screw abutment behaviour is complex and under-researched. Screw abutments flex and shift under strain and stress. A degree of screw torque-tightening is carried out to overcome the friction between the abutment screw head and the abutment-seating surface. Some screw torque-tightening is performed to overcome friction between the threads, and only 10% produces tension [45,46].

Palladium gold can be used (with or without solid lubricant), or the titanium surface can be treated to reduce friction. Teflon should not be used as it decreases the coefficient of friction [47].

A lubricant like minocycline hydrochloride ointment increases the clamping force and increases the fatigue life of the screw, but at high load, the opposite behaviour will be observed, leading to ductile fracture at the first thread. This is the leading cause of failure. While it provides lower de-torque forces, which make the joint easier to loosen, it does not improve the dental implant-abutment grip [48].

Repeated consecutive opening and closing of the abutment screws leads to loss of torque retention [49].

Risk factors:

Risk analysis – the identification of potential risks and their prevention - is one of the keys to successful treatment.

Most people show their incisors and papillae, so replicating natural teeth is essential. While replicating a tooth is complex, replacing soft tissue and multiple teeth is far more complex.

The inter-arch distance may influence the choice of the final restoration: if the distance is less than 10 mm, then a fixed prosthesis is recommended, and if it is more than 15 mm, a removable prosthesis would have fewer complications (figure 9.14). The torque on the implant significantly increases with the added height, and the prosthesis's weight will be a further concern. In these cases, using materials such as BIOHPP - which is PEEK, a ceramic-reinforced polymer - is promising. If the bridge is long enough that it is not in a straight line and is in a tripod position, the torque on each dental implant is reduced, which can be beneficial in scenarios where a high load is inevitable.

Patients have three overriding preferences during implant treatment: comfort, a short chair time during surgical treatment, and acceptable provisional aesthetics between treatment visits. Despite the development of techniques enabling immediate implant placement with immediate restoration, there are still cases where two-stage surgery is recommended, so patient preferences will need to be addressed.

When planning dental implant treatment, the dentist will need to assess a number of factors and take them into account, which are as follows: patient-orientated aesthetics such as the lip line, dental morphology, bone morphology, three-dimensional limitations which govern the operative environment such as the interdental space, ideal implant positioning, optimal surgical approach for handling the soft tissue, the characteristic of the prosthetic crown, as well as the preferred provisional prosthesis.

All these factors are interrelated.

The interdental space should be 5.5mm mesiodistally and 6.5mm buccal-lingually, with 1.5mm made available in the proximal regions to allow for the formation of the gingival papillae. These will determine the dimensions of the future crown.

If the implant axis is the same as the crown axis, then the crown height will be similar to that of the natural crown. If the implant axis has a lingual inclination, then the prosthetic crown's inevitable buccal overextension will jeopardise its aesthetics and subsequent hygiene needs.

If the implant axis has a buccal inclination plus a more apical placement, this will lead to the early emergence of the cervix, necessitating a long prosthetic crown. Now, the cervical area does not align with the adjacent teeth.

The position of the ideal abutment-implant junction is a subject of disagreement. In one study, there was less bone resorption when the junction was placed supracrestally, and the connection extended to the outer circumference of the implant [50].

Another study reported that subcrestal placement of the implant-abutment junction demonstrated less bone resorption, with a tendency towards thicker gingival epithelium and connective tissue [51].

When the diameter of the abutment is deliberately made smaller than that of the implant – this is known as platform switching – the abutment periphery is not immediately adjacent to the bone. This discrepancy has the beneficial effect of decreasing crestal bone loss, promoting soft tissue health by sealing off the abutment-implant junction from the oral environment and producing favourable stress distribution within the implant complex [52].

Dental implant companies have designed dental implants in which the coronal part of the implant flares to accommodate an abutment which is roughly the same diameter as the implant body but narrower than the flared neck. Such a design demands a minimum of 6.5mm of alveolar crestal bone, which is unlikely to be available. If this is the case, using restorative components with a smaller diameter will be necessary.

Comparing different techniques, subcrestal dental implant placement and platform-switching of abutment-implant components encourage bone stability and soft tissue growth at the superior edge of the implant circumference.

The result is a greater degree of papilla-fill and less bone loss. Conversely, Cochran et al. found slightly more bone loss if platform-switched implants were placed 1mm subcrestally, compared with those placed 1mm supracrestally. Veis disagreed and concluded there was less bone loss [53, 54].

Subcrestal placement has aesthetic advantages by providing a minimum of 3mm extra height to allow an anatomical emergence profile.

Several procedural options affect the peri-implant gingivae:
• The application of a template for the optimal implant position,
• The application of the implant-supported provisional prosthesis,
• The size and form of the restorative platform,
• The abutment material,
• The final prosthetic mode of retention of the final prosthesis.

While the effectiveness of the surgical guide or template is arguable in the buccal-lingual position, it must be remembered that the facial position of the implant can certainly influence gingival recession.

Unfortunately, no published studies have a comparison of the aesthetic outcome of the provisional prosthesis as their primary experimental focus. Papilla regeneration has been seen in most cases. Even though, because of a lack of data, no firm conclusion can be drawn, it seems that horizontal offset designs have resulted in stable or even a slight gain of the midfacial mucosal height [55].

Definitive Restorative Material

Screw-retained all-ceramic restorations demonstrate no difference in papilla regeneration when compared with metal-ceramic restorations. However, while the crown morphology, colour, and mucosal discolouration were no different, the all-ceramic restoration had superior aesthetics.

A comparison of all-ceramic definitive restorations shows whether cement- or screw-retained, showing that the gingival tissue's colour was the same in both groups. Customised ceramic abutments with an all-ceramic restoration did not improve marginal soft tissue volume compared to those produced by standard prefabricated abutments with metal-ceramic crowns.

Even though there are some standard gauges for papillae evaluation, there is little agreement in the literature to allow a standardized judgement on the aesthetic outcome of different restorative procedures [56].

Because both the internal thread of the dental implant and the external thread of the abutment cannot be machined perfectly smooth, as the surface irregularities seen under the SEM demonstrate, a part of the initial torque applied is used to overcome the resultant friction rather than drive down the screw [57].

A lower predetermined torque value will be achieved, and a settling of the engaged surfaces will be observed after final screwing and preloading. Thus, a second torquing should be applied to limit the settling effect. It is documented that, during both abutment screw insertion and removal, frictional resistance can be affected by metal debris. It is strongly suggested, therefore, that the complete removal of debris will improve the preload maintenance of the abutment screw complex [58].

The re-use of trans gingival healing abutments (Gingival formers) used to be recommended by dental implant manufacturers. However, adhering strictly to varying cleaning and sterilisation protocols is essential when removing biological debris from reused healing abutments to ensure successful re-attachment of subgingival connective tissue. For instance, protocols can include cleaning with detergent and either ultraviolet light, steam autoclaving, or a combination of the preceding with plasma cleaning. Plasma cleaning and Ultraviolet sterilisation can be effective, but autoclaving alone is inadequate if organic and inorganic debris has not been removed beforehand [59]. It must be added that in some countries, the re-use of healing abutment is not legal.

It must be emphasised that no matter what sterilising technique is applied, a clean, non-contaminated abutment should be placed in the dental implant. It needs to be decontaminated after handling the abutments in the dental laboratory. Exposure to saliva at placement can inhibit the adhesion of gingival fibroblasts and induce epithelial down-growth. The presence of an amino alcohol film will prevent re-integration from occurring at the implant-tissue interface. H_2O_2 5% does not remove the amino alcohol, but exposure to ozone does.

Note that repeated abutment disconnection and reconnection after alcohol disinfection can induce both apical repositioning of the soft tissues and marginal bone resorption [60]. However, a single repositioning of the healing abutment led to no marginal bone loss [61].

When the company recommends the single use of healing abutments, it is illegal for them to be reused.

Clinical studies have demonstrated that "one abutment - one-time" results in significantly less marginal bone loss than conventional techniques [62].

Intraoral radiography can help check the accuracy of fit of the abutment to the implant at the junction. This depends on accurate beam alignment with the implant-abutment junction, and the co-incidence of the angle of the collimator to that of the implant is critical. The clarity of the threads on the film also determines the diagnostic value of the radiographs.

It has been shown that the use of a paralleling device will help the clinician more accurately assess the

the implant-abutment junction where there are 50- and 100-mm gaps [63].

From his experience, the author recommends the following clinical steps as providing the most straightforward and convenient approach for both patient and dentist:
- place a standard abutment instead of a gingival former,
- prepare intra-orally,
- then place the provisional bridge to make sure that the aesthetics are acceptable, and the occlusion is correct,
- after that, plan to make final impressions at the abutment level and then insert the permanent bridges.

9.4. Dental Implant Impression

These are classified into two main groups: direct and indirect. Direct impressions are those to be made directly from the abutment, and indirect are made when the position of the implant has to be transferred to the cast for the addition of another component.

Conventional three-piece dental implant impressions

The position of the dental implants must be accurately transferred to the cast (or via other means if appropriate) to produce the dental prosthesis.

All dental impression techniques work, and each has advantages and disadvantages. While the dentist chooses which technique will be used, the best results come when the dentist and technician work together, perhaps even training together.

The first point to consider will be whether the abutment will be placed directly in the mouth immediately after dental implant placement or at the second stage of surgery, whether the abutment will be prepared in the patient's mouth or be prepared by the technician, or a mix of the above.

When the level of the dental implant is more than 2 mm below the gingival margin, the ability to take a successful impression at the dental implant abutment level will be a challenge. In the author's view, any recommendation to obtain a dental implant level impression is not generally justified as there may be abutments of different gingival heights available, depending on the system being used, although the option is not guaranteed.

In the mixed technique, the dental technician does the abutment selection, customisation, and preparation of the finishing margin supragingival. This is then cleaned and sterilised so the dentist can place the semi-customised abutment in the implant instead of placing the temporary trans gingival extension (Gingival Former or healing abutment). The final finishing margin is prepared after the complete healing of the soft tissue has taken place.

If the abutment is to be placed inside the dental implant, it may make impression-taking uncomfortable for the patient. This would be so if the gingivae have encroached on the abutment space through overgrowth. The degree of discomfort will depend on the degree of overgrowth. Furthermore, the thicker the soft tissue, the greater the chance of not placing the abutment in the correct position.

Accordingly, the greater the number of dental implants to be placed, the greater the unpredictability at each session and placing the abutments in the correct position at the um level.

Indirect (implant level or abutment level) impression:

Open tray impression:

In this technique, a long screw fastens the impression coping or post to the dental implant, with its proper seating being confirmed by a bitewing X-ray. A special tray is used, although a stock plastic tray with an appropriate hole is possible. The dentist must ensure that the long screw, as it passes through the tray, does not touch the surface of the impression tray at all. Careful control of the impression tray must be maintained to ensure that the patient can open his mouth for the procedure.

It is also important to note that before the impression has been set, the dentist must make sure that all the tips of the long screws (if more than one is used) are visible. If they are not, remove the unset impression material with a spatula to expose the tips of the long screws. If the dentist forgets this simple

point, removing the impression without sectioning the tray, cutting the impression material, and removing the sectioned pieces will be impossible. This is hazardous, will take a long time, and the impression will need to be repeated.

After taking the impression using polyether, polyvinylsiloxane, or polyvinyl sulfide, the impression post is unscrewed completely, and the impression is removed, which the impression post would be pickup simultaneously with the impression. A dental implant analogue (which is a replica of the implant with the same dimensions as the inner part of the implant) is screwed to the impression post.

The use of square sandblasted impression copings does not produce a significant difference in the abutment-framework interface gap but significantly reduces the chances of the accidental displacement of the direct impression (implant) copings [64].

Splinting the impression post has been recommended, but it remains a personal preference rather than being evidence-based. The use of metal-splinted impression copings was found to significantly affect the better accuracy of the abutment-framework interface gap compared to that found with the use of Duralay-splinted impression copings [65].

We do not recommend using pattern resin to splint the impression posts, and we much prefer using composite in two layers. First, make a rectangular shape (block) composite around each impression post, leaving a space of 1mm between each block. At a separate stage, the 1mm gap will be filled with fluid composite, the shrinkage of which will be minimal. This may become tricky if the implant position is altered.

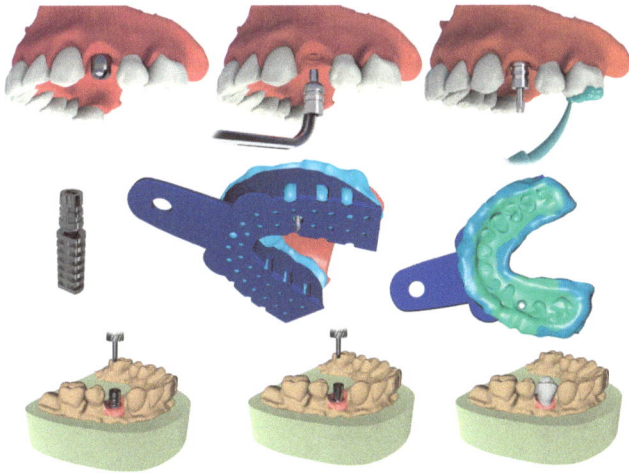

Figure 9.12a Steps of the open tray impression. The gingival former is removed, and an impression post with a long screw is placed. The stock tray is perforated. After setting of impression, the long screw is removed, and the impression post, which is set in the impression, comes out of the patient's mouth. The implant analogue is fastened by putting back the long screw and sent to the laboratory. The impression post is removed at the laboratory, an abutment is placed and prepared, and the crown is fabricated.

We do not recommend using pattern resin to splint the impression posts, and we much prefer using composite in two layers. First, make a rectangular shape (block) composite around each impression post, leaving a space of 1mm between each block. At a separate stage, the 1mm gap will be filled with fluid composite, the shrinkage of which will be minimal. This may become tricky if the implant position is altered.

Close tray impression:

When the screw is short (at most at the level of the impression post when it is unscrewed), the impression post is fastened to the implant analogue, and then the entire unit is inserted into the impression in the proper orientation. After removing the impression, the short screw is unfastened and removed. The impression post is removed, placed in the implant analogue, the screw is placed and fastened. The complex implant analogue, screw and the impression post is placed in the impression.

Both techniques work and have their own limitations, but the open-tray technique seems more accurate. Also, a polyether impression of soft, medium consistency has better dimensional accuracy compared to that of a vinyl polysiloxane. The relative gaps will be 31.5um and 151um, respectively [66].

The indirect technique has the advantage that the stone master cast can be more easily adjusted as the technician fabricates the soft tissue model.

A study was conducted by Berri et al. to examine the effectiveness of communications between dental technicians and dentists. It was central to the study for the needs of both technician and dentist to be considered as a team project.

Even though most of the data was collected from memory, it was still found that the catalogue of poor practices is shared equally between laboratories and practices.

Impressions were not clearly labelled as having been disinfected; about 65% of impressions for the fabrication of prostheses were disinfected by the lab before being poured, and 60% of impressions were taken using full arch plastic or metal custom trays or dual arch impression (triple tray technique), or quadrant plastic or metal trays, while custom tray use was of a lower percentage.

The leading causes of poor impressions were bubbles or voids, deformation of the impression material, and defects at the preparation margins.

Most laboratories used semi-adjustable, simple hinges or static articulators with only an up-and-down motion. Only 11% of occlusal records sent to the laboratories were satisfactory, and only 5% of the dentists provided a design guide to help the tech-

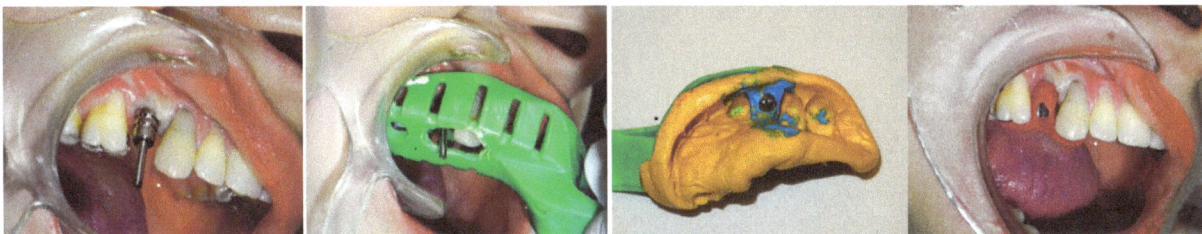

Figure 9.12b. The clinical steps of open tray impression. When the abutment is inserted, it is wise to use the laboratory jig to ensure it is sitting properly.

202

nician in the fabrication of the definitive prosthesis, such as a diagnostic wax-up or a tooth preparation guide for an impression of the provisional prosthesis.

The crown's shape and size need to be transferred to the laboratory by diagnostic wax-ups, written instructions, drawings, and/or contour guides such as a putty index and photographs. In most cases, the dentist detailed the type of the material to be used, with half of the requests being metal-based and the other half being palladium alloy, low gold content, or high gold content. About 70% were metal-ceramic in the anterior region, with almost 30% all-ceramic and a small number of metal-composite. About 70% of requests in the posterior region were for metal-ceramic, 20% were for metal only, and only 8% all-ceramic. In a small percentage, poor communication meant it was left to the technician to decide both the surface material and the veneering material [67].

No reports comment on how often implant analogues and impression posts can be used, but it is clear that they should be used singly for accuracy.

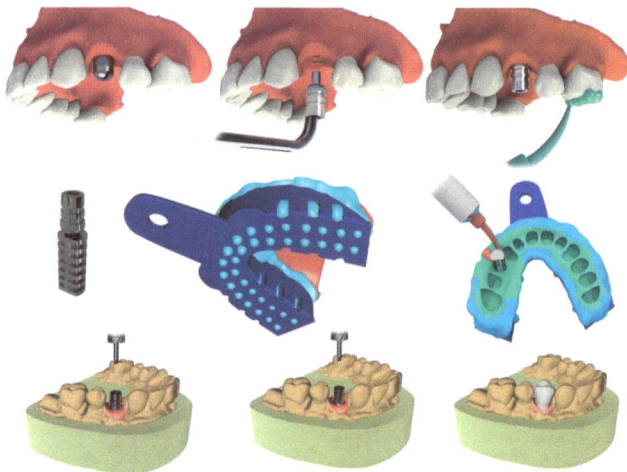

Figure 9.13 Steps of the close tray impression. The gingival former is removed, and an impression post with a long screw is placed. The stock tray is Not perforated. After setting of impression, the impression is taken out; then, the short screw is removed with the impression post, which is left in the mouth while taking the impression out. The implant analogue is fastened to the impression post and put back manually; the complex of impression post, short screw and implant analogue and sent to the laboratory. The impression post is removed at the laboratory, an abutment is placed and prepared, and the crown is fabricated.

Direct (abutment level) impressions
Intra-oral abutment preparation:

Abutment preparation must maximise height and be tapered to provide resistance and retention. When all the prepared surfaces are viewed from above, all the margins and internal line angles must be clearly visible.

Ideally, a single path of insertion should be achieved. Avoid the potential overhang of the adjacent teeth over the margins of the prepared abutment, where it could impinge on the path of insertion or withdrawal of the definitive crown.

The opposing wall in the gingival half of the preparation should be near parallel and the rest more tapered, leaving a minimum of 2mm of occlusal space.

Two factors are responsible for the smoothness of a marginal preparation: the rotating instrument and the handpiece used. For all diamond tools, the surface roughness of the samples is directly proportional to the size of the diamond grains of the bur. The elastic aluminium oxide fibres of the dura white stone can polish a surface to a certain degree.

Whenever possible, the preparation margin should be supragingival, following the natural contour of the gingivae. Chamfers and shoulders have definite finish margins, which can be identified in preparations, provisional crowns, and dies.

The impression material's ability to access the preparation margins should be evaluated.

The capture by the impression material of the margins of the abutment preparation may require the careful clearance of blood and debris, careful haemostasis, and gingival retraction.

There are several ways to retract soft tissue. For instance, put a small amount of topical anaesthetic on the end of a cotton roll and use finger pressure push till the end of the cotton roll reaches the finishing margin and soft tissue around it. Keep it there for 3 minutes. This will expose the margins of the abutment.

A pre-selected pressure kit that does just this is available. Expasyl (Kerr, CA), a clay-like material consisting of Kaolin and Aluminium chloride, is injected through a narrow blunt needle and works only by expansion. The material is left for 2 minutes and then rinsed off. The sulcus is ready for the impression.

Injection of the clay expands and does not need haemostatic solutions, which claims it saves chair time, avoids tearing gingiva and is more comfortable for the patient. It also absorbs excess crevicular fluid. However, the author's experience is not as good as mentioned.

Difficulty in placement and removal and in not controlling the bleeding.

Magic Foam Cord is another non-haemostatic vinyl polysiloxane that retracts the gingiva. The material is injected into the margin and pressured with a putty impression material in a stock tray. The material is expanded, and after 5 minutes, the impression can taken. It does not help to control bleeding.

The default method is the use of a retraction cord, followed by the detachment of the pseudo-attachment. Subsequent gingival recession has been reported. Usually, if the finishing margin is no more than 1mm in the gingival sulcus, pressure by the silicone putty or Impregum will take the impression of the finishing margin without any retraction device.

Where there is the possibility of poor marginal adaptation of the provisional prosthesis because of gingival overgrowth, removal of marginal soft tissue is indicated.

The author's experience with soft laser is that it can provoke a gingival recession. He believes the best results are achieved with the ceramic soft tissue trimmer in a high-speed handpiece (rpm:200.000-500.000) without irrigation. For contouring and cutting the gingiva, a 45-degree angle is recommended. For widening the sulcus to provide access to the impression material, an angle of 10-20 degrees is best. The ceramic trimmer also has a coagulating effect.

Put 3% hydrogen peroxide at the end of a cotton roll, and using finger pressure, press the roll over the preparation until the end reaches the finish margin and surrounding soft tissue. With a rotating movement, clean the abutment finish margin. Please do not use the dental air/water spray as it will promote bleeding. Hydrogen peroxide can halt minor bleeding and help prevent infections from setting in. It (H_2O_2) is the only germicidal agent composed only of water and oxygen - it kills disease organisms by oxidation. Although there is a common belief that H_2O_2 slows down healing, the author has not seen any evidence to support this, certainly for a single use.

The author believes that an impression at the direct abutment level is the most accurate and least complicated - especially in the maxillae, where the lack of parallelism is inevitable.

The author recommends a modified resin (acrylic) transfer coping technique in complex cases.

a) A primary impression is needed so the laboratory can provide a pattern resin frame. At the chairside, the pattern resin frame is adjusted on the abutments, and then a pick-up impression is provided using light body PVS and putty.

b) An alternative would be, if the finishing margin is short, the dentist can add the resin incrementally until a good margin is formed. Clinical adjustments of the resin framework may well have left internal discrepancies within the framework, which must be located and smoothed out. It is highly recommended that these be located using loupes and removed in the laboratory after casting.

c) Another approach would be to construct individual resin cuffs by incrementally applying the resin to the margins (do as much as possible on the model you already have) until you get a good margin. Add retention points to the exterior, then place silicone adhesive on the inside as well as all over the exterior, place light-body polyvinyl siloxane (PVS) material within them, place them in position, and then take a wash impression with light-body and putty.

d) Scribe a line at the soft tissue level or 1mm below the emergence point on the dental implant abutment. If the soft tissue is thick, ensure that the abutment's gingival height, or one-piece implant, has been selected accordingly. An appropriately sized copper band is selected. This needs to be annealed by heat. Using college tweezers or pliers, heat it till it gets red and then rub it with alcohol so it is soft and sterilised with no spring. The band should now slip neatly around the abutment without trapping any soft tissue, but you must ensure that this is so. If bleeding is observed, the tissue will re-attach without gingival recession. With a pencil, mark the abutment at the gingival margin, then trim the band with crown scissors and polish it with composite-polishing stones. The incisal end remained for retention within the overall impression with medium or heavy silicone.

Advantages:

With this approach, the potential errors of using an implant analogue, errors possible when transferring the impression post to the mouth, or the errors possible when casting, all the preceding, are eliminated.

Tolerances between the implant and the impression copings, analogue and abutments are between 0.022 and 0.1 mm 68.

This is especially so when the angles of the implants are not parallel. The tolerances of the manufacturing process become too many as each piece has dimensional tolerances, and the variability inherent in the transference of the implant position from the mouth to the cast is increased. This will be avoided when the abutment is placed in the dental implant: the model must exactly replicate its position in the mouth.

Because of the reduced number of pieces, the lab will treat it as a standard crown, applying a minor additional surcharge for the soft tissue model and alloy as the abutments are smaller than the naturally prepared crown.

A provisional crown can also be provided to protect against soft tissue growth and provide a fixed provisional prosthesis.

Indirect- direct impression

This approach may be recommended for implants with divergent angulation, which needs significant abutment preparation. An indirect impression is first provided, and then the dentist places the abutments, but a further impression (e.g. direct coping impression) will increase procedural accuracy.

Digital Impression (computer-aided design):

Patients do not like having dental impressions taken, and dentists do not like it when patients gag. When both these scenarios lead to the need for the correction of minor imperfections in the impression, it can be very frustrating. Hence, there is a current interest in digital impressions.

Digital implant impressions using intraoral scanners (IOS) have been continuously developed. It relies on technologies such as triangulation, confocal lasers, and active wavefront sampling to determine the relative position of the implant. IOS impressions can simplify the workflow and reduce time and material costs compared to traditional impressions. Theoretically, it may reduce the model deviation accumulated by traditional impression technology (such as impression material mixing, impression disinfection, impression storage, impression transportation, and gypsum model pouring) and can improve the accuracy and suitability of the final restoration.

Computer-aided design and computer-aided manufacturing (CAD-CAM) eliminate a series of current problems, but as with any new technology, it can present new challenges.

Digital intra-oral impression can be used when the finish line is clearly visible, and it is possible to keep it dry [69].

As the implants are placed subgingivally, a perfect transfer of the image of all parts of the implant is needed; there is a need for the perfect manufacturing and a perfect fit of the bodies within the implant.

Despite advertising claims that only 1.5 minutes is necessary

for a single unit impression and less than 1 minute for an impression of the opposite arch, there are still debates over the usefulness of digital impressions.

A single tooth impression can take about 6 minutes, and a full arch can take 21 minutes. These timings may be variable between different scanners [70].

The accuracy is a composite of trueness and precision. According to ISO standards, Trueness is defined as the proximity of measurement to the actual dimension, and precision is the repeatability of measurements. Operator experience, design of scan bodies, position, number and angle of dental implants, scan and strategy affect the Shape, colour, material, and alignment between the captured mesh and STL file used in the software, affecting the correct acquisition position of the dental implants.

Proper training and clinical experience may well increase the popularity of digital impression-taking. The digital impression of the subgingival margin is the most difficult to obtain accurately. It requires carefully isolating the surrounding soft tissues before the impression can be taken.

For undergraduate students with less experience, digital impressions are claimed to be more efficient than conventional impressions [71].

Most of the intra-oral scanners employed in vitro provided acceptable accuracy (below a threshold of 150 μm). The main parameters identified for their influence on precision were interim plant distance, body scan design, scanning pattern and operator experience. Even though the literature is limited, significant differences emerged between the different models of intra-oral scanners evaluated in the studies considered within this review [72].

The clinical threshold of displacement is 100 um, and the accuracy of IOS impressions of implant-supported restorations varied greatly depending on the scanning strategy.

The linear displacement of the IOS impressions produced is 360 μm 3D linear displacement, but the pick-up impression is 160 μm. However, a 3D deviation of 27 um also has been reported. Different evaluation methods, distribution of implants, IOS devices, operator experience, and scan strategies probably caused unreliable results.

The primescan system, compared to Trios **4** and 3, demonstrates the slightest standard deviation, which statistically showed a significant difference [73].

In the completely edentulous arch, the image scan body is comparable to digital scanning; however, increased angulation (10 degrees) and increased distance of 10 mm reduced the accuracy of the impressions [74].

The 3D accuracy of different scanning strategies using TRIOS 3 intraoral scanner, compared with conventional open-tray splinted implant-level impressions, was inferior, even with 0 degrees angulation. The standard deviation of the conventional method was 91 um, but the digital method was 183 um, with an angular distortion of up to 0.69 um [75].

Another impression system in which the gingival former serves as a scan body is offered by Zimmer Biomat, which prevents abutment changes.

However, it is not advised to apply an elastomer impression of the coded healing abutment, cast it, and use the implant analogue in the master cast as the company recommends.

Even though some clinics prefer to use IOS impressions, many dentists prefer to wait for more improvement in precision [77].

Conventional and digital impressions have comparable accuracy; significant differences are in fossae and vertical displacement of the implant position from the gypsum and digitally milled model compared to the reference model. This displacement is more apical in the cast, and in milled models, the displacement is more coronal. Thus, the restoration from the conventional impression is hyper-occluded, which needs reduction and adjustments. However, the digital milled model restoration does not have occlusal contacts. The error of the conventional impression is due to numerous potential sources during placement of implant analogue, which can be reduced by direct impression; however, the error from the scanning system is systematic [78,79]. Scanners vary in their accuracy. There is a deviation pattern between single-shot captures, which can exhibit greater deviation at the tooth surface and high frame rates in the gingival margins.

As the distance between intra-oral scan bodies increases, the precision decreases. This is not observed when laboratory scanners are tested. Furthermore, detachment and repositioning of the scan bodies do not influence the precision of impression [80].

In private clinical practice, the high cost involved and the variabilities in the accuracy of digital scanners indicate the need for more research to explain the procedural discrepancies in the results obtained hitherto from the use of intra-oral scanners and digital dental impressions. Only when the causes of the discrep-

ancies have been ascertained can proper training be instituted. Remember that the increase in the cost of treatment should be justified, and increasing the cost will deprive a series of patients of dental implant treatment.

One-Piece Dental Implant impression:
Indirect:

If the abutment of the one-piece implant needs minor preparation, but the finishing margin does not need modification, then a putty and wash silicon impression can be taken, and a one-piece implant analogue of the same type and dimensions is placed in the impression tray. This can now be sent to the laboratory. After the impressions have been cast, the technician prepares the abutment and provides a jig for the dentist to use intra-orally. The dentist will reproduce the preparation in the patient's mouth by using the jig until it fits at the margins. This confirms that the preparation needed has been achieved.

Direct:

The same procedure is used for the direct impression of a three-piece dental implant.

The patient's maxilla–mandibular relationship is established and recorded in centric relation. The dental casts from the intraoral impressions are then mounted on articulators. We recommend using a face bow in the case of a partial fixed bridge where there are no natural teeth and occlusal stops are not available. Establish tooth set-ups with anterior and cuspid guidance in laterotrusion.

The wax-up is pattern resin with wax build-up. This is now tested for fit intra-orally, and following dentist and patient approval, it is indexed for final reconstruction. The passive fit test is performed by pressing the most distal end. Inaccuracies are adjusted by cutting and welding the resin wax pattern until a passive fit is achieved.

The processed prosthesis is adjusted to fit with the occlusion using articulating and/or Shimstock foil.

In the laboratory, burn-out copings placed over the implant analogues or directly onto the stone cast are adapted to the cast and connected by wax sticks. A passive fit on the cast is not required as it has been tested in the clinic, where the precision of its fit is greater than that on the cast. Sprue the wax models and invest them using investment materials compatible with the alloy. Cobalt-chromium alloys are cast in one piece and ground to the required shape. Heat the invested sprues to the required head using the company IFU and transfer them to the plasma machine. The molten alloy is injected into the mould under the required vacuum pressure.

The temperature and pressure need to be under control. After casting and cooling, the divested framework is sandblasted. Make sure that the area of the implant cylinder platform is not damaged. Examine its passive fit with an optical stereomicroscope at 15 magnifications. Because of technical complexities, some believe in order to provide a satisfactory fit, it has been recommended that it first be cast without the burn-out copings and then welded with a prefabricated gold cylinder using a laser-welder, but it is not necessary. The required adjustments have already been made by controlling the resin wax and trying it clinically.

9.5. Cementation Techniques

It has been recommended that a gingival retraction cord be used during cementation to prevent the cement from being contaminated by tissue fluid. In the aesthetic region, if the finishing margin of the crown is deeper than 2 mm, cord placement and removal will be difficult.

The finishing margin must follow the contour of the soft tissue. If the finishing margin is not in an ideal position, non-adhesive cement like zinc phosphate has been recommended. As an alternative, a screw-retained prosthesis can be employed.

A videoscope has been proposed to confirm the total removal of the cement remnants from the gingival sulcus. Some operators prefer to cure the resin for a very short time, three seconds and then remove excess resin as they find that the material peels away from the tooth more cleanly. Despite the earlier warning contraindicating subgingival preparations, should these occur, the latest research suggests that the use of resin-modified glass-ionomer cement leads to significantly less microleakage at the enamel margins compared to self-cure or dual-cure resin cement. However, there is no data regarding the titanium surface.

While the goal is to reduce the amount of finishing required to a minimum, there will always be situations where some are necessary. Using a series of finishing grit diamonds followed by a 30-fluted carbide bur and polishing pastes will produce highly satisfactory results. Polishing underwater spray has also produced a smoother surface than dry polishing. Despite these apparently reassuring findings, the general consensus is that the less finishing that needs to be done, the better.

9.6. Cement-retained versus Screw-retained

Microbial ingress has been observed in both cemented and screw-retained prostheses, with the cemented group presenting higher bacterial loads in the peri-implant sulcus but lower bacterial loads at the inner portion of the implant connection 81.

Cement-retained prosthesis:

Prefabricated or custom abutments are available. Zirconia and titanium abutments are on the market and can be prepared and customised intra-orally by the dentist or extra-orally by the laboratory. The abutment can be prepared using carbide or diamond burs with copious irrigation.

The custom abutments are ceramic, metal, or metal connected to ceramic.

The factors that influence the clinical choice are the intra-oral position of the dental implant, the soft tissue profile, the adjacent teeth or crowns, the opposing arch, the inter-arch space, and the school of thought that the operator favours.

Screw-retained prosthesis:

These are classified as horizontal or vertical screw-retained prostheses.

One-piece restorations can be classified as screw-retained, as the abutment and crown are all in one piece. In addition, the abutment can be tapped, and then a screw is used to fasten the final restoration to the abutment from a different position. Alternatively, a short screw can fasten the abutment to the implant, while another screw can fasten the prosthesis to the abutment. This is then called a horizontal (again from different positions) screw-retained prosthesis.

How can we cover the implant's titanium surface with an opaque layer – and why?

When the angulation of the alveolar ridge is adversely influenced by any inclination imposed by bone grafting, it can force the implant and abutment to be placed too buccally. This will reduce the space available buccally, which will, in turn, restrict the space needed to provide for good crown aesthetics. This is most readily seen in the upper anterior maxillae. Significant implant deviation from the optimum angulation can most easily be predicted by looking at the abutment or post. Where a compensating angle is needed, one answer can be a one-piece custom abutment/crown. However, the screw entry hole will be through the facial or incisal portion of the crown.

How to hide screw hole opening?

The Bisco repair kit, or other similar material, is compelling. Place a dry cotton, plumber's Teflon tap, gutta percha or any soft material in the depth of the hole. Place opaque from the kit over the soft material. Sandblast the internal surface and surroundings of the opening. Place silane and bonding agent, proper resin, and finish the margin. Another option would be to manufacture a metal or zirconia framework to position access holes that align with the locations of the implants. By utilizing screws, the framework is affixed to the implants. Individual ceramic or porcelain crowns are permanently bonded onto the framework. Each crown is securely attached to the framework at the designated position to effectively replace the missing tooth or teeth. Traditionally, this name was associated with a fixed metal bridge featuring acrylic teeth. However, more recently, "hybrid bridge" may refer to implant-supported restorations combining different materials and technologies to achieve optimal function and aesthetics.

Trends in Dental Implant Prostheses
Global Trends:

In dental implantology practices worldwide, clinicians often have the option to choose between cement-retained and screw-retained prostheses based on various clinical factors and practitioner preferences. While the prevalence of each type may vary by country, both options are commonly utilised to address patient needs and treatment objectives.

Cement-Retained Prostheses:

Cement-retained prostheses are favoured in many countries, including the United States, Canada, and the United Kingdom. These prostheses offer advantages such as enhanced esthetics and ease of fabrication, making them popular for clinicians seeking predictable outcomes in restorative dentistry.

Screw-Retained Prostheses:

Conversely, screw-retained prostheses are preferred in countries like Germany, Switzerland, and the Nordic countries (Sweden, Norway, and Denmark). These prostheses emphasise retrievability, ease of maintenance, and long-term stability, particularly in complex rehabilitative cases and scenarios where precision and passive fit are paramount.

Trends in the United Kingdom:

In the United Kingdom, dental implantology practices align with global trends, offering both cement-retained and screw-retained prostheses to address patient needs and clinical indications. However, recent observations suggest a growing preference for screw-retained prostheses, particularly in cases of full-mouth rehabilitation.

Factors Influencing Trends in the UK:

Several factors contribute to the increasing adoption of screw-retained prostheses in the UK. These factors include the emphasis on retrievability, ease of maintenance, and long-term stability, which align with the evolving standards of care and patient expectations in modern dentistry.

Clinical Considerations in the UK:

In clinical practice, the UK's choice between cement and screw-retained prostheses is influenced by factors such as esthetics, occlusal forces, implant position, and practitioner preferences. While both options offer distinct advantages, clinicians must carefully evaluate patient-specific needs and treatment objectives to determine the most appropriate prosthesis for each case.

Education and Training Programs:

Dental education and training programs in the UK provide clinicians with comprehensive training in both cement and screw-retained prostheses, equipping them with the necessary skills and knowledge to make informed clinical decisions and deliver high-quality patient care.

In conclusion, while the choice between cement and screw-retained prostheses may vary by country, dental implantology practices in the United Kingdom reflect global trends, offering both options to address diverse patient needs and treatment objectives. The increasing adoption of screw-retained prostheses in the UK underscores the importance of staying abreast of evolving standards of care and incorporating evidence-based practices into clinical decision-making processes.

Marginal accuracy of fit

Fit accuracy is considered one of the most important clinical quality and success criteria. Increased marginal discrepancy presents a greater risk for cement dissolution, subsequent microleakage, and heightened plaque retention. Ultimately, these factors can lead to the displacement of the crown from the abutment.

. Marginal openings not visible to the naked eye and undetectable with a sharp explorer are clinically acceptable.

The most considerable acceptable marginal discrepancy in visually accessible surfaces was 39 microns, according to Christensen and Lofstrom, who used a scanning electron microscope to measure the supragingival margins of crowns that were considered clinically well-fitting. Marginal discrepancies of 7 to 65 microns were observed [82,83].

The use of CAD/CAM did not increase the accuracy of the finishing margin, and 64-83 microns of leakage have been reported [84].

The author recommends using light wash silicone material at every trial step, comparing the frame, resin frame, and frame with porcelain. This should be done before cementation and should always be cut 360 degrees around the prosthesis. The average accuracy of fit will be less than 0.03 mm or 30 microns, with a tolerance of 10 microns.

Using a Coordinate Measuring Machine, the author measured the tips of the dental probe, which showed that the tip is in variable sizes and the average is 0.24 mm (240 microns) and demonstrates there is no clinical instrument to measure the gap between the crown margin and abutment. The tip of the probe is not standardized, and the dimensions of the tip would change after clinical use. Also, using probes in proximal surfaces is not possible. The author does not believe that a dental probe is an accurate and appropriate instrument to study the leakage between the margin of the crown and the abutment margin.

The author recommends using light body wash of additional polyvinyl siloxane impression material. Using this method demonstrates the proximal finishing lines and where they are not accessible. The author used the material and demonstrated an acceptable finishing margin when cutting the impression material. Using a Coordinate Measuring Machine, the margin of the impression cut was measured, and the thickness was between 0.025 mm (25 microns) and 0.038 (38 microns). This measurement should be applied in every step from resin frame,

frame only, frame with porcelain and after glaze before cementation (figure 9-14).

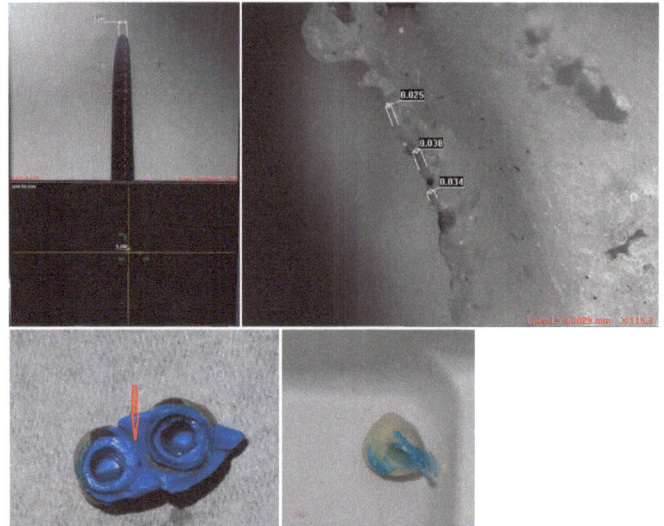

Figure 9.14 Upper left: the tip of the dental probe is 0.24 mm, and the upper right demonstrates the margin of the light body wash of additional polyvinyl siloxane impression. Lower left: the red arrow demonstrated that the wash had not been cut through. Lower right: the wash is cut 360 ° around the finishing margin of the crown.

9.7. Overdenture

The conventional complete denture has a low success rate in a resorbed ridge.

There are three options to resolve the issue: fixative, providing adequate depth in the labial vestibular area of the flange and overdenture retained by dental implants.

Denture adhesives:

The efficacy of cream, powder, and strips is not significant; however, the strips are easier to clean as others are messy, and incomplete removal is essential for the stability and hygiene of the denture.

Side effects of the denture adhesive are increased bone resorption development of denture stomatitis or candidiasis, especially in patients suffering from xerostomia. It is crucial to find the cause of the loose denture and not to solve the problem with adhesives as it will accelerate bone resorption. The long-term side effects on the digestive system are not apparent, as constipation has been reported. It used to have zinc, which is toxic and will result in nerve impairment, which was sued, and now it is zinc-free. A long solution of a loose denture is not recommended.

Surgical techniques have been developed to enhance the stability of dentures on a resorbed alveolar ridge. One such technique is vestibuloplasty, which involves deepening the vestibular trough (the space between the lips/cheeks and the gums), as well as altering the positions of the frenum (the small fold of tissue connecting the lips/cheeks to the gums) and muscle attachments. These procedures aim to create a more favourable environment for denture retention and improve the overall fit and comfort of the prosthesis.

The author proposes a modification of the lip-switch technique. If there are bony undercuts, do not remove the bone; instead, fill the undercut with artificial bone substitute particles and, after two months, proceed with vestibulopathy. After split-thickness, a longitudinal incision is made using blade 15 and blunt supraperiosteal dissection, detaching muscle fibres and fibrous bands on the periosteal bed. Before suturing the labial flap, a window with 3 mm of periosteum is removed at the predetermined depth. Thus, most of the periosteum is preserved, and the flap is attached directly to the bone, which prevents the relapse of the labial vestibule depth by healing with scar tissue.

The apical end of the flap is sutured to the lower border of the periosteum of the window. The flap is sutured using Vicryl 4 suture with a reverse triangle needle. The nude labial area is left to heal by secondary epithelisation.

No doubt, fixed restorations feel more natural than overdentures. However, there are circumstances including aesthetic and financial, lack of bone and the need for complicated surgeries, and the need for less complex hygiene procedures, which the patient's age will affect the patient's decision, that the patient requests overdenture.

Overdenture retained by dental implants is a simple and economical option, requiring 2-4 dental implants. However, it has high maintenance, so there would be the need to activate the attachment; attachment replacement and frequent relining are inevitable. Usually, it is used for the mandible and placing two

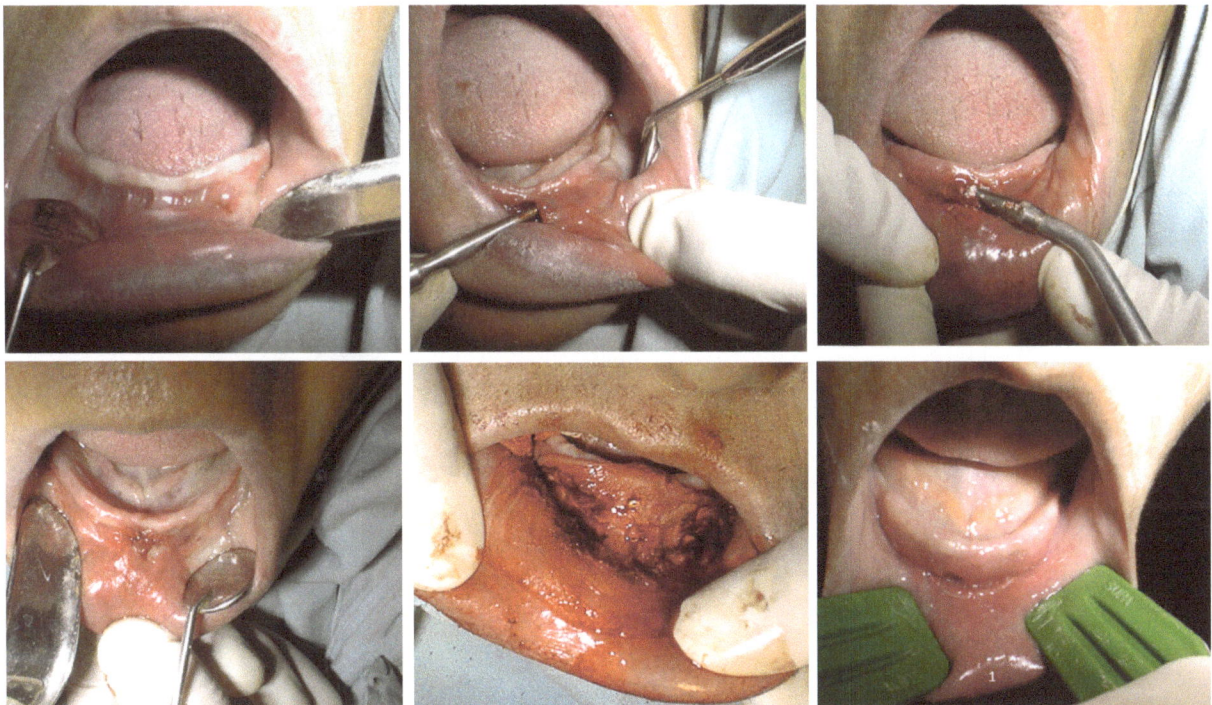

Figure 9.15 up (left to right), undercuts, frenum, and muscle attachments. An incision is made in the midline, and non-resorbable bone substitute particles fill the undercut. Low (left to right): after two months, the undercuts were filled, and a vestibuloplasty was performed, providing an improved base for the new denture.

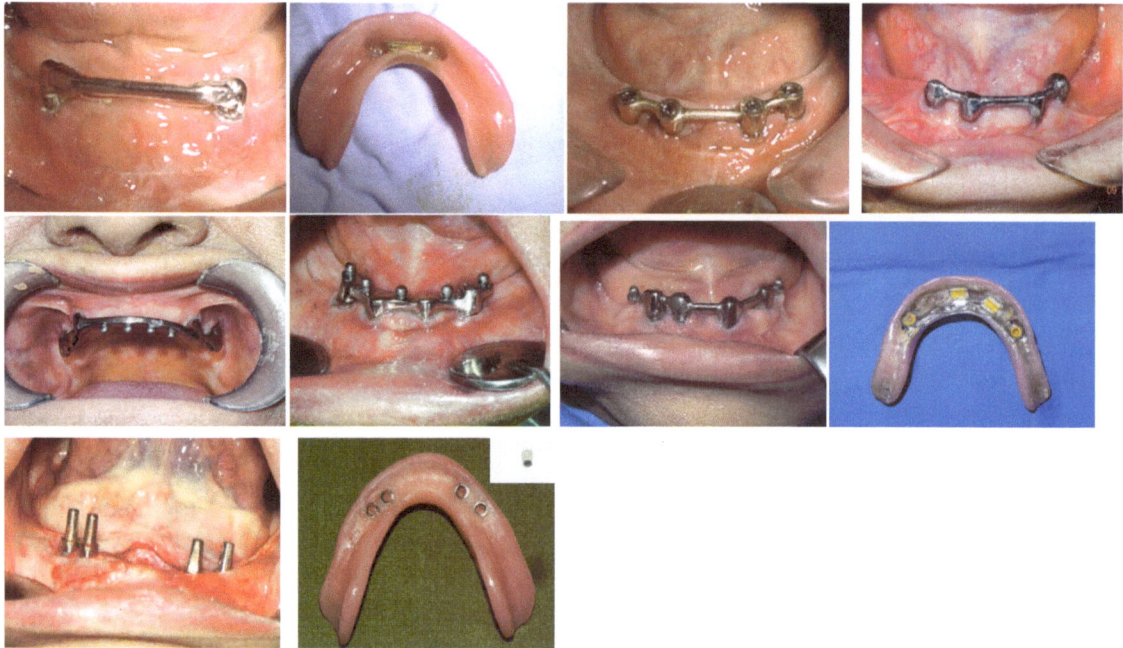

Figure 9.16 Up (left to right): two implants with one cement-retained metal gold bar and clip, screw-retained gold bar and cement-retained semi-precious bar. Middle: different types of studs. Low: four one-piece dental implants and prefabricated titanium telescopic attachment for immediate loading.

implants is the default treatment. If two implants are used in the mandible, they are usually placed in the lateral Incisors or Canines.

The attachment types are so various and many that we cannot mention all of them. The choice type depends on vertical space, the school of thought, and laboratory experience rather than evidence.

The types of implant attachment systems can be classified as free-standing and splinted bars.

The types of implant-supported overdentures can be categorised into two main groups: free-standing and splinted.

1. Free-standing types include:
• Studs (such as ball and socket, locator)
• Magnet attachments
2. Splinted types include:
• Bar attachments (direct retained)
• Studs integrated into a bar
• Offset attachments

These classifications outline the different types of attachments used in implant-supported overdentures based on their design and configuration.

The minimal interocclusal space for a bar is 13 mm, ball at-tachment is 10 mm, and locators are 8.5 mm, which can be estimated using CBCT and oral examination. Lack of space can provide a step on the overdenture's lingual surface and reduce the tongue space. Some patients may get used to it, and some would not tolerate it, especially those with a big tongue or sensitive patients.

The bar attachments are more rigid, and fewer movements are expected than free-standing attachments in which soft tissue loading is minimised by a bar. The bar has less frequent maintenance but is more demanding for cleaning.

During zygomatic implants, using bar attachment is the only treatment option. However, more cost and hygiene dexterity is the limitation. It also needs more space, which is usually available due to vertical bone loss. Bars can be used as direct retainers or indirect retainers, in which stud attachments are used. Also, offset attachments such as Plunger Loc can be used when redoing the bur is necessary, and instead of redoing, a hole is prepared in the bar, and the attachment (a small rod) is placed. Free-standing attachments are partially soft tissue-supported and have easier hygiene maintenance. The main ones are studs (ball attachments, Locator attachments), telescopic attachments and magnets.

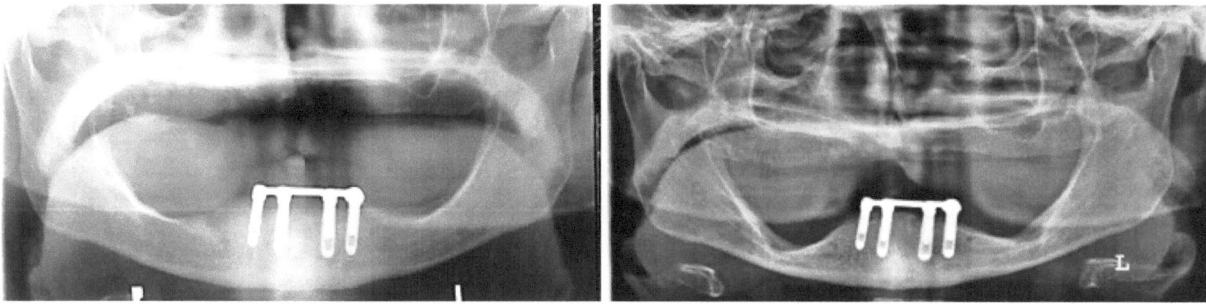

Figure 9.17 Overdenture after 25 years (the right DPT), bone loss in the posterior region is eminent.

Free-standing attachment is associated with lower microstrain values around the implants after vertical loadings [85].

The stud attachment is fitted into the implant, and the housing is in the overdenture. The studs are more vertically resilient, and the locator is more rotationally resilient; thus, some dentists prefer to use Studs (e.g., ERA system) for dental implants and locator for teeth.

Magnet retention wears off and needs replacement; however, as self-locating is more straightforward, it may help patients with limited manual adeptness. There has been a report of magnetic interference with MRI. The mandibular overdenture on two implants and more than two implants does not affect the masticatory efficiency [86].

However, the author believes 3 or 4 implants will provide more stability and retention to a denture, especially when the ridge is flat.

Maxillary overdentures are more prone to mechanical complications. Bar retention is the most successful, followed by ball- and magnet-based retention, which is the least successful. Passive fit of framework on abutments, adequate abutment screw tightening (use the company recommendation), application of internal hex instead of external hex and fabrication metal framework or overdentures and addressing precise occlusion adjustment is highly recommended in the maxillary overdentures [87].

Customised and prefabricated telescopic attachment has been used. Telescopic attachments are a good option for immediately loading fixed or removable prostheses. The application of frictional varnish can increase the retention of the overdenture, and freplacing it after fatigue is easy and affordable [88].

As a guide, the author recommends that 4 one piece implants and telescopic overdenture with frictional varnish is an ideal treatment plan if immediate loading is the plan. If the plan is delayed loading, four implants are retained by a bar and bilateral distal ball attachments to maximise the stability and minimise the soft tissue support and loading (figure 9.16).

There are controversies about the benefit of overdentures in preventing bone loss in the posterior region. However, on the basis of the author's experience, a successful overdenture does not prevent bone loss in the posterior region (figure 9.17).

References:

1. Hyung Joo Lee, Ivete Aparecida de Mattias Sartori, Paola Rebelatto Alcântara, Rogéria Acedo Vieira, Dalton Suzuki, Flávia Gasparini Kiatake Fontão and Rodrigo Tiossi: Implant Stability Measurements of Two Immediate Loading Protocols for the Edentulous Mandible: Rigid and Semi-rigid Splinting of the Implants. IMPLANT DENTISTRY /VOLUME 21, NUMBER 6 2012, 486-9.

2. Ross SB, Pette GA, Parker WB, Hardigan P: Gingival margin changes in maxillary anterior sites after single immediate implant placement and provisionalization: a 5-year retrospective study of 47 patients. Int J Oral Maxillofac Implants, Jan-Feb 2014;29(1):127-34.

3. Nik S, Golab K: Immediate aesthetic rehabilitation with one-piece implants. IDT, July 2015,1-3.

4. Anastassiadis PM, Hall C, Marino V, Bartold PM. Surface scratch assessment of titanium implant abutments and cementum following instrumentation with metal curettes. Clin Oral Investig. 2015 Mar;19(2):545-51.

5. Bohra PK, Ganesh PR, Reddy MM. Colour stability of heat and cold cure acrylic resins. J Clin Diagn Res 2015;9:12-15.

6. Balshi TJ, Wolfinger GJ: Conversion prosthesis: a transitional fixed implant-supported prosthesis for an edentulous arch—a technical note. Int J Oral Maxillofac Implants 1996;11: 106-111 N Y State Dent J 1997;63:32-35.

7. Cibirka RM, Linebaugh ML: The fixed/detachable implant provisional prosthesis. J Prosthodont 1997;6:149-152.

8. Babbush CA: Provisional implants: surgical and prosthetic aspects. Implant Dent 2001;10:113-120.

9. Ivanoff CJ , Gröndahl K, Sennerby L, Bergström C, Lekholm U: Influence of variations in implant diameters: a 3- to 5-year retrospective clinical report. Int J Oral Maxillofac Implants. Mar-Apr 1999;14(2):173-80.

10. Klongbunjit D, Aunmeungtong W, Khongkhunthian P: Implant-abutment screw removal torque values between customized titanium abutment, straight titanium abutment, and hybrid zirconia abutment after a million cyclic loading: an in vitro comparative study. Int J Implant Dent. 2021 Oct 4;7(1):98.

11. García-González M, González-González I, García-García I, Sergio Blasón-González , Lamela-Rey MJ, Alfonso Fernández-Canteli, Álvarez-Arenal A: Effect of abutment finish lines on the mechanical behavior and marginal fit of screw-retained implant crowns: An in vitro study. J Prosthet Dent 2022 Feb;127(2):318.

12. Ramzy NA, Azer AS, Khamis MM. Evaluation of the marginal adaptation and debonding strength of two types of CAD-CAM implant-supported cement-retained crowns. BMC Oral Health. 2023 Dec 5;23(1):967.

13. Seferis JC: Polyetheretherketone (PEEK): Polyetheretherketone (PEEK): processing-structure and properties studies for a matrix in high performance composites. Polymer Composites 1986;7:158-169.

14. Rivard CH, Rhalmi S, Coillard C: In vivo biocompatibility testing of peek polymer for a spinal implant system: a study in rabbits. J Biomed Mater Res 2002;62:488-498

15. Adler S, Kistler S, Kistler F. Compression-moulding rather than milling: a wealth of possible applications for high performance polymers. Quintessenz Zahntechnik2013;39:376-384

16. Neugebauer J, Adler S, Kisttler F: The use of plastics in fixed prosthetic implant restoration. ZWR- German Dent J 2013;122:242-245

17. Siewert B, Parra M: A new group of material in dentistry. Peek as a framework material used in 12-piece implant-supported bridges. Z Zahnarzt Implantol 2013;29:148-159.

18. Zoidis P, Papathanasiou I, Polyzois G The Use of a Modified Poly-Ether-Ether-Ketone (PEEK) as an Alternative Framework Material for Removable Dental Prostheses. A Clinical Report. J Prosthodont 2016 Oct;25(7):580-584.

19. International Organization for Standardization. Dentistry—Polymer-based filling, restorative and luting materials. 3rd edition. Geneva, Switzerland: ISO 4049; 2000.

20. Reis J, Jorge EG, Ribeiro JG, Pinelli LA, Abi-Rached F, Tanomaru-Filho M: Radiopacity Evaluation of Contemporary Luting Cements by Digitization of Image, ISRN Dent. 2012; 2012: 704246.

21. Heinemann F, Mundt T, Biffar R: Retrospective evaluation of temporary cemented, tooth and implant supported fixed partial dentures. J Craniomaxillofac Surg 2006 Sep:34 Suppl 2:86-90.

22. Pasqualini U, Pasqualini ME: Treatise of implant dentistry: The Italian tribute to moderna implantology. Carimate: 2009.

23. Bandela V, Basany R, Nagarajappa AK, Basha S, Kanaparthi S, Ganji KK, Patil S, Gudipaneni RK , Mohammed GS, and Alam MK: Evaluation of Stress Distribution and Force in External Hexagonal Implant: A 3-D Finite Element Analysis. Int J Environ Res Public Health. 2021 Oct; 18(19): 10266.1-9.

24. Maeda Y, Satoh T, Sogo M: In vitro differences of stress concentrations for internal and external hex implant-abutment connections: A short communication. Journal of Oral Rehabilitation 2006; 33(1):75-8.

25. Maior BS, Senna PM, Neto JP, Nóbilo MA, Cury AA: Influence of crown-to-implant ratio on stress around single short-wide implants: a photoelastic stress analysis. J Prosthodont . 2015 Jan;24(1):52-6.

26. Tsouknidas A, Lympoudi E, Michalakis K, Giannopoulos D, Michailidis N, Pissiotis A, Fytanidis D, Kugiumtzis D: Influence of Alveolar Bone Loss and Different Alloys on the Biomechanical Behavior of Internal-and External-Connection Implants: A Three-Dimensional Finite Element Analysis. Int J Oral Maxillofac Implants. 2015 May-Jun;30(3):e30-42.

27. Merz BR, Hunenbart S, Belser UC. Mechanics of the implant-abutment connection: an 8-degree taper compared to a butt joint connection. Int J Oral Maxillofac Implants 2000;15:519-26.

28. Bambini f, Lo Muzio L, Procaccini M. Retrospective analysis of the influence of abutment structure design on the success of implant unit. A 3-year controlled follow-up study. Clin Oral Implant Res 2001;12:319-324.

29. Bambini F, Meme L, Pellecchia M, Sabatucci A, Selvaggio R. Comparative analysis of deformation of two implant/abutment connection systems during implant insertion. An in vitro study. Minerva Stomatol 2005;54:129-38.

30. Goiato MC, Pellizzer EP, da Silva EV, Bonatto Lda R, dos Santos DM. Is the internal connection more efficient than external connection in mechanical, biological, and esthetical point of views? A systematic review. Oral Maxillofac Surg. 2015;19(3):229-42.

31. Mangano C, Mangano F, Piatelli A, Iezzi G, Mangano A, La Colla L. Prospective clinical evaluation of 307 single-tooth morse taper-connection implants: a multicentre study. Int J Oral Maxillofac Implants 2010;25:394-400.

32. Tesmer M, Wallet S, Koutouzia T, Lundgren T. Bacterial colonization of the dental implant fixture-abutment interface: an in vitro study. J Periodontol 2009;80:1991-7.

33. Schwarz MS. Mechanical complications of dental implants. Clin Oral Implants Res 2000;11:156-8.

34. King GN, Hermann JS, Schoolfield JD, Buser D, Cochran DL. Influence of the size of the microgap on crestal bone levels in nonsubmerged dental implants: a radiographic study in the canine mandible. J Periodontol 2002;73:1111-7.

34. Penarrocha-Oltra D, Rossetti PH, Covani U, Galluccio F, Canullo L: Microbial leakage at the implant-abutment connection due to implant insertion maneuvers: Cross-sectional study 5 years postloading in healthy patients. J Oral Implantol 2015;41(6):e292-6.

35. Pittayachawan P, McDonald A, Petrie A, Konwles JC: the biaxial flexural strength and fatique property of Lava Y-TZP dental ceramic. Dent Mater 2007;23:1018-1029.

36. Nakamura K, Kanno T, Milleding P: Zirconia as a dental implant abutment material: a systemic review. Int J Prosthodont 2010;23:299-309.

37. Lops D, Stellini E, Sbricoli L, Cea N, Eugenio R, Bressan E: Influence of abutment material on peri-implant soft tissues in anterior areas with thin gingival biotype: a multicentric prospective study. Clin Oral Imp Res 2017.28, 1283-1268.

38. Ferrari M, Carrabba M, Vichi A, Goracci C, Cagidiaco MC: Influence of abutment color and mucosal thickness on soft tissue color. J Oral Maxillofac Implants 2017;32:393-399.

39. Dede DO, Armagancie A, Ceylan G, Cankaya S, Celik E. Influence of abutment material and luting cements color on the final color of all ceramics. Acta Odonotologica Scandinavica 2013;71(6), 1570-1578.

40. Secinti KD, Özalp H, Attar A, Sargon MF. Nanoparticle silver ion coatings inhibit biofilm formation on titanium implants. J Clin Neurosci. 2011 Mar;18(3):391-5.

41. Kim YS, Ko Y, Kye SB, Yang SM. Human gingival fibroblast (HGF-1) attachment and proliferation on several abutment materials with various colors. Int J Oral Maxillofac Implants 2014;29:969–975.

42. Sailer I, Zembic A, Jung RE, Hammerle CH, Mattiola A. Single-tooth implant reconstructions: Esthetic factors influencing the decision between titanium and zirconia abutments in anterior regions. Eur J Esthet Dent 2007;2:296–310.

43. Happe A, Stimmelmayr M, Schlee M, Rothamel D. Surgical management of peri-implant soft tissue color mismatch caused by shine through effects of restorative materials: One-year follow-up. Int J Periodontics Restorative Dent 2013;33:81–88.

44. Schwitalla A, Muller WD: PEEK dental implants: A review of the literature. J Oral Implant 2013 (6);743-49.

45. Shigley JE, Mechanical Engineering Design, McGraw Hill Kogakusha.

46. Standlee JP, Caputo AA, Chwu MJ, Sun TT. Accuracy of mechanical torque-limiting devices for implants. Int. J. Oral Maxillofac Implants;17(2):220-4.

47. Elias CN, Figueira DC, Rios PR: Influence of the coating material on the loosening of dental implant abutment screw joints. Material Science and Engineering C26, 2006;1361-6.

48. Wu T, Fan H, Ma R, Chen H, Li Z, Yu H: Effect of lubricant on the reliability of dental implant abutment screw joint: An in vitro laboratory and three-dimension finite element analysis. Material Science and Engineering 2017 (C 75):297-304.

49. Weiss EI, Kozak D, Gross MD. Effect of repeated closures on opening torque values in seven abutment-implant systems. J Prosthet Dent . 2000;84(2):194-9.

50. Piatelli, A, Vrespa G, Petrone G, Lezzi G, Annibali S, Scarano A. Role of the microgap between implant and abutment: a retrospective histological evaluation in monkeys. J Periodontol 2003;74:346-52.

51. Welander M, Abrahmsson I, Berglundh T. Placement of two-part implants in sites with different buccal and lingual bone heights. J Periodontol 2009;80:324-9.

52. Baggi L, Cappelloni I, DiGirolamo M, Maceri F, Vairo G. The influence of implant diameter and length on stress distribution of osseointegrated implants related to crestal bone geometry: a three-dimensional finite element analysis. J Prosthet Dent 2008;100:422-31.

53. Cochran DL, Bosshardt DD, Grize L, Higginbottom FL, Jones AA, Jung RE. Bone response to loaded implants with non-matching implant-abutment diameters in the canine mandible. J Periodontol 2009;80:609-17.

54. Veis A, Parissis N, Tsirlis A, Papadeli C, Marinis G, Zogakis A. Evaluation of periimplant marginal bone loss using modified abutment connections at various crestal level placements. Int J Periodontics Restorative Dent

2010;30:609-17.

55. Canullo L, Iurlaro G, Iannello G. Double-blind randomized controlled trial study on post-extraction immediately restored implants using the switching platform concept: Soft tissue response. Preliminary report. Clin Oral Implants Res 2009;20:414–420.

56. Martin WC, Pollini A, Morton D: The influence of restorative procedures on esthetic outcomes in implant dentistry: a systemic review. Int J Oral Maxillofac Implants 2014;29(Suppl):142-154.

57. Khraisat A, Abu-Hammad O, A-Kayed AM, Dar-Odeh N. Stability of the implant-abutment joint in a single –tooth external –hexagon implant system: Clinical and mechanical review. Clin Implant Dent Res 2004;6:222-229.

58. Lee HW, Alkumru H, Ganss B, Lai JY, Ramp LC, Liu PR: The effect of contamination of implant screws on reverse torque. Int J Oral Maxillofac Implants 2015;30:1054-1060.

59. Vezeau PJ, Keller JC, Wightman JP: Reuse of healing abutments: an in vitro model of plasma coating and common sterilization techniques. Implant Dent 2000;9(3):236-46.

60. Abrahamsson I, berglundh T, Wennstrom J, Lindhe J. The peri-implant hard and soft tissues at different implant systems. A comparative study in the dog. Clin Oral Implants Res 1996;7:212-219.

61. Abrahamsson I, Berglundh T, Sekino S, Lindhe J. Tissue reactions to abutment shift: an experimental study in dogs. Clin Implant Dent Relat Rex 2003;5:82-88.

62. Canullo L. Bignozzi I, Cocchetto r, Cristali MP, Iannello G: Immediate positioning of a definitive abutment versus repeated abutment replacement in post-extractive implants: 3 years follow-up of a randomized multicenter clinical trial. Eur J Oral Implantol 2010;3:285-296.

63. Lin KC, Wadhwani CPK, Cheng J, Sharam A, Finen F: Assessing fit at the implant-abutment junction with a radiographic device that does not require access to the implant body. J Prosthet Dent 2014;112:817-823.

64. Wee AG. Comparison of Impression Materials for Direct Multi-Implant Impressions. Journal of Prosthet Dent, 2000; 83, 323-331.

65. Del Acqua MA, Chavez AM, Castanharo SM, Compagnoni MA, Mollo Fde A Jr. The effect of splint material rigidity in implant impression techniques. Int J Oral Maxillofac Implants. 2010 Nov-Dec;25(6):1153-8.

66. Del'Acqua MA, Chávez AM, Amaral AL, Compagnoni MA, Mollo Fde A Jr. Comparison of impression techniques and materials for an implant-supported prosthesis. Int J Oral Maxillofac Implants. 2010 Jul-Aug;25(4):771-6.

67. Berry J, Nesbit M, Saberi S, Petridis H. Communication methods and production techniques in fixed prosthesis fabrication: a UK based survey. Part 2: Production techniques. Br Dent J. 2014 Sep;217(6):E13.

68. Ma T, Nicholls JI, Rubenstein JE. Tolerance measurements of various implant components. Int J Oral Maxillofac Implants. 1997; 12(3):371–375.

69. Lee JS, Gallucci GO: Digital vs conventional implant impressions: efficacy outcomes. Clin Oral Impl Res 2012, 24:111-115.

70. Patzelt SB, Lamprinos C, Stampf S, Att W. The time efficiency of intraoral scanners: an in vitro comparative study. J Am Dent Assoc. 2014 Jun;145(6):542-51

71. Lee JS, Gallucci GO: Digital vs conventional implant impressions: efficacy outcomes. Clin Oral Impl Res 2012, 24:111-115.

72. De Rubertis C, Ferrante F, Stefanelli N, Friuli M, Madaghiele M, Demitri C, Palermo A. The accuracy of intra-oral scanners in full arch implant rehabilitation: a narrative review. Br Dent J. 2023 Dec;235(11):887-891.

73. Meneghetti PC, Li J, Borella PS, Mendonça G, Burnett Jr LH. Influence of scanbody design and intraoral scanner on the trueness of complete arch implant digital impressions: An in vitro study. PLoS One. 2023 Dec 19;18(12): e0295790. doi: 10.1371/journal.pone.0295790.

74. Jeong M, Ishikawa-Nagai S, Lee JD, Lee SJ. Accuracy of impression scan bodies for complete arch fixed implant-supported restorations. J Prosthet Dent 2023 Dec 12:S0022-3913(23)00766-7.

75. Blanco-Plard A, Hernandez A, Pino F, Vargas N, Rivas-Tumanyan S, Elias A. 3D Accuracy of a Conventional Method Versus Three Digital Scanning Strategies for Completely Edentulous Maxillary Implant Impressions. Int J Oral Maxillofac Implants 2023, Dec 12;38(6):1211-1219.

76. Talesara V, Bennani V, Aarts J, Ratnayake J, Khurshid Z, Brunton P. Accuracy of digitally coded healing abutments: A systematic review. Saudi Dent J. 2023 Dec;35(8):891-903.

77. Ma J, Zhang B, Song H, Wu D, Song T. Accuracy of digital implant impressions obtained using intraoral scanners: a systematic review and meta-analysis of in vivo studies. Int J Implant Dent. 2023 Dec 6;9(1):48.

78. Lee SJ, Betensky RA, Gianneschi GE, Gallucci GO: Accuracy of Digital vs. Conventional Implant Impressions. Clin Oral Implants Res. 2015 Jun; 26(6): 715–719.

79. Ender A, Zimmermann M, Attin T, Mehl A. In vivo precision of conventional and digital methods for obtaining quadrant dental impressions. Clin Oral Investig. 2016;20(7):1495-504.

80. Flügge TV, Att W, Metzger MC, Nelson K: Precision of Dental Implant Digitization Using Intraoral Scanners. Int J Prosthodont . 2016 May-Jun;29(3):277-83.

81. OltraDP, Bello AM, Maria Diago MP, Barquero JAP, Botticelli D, Canullo L: Microbial Colonization of the Peri-Implant Sulcus and Implant Connection of Implants Restored With Cemented Versus Screw-Retained Superstructures: A Cross-Sectional StudyJ Periodontol 2016;87(9),1002-1011.

82. Christensen GJ. Marginal fit of gold inlay castings. J Prosthet Dent. 1966;16:297–305.

83. Lofstrom LH, Barakat MM. Scanning electron microscopic evaluation of

clinically cemented cast gold restorations. J Prosthet Dent. 1989;61:664–669.

84. Boening KW, Wolf BH, Schmidt AE, Kastner K, Walter MH. Clinical fit of AllCeram crowns. J Prosthet Dent 2000, 84: 419-24.

85. Ameen NM, El-Khodary NM, Abdel-Hamid AM, Fahmy AE. A comparative study to evaluate microstrain of low-profile attachment associated with and without bar connection in implant assisted mandibular overdenture (in vitro study). BMC Oral Health, 2023 Dec 8;23(1):982.

86. Abou-Ayash S, Fonseca M, Pieralli S, Reissmann DR. Treatment effect of implant-supported fixed complete dentures and implant overdentures on patient-reported outcomes: A systematic review and meta-analysis. Clin Oral Implants Res . 2023 Sep:34 Suppl 26:177-195.

87. Verma A, Singh SV, Arya D, Shivakumar S, Chand P. Mechanical failures of dental implants and supported prostheses: A systematic review. J Oral Biol Craniofac Res . 2023 Mar-Apr;13(2):306-314.

88. Nik SN, Nejatian T. One-Piece Implant-Retained Mandibular Overdentures by Pre-Fabricated Titanium Telescopic Attachments and Frictional Varnish: A Two-Year Prospective Study. Eur J Prosthodont Restor Dent. 2016 Dec;24(4):215-221.

CHAPTER TEN:

BIOMECHANICS AND OCCLUSION

10. BIOMECHANICS AND OCCLUSION

Aim:

To explore the biomechanical factors influencing abutment screws and abutment failures in dental implantology, with a specific focus on understanding the impact of parafunctional habits on implant treatment outcome.

Necessary Knowledge:

At this stage, you are assumed to have a general knowledge of bone biology, biophysics, oral anatomy and physiology, dental implant surgery, and prosthetics.

Learning Outcome:

After completing this module, the reader will have gained a basic knowledge of the biomechanical abutment screw and abutment failure and the role of the parafunction related to dental implant treatment.

> The delayed fracture of titanium dental implants is due to accelerated corrosion and fatigue.
>
> If the occlusion is not respected, then early implant failure, early crestal bone loss, screw loosening or implant fractured is expected.
>
> Tripodization is recommended in order to compensate for 'bending overload' which can be caused when posterior teeth are being replaced.
>
> There are different forms of inter-occlusal parafunction. These include bruxism, thumb sucking, lingual interposition.

The trilogy of biomechanical failure is not well defined, and there is altogether too much argument. If we are to understand the principles, we need to consider the risk factors and see them as part of a coherent system. Less ideology, more a blend.

The delayed fracture of titanium dental implants is due to accelerated corrosion and fatigue. From analysis of the fractured surfaces of retrieved titanium screws, it has been shown that a shear crack is initiated at the root of the thread and propagated into the inner section of the screw. The solution to the problem lies in the grain structure of the titanium screw, which absorbs hydrogen, and this process may delay its fracture [1].

Many factors influence load distribution in implants: Geometry, number, dimensions, axis of the implant, prosthetic design, material, force magnitude, bone density, and food density.

Other factors involved are the strain on the abutment and implants induced by a misfit between restoration and implant and occlusal contacts inducing occlusal overload by any given amount and vector.

A systematic search of the literature related to overload and the biological consequences for osseointegrated dental implants produced no answers, thanks to the poor quality of the studies. This was partly because the term 'overload' is not defined in the papers but also because prospective clinical trials could induce harm, which would be unethical. Nonetheless, the conclusion was drawn that overload, or supra-occlusal contact, in the presence of inflammation significantly increases any plaque-induced bone resorption [2].

Occlusal load stress will result in the deformation of bone, already defined in long bones as the relative change in the length - shortening or lengthening - which is measured as 'microstrain', with 1000 microstrains equal to 0.1% deformation.

Frost classified four levels of microstrains [3]:

1. 50-100, with disuse atrophy as a consequence of bone loss
2. 100-1500, steady state
3. 1500-3000, mild overload
4. More than 3000 fatigue failure

The stress is at the neck of the implant, and the length of the osseointegrated implant does not affect the stress point. One-piece dental implants in young patients in the lower molar position are susceptible to fracture under the bone margin [4].

One of three types of occlusion need to be identified: balanced occlusion, group function occlusion, and canine-protected occlusion.

If the occlusion is not respected, then early implant failure, early crestal bone loss, screw loosening or implant fracture is expected.

The highest stress is always the first contact when two materials meet.

Not only does centric occlusion need to be adjusted, but also the disocclusion of the posterior teeth in protrusion and the disocclusion of posterior teeth on the balancing side. This needs to be visually checked. There should be no posterior teeth working side contacts in a lateral excursion on the working side.

During mastication, the movement of the natural tooth is very different from that of the dental implant. The apical or vertical movement of the naturally healthy tooth is 25-100 um, while that of the implant is a mere 3- 5 um. The horizontal movement of the healthy natural tooth is 56-108 um, while that of the implant is 10-50um – and that is due to flexure of the implant abutment and screw, combined with the elastic deformation of the bone tissue. Above all, premature occlusal contact must be avoided.

The articulating papers are made of silks, papers and foils. Silk is usually used in the laboratory because of its composition; it has a high colour reservoir capacity and can be used many times. Papers are ideal only for static occlusion, in which, in heavy contact, the colour squeezes out of the sponge structure and is released. The lighter the bit, the lighter the mark, and the harder the mark, the darker it is. Thus, dark colours imply high pressure and low colours mean low pressure. The high-pressure area (premature contact) is marked as a target, and the dark surroundings show no occlusal contact, but the white centre shows the actual contact. So usually, the first step uses articulating paper (100 um), and the second step uses 12

um foil, which offers high density, is tear-resistant, and marks a moist occlusal surface. The foil is used in static and dynamic occlusion.

The dentist should not take the guesswork, and the author recommends using 12-um double-sided articulation foil to grind down the crown surface, but the 100 um should demonstrate the occlusion contacts.

The thin 12 um is used for contact points; a maximum of one layer should pass, and if folded one passes the contact point, it should be sent back to the laboratory. If the crown is not sitting in its final position, a high-spot indicator or occlusion spray that provides a thin film of 3 um can be used to find a high spot.

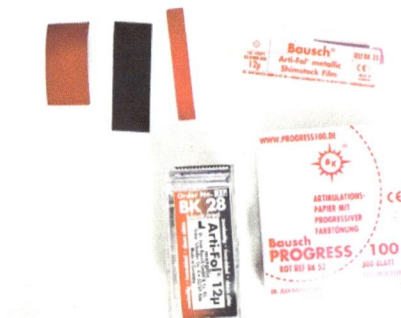

Figure 10.1 The articulating papers are needed to adjust the occlusion.

To minimise the transmission load on a prosthesis in any vulnerable region, the dentist should consider the possibilities of the following steps: placement of additional implants, ridge augmentation and increasing the implant diameter, or reducing the crown height or using lighter dental prosthetic material as BIOHPP [5].

Tripodization is recommended to compensate for 'bending overload', which can be caused when posterior teeth are replaced. If placed along a straight-line lateral force, it induces adverse bending of the implants. Triangles are one of the best shapes for distributing force as a single point force is distributed across a broad base and provides better resistance to lateral forces 6 (figure 3.8).

This treatment plan has been recommended where the butt-joint implant–abutment junction needs extra protection. This applies as the abutment screw is the only piece securing the abutment to the implant assembly, and it must not be stressed. Strains on prostheses retained by dental implants, beyond the physiological limit of bone, can induce bone loss around implants and subsequent implant failure. Providing an occlusion scheme that minimises the stresses applied to the implant without compromising the function and aesthetics is essential.

A protected occlusion scheme was recommended by Dr Misch, which was summarised as follows:

1. No premature occlusal contact

2. Sufficient area to withstand the load and, if needed, increase the number of dental implants, reduce crown height, or increase implant width with different types of bone graft.

3. Mutually protected articulation. When a natural canine is present, canine guidance is recommended. The anterior guidance should be shallowed.

4. The cusp angle of the crown and occlusal contact should be reduced on a flat surface perpendicular to the implant body by increasing the width of the central groove in the posterior implants.

5. As implants are designed to tolerate long-axis load, the occlusal load should be in the axis of the dental implant as much as possible.

6. Crown height will increase the load and can be compensated by increasing the number of dental implants or using lighter and more resilient material such as PEEK (BIOHPP).

7. Try to avoid cantilevers as they have detrimental effects.

8. Occlusal contact position: There are different concepts, from tripod contact on each occluding cusp, marginal ridge, and central fossae to reducing the occlusal contact in molars. However, it is not consistent with the whole excursion path. In theory, 15-18 individual occlusal contacts on molars with tripodal contact on each contact in the cusp, marginal ridge and central fossa are recommended.

9. Occlusal material, from PMMA, PEEK, metal (high gold, NPG), zirconia, and porcelain, has affected the lightest to most harmful.

Occlusion schemes and excursive position impact the peri-implant strains; however, the latter has more influence. At maximal intercuspation, group function has the least strain, followed by canine-guided and long-centric occlusion, which has the most detrimental effect. Shallow canine palatal morphology reduces strain at MI[7].

The location of the load is more critical than palatal morphology; thus, changing the lateral contact pattern is more important than morphology and cusp inclination. The group function is more comfortable due to less restricted mandibular movements[8].

However, the chance of grinding will increase, and implant-protected occlusion by eliminating lateral contacts on implant prosthesis is likely the best option. Even though many believe no specific occlusion scheme should be selected for all implant prostheses, only the dentist's objective should be to reduce occlusal contact in excursive positions.

Canine guidance, which allows the teeth to distribute horizontal load during an excursion and the posterior teeth to disclude, is not recommended for any dental implant prosthesis. From different schemes, such as canine-guided, group function, long-centric, and implant-protected occlusion, the peri-implant shear strain of the group function has the slightest strain.

The dental prosthesis should not make contact with the opposing teeth when the jaw moves sideways (during lateral excursions) on the opposite side or when the jaw moves forward (during protrusion). This ensures proper alignment and function of the prosthesis without interference during normal jaw movements[9].

The cuspal inclination should be another concern. Every 10° increase in cusp inclination produces approximately a 30% increase in torque. The width of the central groove in the posterior implant crowns should be increased to 2-3mm, and the opposing cusp should occlude into the central fossa[9].

The natural inclines of the occlusal table increase their cantilever effect on the crown, but there is disagreement over whether or not the occlusal table should be reduced. It is a case of theory versus the patient's aesthetic expectations – what would the patient think of the occlusal reduction?

The choice of a straight abutment on an anterior maxillary dental implant produces a 15% increase in bone strain in the adjacent bone when compared to that produced by an angulated abutment on the same implant[11].

When replacing six anterior teeth, a minimum of 3 implants should be placed, of which two should be in the canine positions. If greater risk is anticipated, then four implants should be placed and splinted together[11].

The pathological force of the lever arm is always a threat. The longer the distance, the greater the bending moment will be. Over 4000 microstrains are pathological; bone-implant interface micro-fractures can be expected. This may lead to failure [13].

When parafunction is encountered, we must compensate for its major clinical features – the magnitude of the force involved, its duration, and its direction. Compensation can involve ridge augmentation, crowns of a reduced height, or the use of more implants of greater diameter. If this is not possible, Misch recommended changing a treatment plan that had envisaged a fixed prosthesis to one using a removable one. However, if the patient's expectations or lifestyle demands a fixed prosthesis retained by a dental implant, then the author recommends BIOHPP, which may present a better alternative.

In the case of the weight of an upper PFM full mouth bridge, the author weighed a full mouth PFM bridge with 117 grams, but the same patient, the BIOHPP, weighed 38 grams.

At the other extreme, a lack of mechanical loading resulting from extremely low intra-osseous strain below 100 microstrains may induce bone resorption.

The crown/root ratio relates to the boundary between the implant shoulder and the clinical crown. In dental implantology, it is usually referred to as the C/I ratio. The ratio measures the length of the crown from that boundary line against the length of the implant from its shoulder to its apex. The C/I ratio influences the implant success rate and marginal bone loss (MBL). Most studies confirm an increase in bone loss the longer the crown is relative to the length of the implant. Surprisingly, the opposite effect has also been reported [14] (figure 9.4).

There is a belief that an angulated implant increases the risk of bone loss, but high success rates have been published, and it seems to provide a better option than that offered by grafting procedures.

The ideal Implant-abutment connection does not exist.

The implant-abutment connection in a three-piece dental implant complex comes in one of three forms: cemented, screwed, or conometric. In Sweden, the screw is the most popular, whether with an internal hex or an external hex. Other classic geometries have been developed, such as the octagon. Problems arise from the misfit of the implant-abutment connection and are both mechanical and biological. The immediate problems arise from pre-load loss or screw fracture, which can allow bacterial penetration. This leads to the build-up of bacterial endotoxins, which seep into local tissue and can affect both gingiva and bone.

Conometric attachments with perfect implant-abutment fit provide the best seal because they prevent bacterial penetration. Compared to other connection types, such as external or internal hex, they provide a more central interface with the implant platform. Nonetheless, zero leakage can only be provided by the one-piece dental implant.

Most studies are undertaken in static conditions, and few assessments of the effects of temperature and chewing stresses are available. While studies have been carried out during mastication, they have shown that the perfect seal does not exist but would need to be less than 10 um [15,16].

The distribution of occlusal forces, mainly from eccentric occlusal loading, is better tolerated by the conometric connection because it is better distributed than the two flat surfaces characterised by contact surfaces with vertical components inside the implant body [17].

The Morse taper design has a reduced micro-gap and biofilm, and this presents greater resistance to peri-implantitis and bone resorption. The resultant biologic width is generated more apically and laterally, and it encourages increased thickness of connective soft tissue around the abutment.

Thanks to the biconical system, torque, stability, and surface area contact are high, reducing the implants' micro-movements. Therefore, the need for an additional screw-retained connection is eliminated. It has also been shown that the narrower profile occupies less space. With this configuration, the distance between dental implants of only 1,2 or 3 mm no longer has statistically significant effects on bone resorption [18].

The above studies do not apply directly to one-piece implants or the way they behave. While they do not have separate components so that no leakage or reservoir can promote bacterial growth, we can assume their biomechanical behaviour will not significantly differ.

Morse abutments, with their small diameter, demonstrate clinically acceptable strain, but as the diameter increases, the strain around the internal and external walls of the cervical region reduces significantly [19].

Parafunctional habits

There are different forms of inter-occlusal parafunction. These include bruxism, thumb sucking, lingual interposition and abnormal mandible-maxillae relationship.

Bruxism is characterised by tooth grinding, clenching, and constant and repetitive occlusal contacts of increasing magnitude and frequency. The force applied can potentiate flexion, bone loss and/or fracture of any prosthesis or component of a dental implant complex.

The unpredictability of success and any complications involving any implant-supported prosthesis can result in a higher number of implant failures. It was mentioned that the guidelines produced are not based on scientific evidence; improved clinical pathways are needed to enable better treatment for patients suffering from bruxism and needing implant placement [20].

References:

1. Yokoyama K, Ichikawa T, Murakami H, Miyamoto Y, Aaoka K: Fracture mechanisms of retrieved titanium screw thread in dental implant. Biomaterials 2002,23(12), 245902465

2. Naert I, Duyck J, Vandamme K. Occlusal overload and bone/ implant loss. Clin. Oral Implants Res. 23(Suppl. 6), 2012, 95–107.

3. Frost, H.M. (2004) A 2003 update of bone physiology and Wolff's Law for clinicians. Angle Orthodontist 74: 3–15.

4. Fujii Y, Hatori A, Minami S, Kanno Y, Hamada H, Miyazawa T, Chikazu D. Characteristics and Risk Factors for the Fracture of One-Piece Implants. J Maxillofac Oral Surg. 2023 Dec;22(4):1091-1098.

5. Rangert B, Krogh PH, Langer B, Roekel VN , Bending overload and implant fracture: a retrospective clinical analysis, Int J of Oral Maxillofac Implants,1995; 10(3):326-34.

6. Weinberg L, Kruger B. An evaluation of torque (moment) on implant/prosthesis with staggered buccal and lingual offset. International Journal of Periodontics and Restorative Dentistry 1996;16:252–65.

7. Lo J, Abduo J, Palamara J: Effect of different lateral occlusion schemes on peri-implant strain: A laboratory study. J Adv Prosthodont 2017;9:45-51.

8. Belser UC, Hannam AG. The influence of altered working side occlusal guidance on masticatory muscles and related jaw movement. J Prosthet Dent 1985;53:406-13.

9. Weinberg LA, Kruger G, A comparison of implant prostheses loading for clinical variables, Int J Prosthodont,8, 1995, 421-433.

10. Y Y Chen, C L Kuan, Y B Wang, Implant occlusion: biomechanical considerations for implant supported prostheses, J Dent Sci, 3(2), 2008, 65 -74.

11. Saab XE, Griggs JA, Powers JM, Engelmeier RL. Effect of abutment angulation on the strain on the bone around an implant in the anterior maxilla: A finite element study. J Prosthet Dent, 97: 85-92, 2007.

12. Misch CE, Bidez MW. Implant-protected occlusion: a biomechanical rationale. Compendium 1994, 15: 1330-1344.

13. Roberts WE. Fundamental principles of bone physiology, metabolism and loading. In: Naert I, van Steenberghe D, Worthington P, editors. Osseointegration in oral rehabilitation.

14. Lee KJ, Kim YG, Park JW, Lee JM, Suh JY. Influence of crown-to-implant ratio on periimplant marginal bone loss in the posterior region: A five-year retrospective study. J Periodontal Implant Sci 2012;42:231-236.

15. Tsuge T, Hagiwara Y, Matsumura H. Marginal fit and microgaps of implant-abutment interface with internal anti-rotation configuration. Dent Mater J 2008;27(1):29-34.

16. Coelho AL, Suzuki M, Dibart S, Da Silva N, Coelho PG. Crosssectional analysis of the implant-abutment interface. J OralRehabil 2007;34:508-16.

17. Deborah Meleo, Luigi Baggi, Michele Di Girolamo, Fabio Di Carlo, Raffaella Pecci, and Rossella Bedini: Fixture-abutment connection surface and micro-gap measurements by 3D micro-tomographic technique analysis. Ann Ist super Sanita. 2012 | Vol. 48, no. 1: 53-58.

18. Platform switching: The new paradigm in oral implantology. José Paulo Macedo, Jorge Pereira, [...], and Júlio C. M. Souza, Eur J Dent. 2016 Jan-Mar; 10(1): 148–154.

19. Castro CG, Zancope K, Verissimo C, Soares CJ, das Neves FD. Strain analysis of different diameters. Morse taper implants under overloading compressive conditions Braz Oral Res [online]. 2015;29(1):1-6.

20. Toracato LB, Zuim PRJ Daniela Atili Brandini DA, Falcon-Antenucci RM: Relation between bruxism and dental implants, RGO, Rev Gaúch Odontol 2014, Porto Alegre, v.62, n.4, p. 371-376, out./dez.

CHAPTER ELEVEN:

PERI-IMPLANTITIS AND MAINTENANCE

11. PERI-IMPLANTITIS AND MAINTENANCE

Aim:

Provide a comprehensive understanding of the causes (aetiology) of peri-implantitis and explore the various treatment options available for managing this condition in dental implantology.

Necessary Knowledge:

It is assumed that at this stage, you have a general knowledge of bone biology, biophysics, oral anatomy and physiology, dental implant surgery prosthetics, and biomechanics related to dental implants.

Learning Outcome:

After completing this module, the reader will have gained a basic knowledge of the aetiology and treatment options of peri-implantitis.

> Peri-implant mucositis is the presence of inflammation of the peri-implant mucosa without signs of supporting bone loss, while peri-implantitis itself was defined as the presence of inflammation of the mucosa plus supporting bone loss.
>
> Peri-implant probing is essential for establishing a diagnosis of peri-implant disease.
>
> Caution should be taken with implantoplasty due to the limited thickness of the conventional implant with an internal connection.

Oral hygiene recommendations for the care of natural teeth have been recommended for the care of prostheses retained by dental implants – but without adequate research or assessment showing that they are suitable [1].

The effect of different factors on the reasons for implant failure has been studied.

The patient must carry out regular and effective oral hygiene.

Powered toothbrushes produced an improvement within clinical parameters. Elderly patients showed the most remarkable improvement, which could be due to compensation and intelligence.

The bioelectric integrated toothbrush has a biofilm cleaning effect, which is effective in areas that generally bristles do not reach, like deep pockets interproximal and lingual surface, with direct electric current propagating through saliva (as media) [2].

Interdental brushes are effective, but patients must be shown how to use them properly. Patients find water jet device-powered brushes easier, but not all patients can afford the cost. The author believes that corded electric Waterpik helps remove plaque debris under the bridge and in the interdental spaces; however, the cordless is not effective.

Peri-implant mucositis is the presence of inflammation of the peri-implant mucosa without signs of supporting bone loss, while peri-implantitis itself is defined as the presence of inflammation of the mucosa plus supporting bone loss. The critical feature of peri-implant mucositis is the presence of bleeding upon probing, while the key features of peri-implantitis are changes in bone crest level plus bleeding upon probing.

Peri-implant probing is essential for establishing a diagnosis of peri-implant disease. Under appropriate pressure conditions, conventional peri-implant probing, such as 0.25 N, does not cause tissue damage. Such a probe is an essential instrument for the proper diagnosis of peri-implantitis. The probes are plastic or titanium [3].

In addition, parallelized intraoral X-rays should be taken of all dental implants to determine possible marginal bone loss. These need to be taken in the first week after implant placement and the first week after prosthesis delivery in order to be available for comparison with the X-rays obtained at the periodic patient reviews.

Bacteria-induced peri-implant disease has been classified as either mucositis or peri-implantitis.

Peri-implant mucositis is a reversible inflammatory process, the signs of which are mucosal redness, swelling, and bleeding on periodontal probing. Peri-implantitis is a poly-microbial, anaerobic infection accompanied by bone resorption, pocket formation and pus. It is irreversible.

Peri-implantitis microbiota is not the same as those associated with periodontitis, most notably Staphylococcus aureus, which has an affinity for titanium.

There are different types of bone resorption classifications around dental implants. The author recommends Spiekermann, which can reflect the type of treatment which as follows [4]:

Class 1: Horizontal

Class II: I-shaped

Class IIIa: funnel-shaped

Class IIIb: gap-shaped

Class IV: horizontal-circular

The simplest is to classify it as 'early' implant loss if it has arisen within one year of implant insertion and 'delayed' implant loss if it has occurred at least one year after insertion. This classification does not help one assess the speed of disease progression or its prognosis or decide on the best treatment path.

However, concluding progression and prognosis criteria from these classifications is impossible.

Rough surfaces demonstrate greater bacterial attachment than smooth surfaces. A roughness average of 0.088 um inhibits the accumulation and maturation of plaque. TiN and ZrN coatings reduce the number of initially adherent bacteria and minimise plaque biofilm formation and inflammation.

Subgingivally, rough abutment surfaces harboured nearly 25 times more bacteria, with a slightly lower density of coccoid organisms. Surface roughness of Ra 0.2um prevents microbial accumulation, and less than 0.2 um has no further effect, even after 12 months [5].

11.1. Biofilm Formation on Implant Surfaces

After 4 hours, Streptococci predominate, and Actinomyces species provide an ecosystem in which pathogens such as Fusobacterium species bind to Streptococci, producing the unhappy consequence of peri-implantitis. Endotoxins such as collagenase, hyaluronidase, and chondroitin sulfates produce a reflexive inflammatory response along with bone resorption. The abutment surfaces should be chosen and prepared to prevent initial microbial adherence. Aetiology of peri-implantitis is bacteria, but the pathogenesis is inflammatory, which is the interaction of bacteria and defence mechanisms. Saliva will be a good source of biomarkers of peri-implantitis in the future.

There are risk factors for peri-implantitis which, though linked to the disease and do not cause it directly, nonetheless predispose the implant site to it. These factors are:

11.2. Peri-implantitis predisposing factors

Smoking increases the failure rate of dental implant treatment.

Interleukin 1 genotype polymorphism describes a group of 11 cytokines, which play a central role in regulating immune and inflammatory responses to infections or sterile insults. It is a pro-inflammatory cytokine that plays a vital role in the pathogenesis of periodontitis, so it might be useful for detecting high-risk cases of peri-implantitis.

It has been reported that IL-1 polymorphisms plus a smoking habit have a mutually synergistic effect, which increases the chances of peri-implantitis [6].

An existing bacterial profile, plus a genetic predisposition, may combine to produce the related host response, which could explain the initiation of the disease process.

A meta-analysis concluded a study that smoking is the leading systemic risk factor with which interleukin gene polymorphism and poor oral hygiene will combine to exacerbate the condition [7].

However, controversial research claims otherwise - that IL-1 genotypes do not seem to be good predictors of peri-implantitis in the great majority of smoking patients. The treatment of peri-implantitis could have a worse prognosis in IL-1-positive genotype patients.

Furthermore, no synergistic effect was found in IL-1 genotypes who were heavy smokers. Patients with a previous history of periodontitis were more prone to peri-implantitis [8].

The role of these genetic polymorphisms in the aetiology and progression of peri-implant diseases is still unclear.

With a sterile cotton swab, epithelial cells were removed, transferred by sterile spatula to a snap tube, and sent to the laboratory, which used a PCR Kit for the IL1 genotype. Genetic polymorphism can arise in homozygosity or heterozygosity; the sum is a positive genotype.

However, systematic genetic testing to assess the risk of peri-implantitis cannot be recommended as a standard of care. Thus, who committed murder? Was it the maid or the gardener? The presence of periodontitis or cigarette smoking increased the risk for periimplantitis by up to 4.7-fold, as reported.

Although bacteria may be considered the initiating factor of periodontal disease, other aspects, like genetic factors, may be fundamental. The bacterial profile combined with a host response, which includes a genetic predisposition, is supposed to explain the relationship of periodontitis with smoking as the major risk factor for peri-implantitis. The prevalence rate of peri-implantitis can increase from 11.2% to 53.3 % in the presence of smoking habits and periodontal disease history [9,10].

The effect of soft tissue quality on dental implants is controversial. The author recommends that the lingual surface must have the benefit of an attached mucosa, and in the posterior mandible, a minimum of 3 mm of non-mobile gingival mucosa (keratinized or non-keratinized) is essential for prevention of peri-implantitis. Maxillary implants with thick connective tissue are more prone to peri-implantitis than mandibular implants [11].

Residual dental cement can be another risk factor. After it has been removed, the clinical signs, in most cases, resolve and disappear. Where the patient has a history of periodontal disease, the remnants of dental cement remaining in the gingival sulcus can significantly exacerbate the signs and symptoms of peri-implantitis [12].

Poor oral hygiene greatly impacts the development and progression of peri-implantitis.

Uncontrolled systemic diseases like diabetes mellitus, cardiovascular disease, immunosuppression and drug therapies like bisphosphonates or corticotherapy have a significant effect on peri-implantitis.

Other iatrogenic factors, such as the inadequate seating of restorations or the over-contouring of restorations, implant mispositioning and overloading, can exacerbate peri-implantitis.

Poor bone quality is the last risk factor that needs to be emphasised.

To avoid continuous alveolar bone loss, all failing dental implants must be speedily identified to prevent the need for replacement. At the worst, they can be replaced. Nevertheless, late identification of failed implants can make their replacement difficult or impossible.

11.3. Prevention and Treatment

Treatment planning starts with the clinical examination.

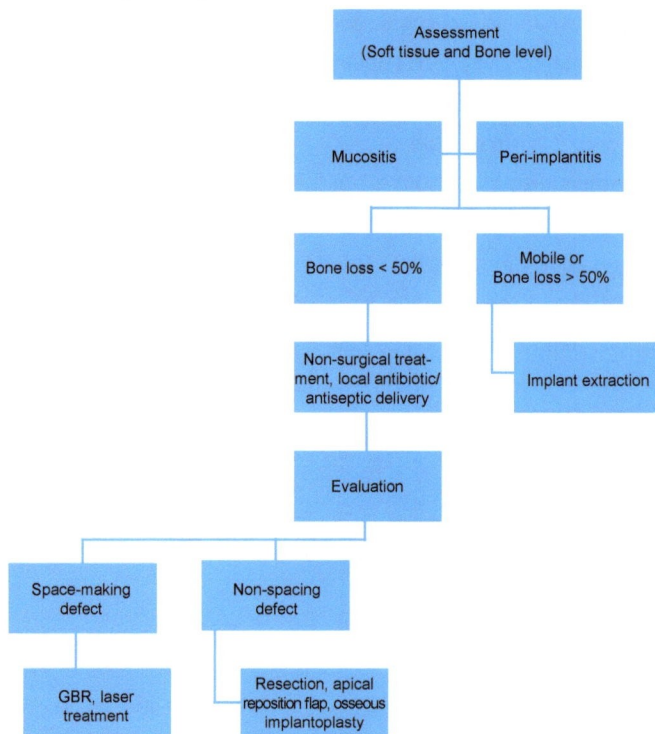

Figure 11.1 The hierarchy of the treatment of peri-implantitis.

Assess the risk factors: can they be minimised? Can their likely clinical effects be minimised or countered? If so, how?

Plan the actual treatment and implement a step-by-step approach: regular appointments with non-surgical therapy followed by surgical treatment if necessary.

Non-surgical therapy:

Mechanical implant cleaning instruments, such as titanium or manual plastic curettes, ultrasonic or air polishing, are used. Local antiseptics, chlorhexidine gluconate, hydrogen peroxide, sodium percarbonate, and povidone-iodine have all been recommended.

Even though papers have been published that maintain there are no benefits in attempts at pocket reduction, the author has observed a reduction in signs and symptoms following the use of intra-pocket irrigation with the Waterpik combined with oral hygiene training [13].

Conventional curettes are harder than titanium and roughen the surfaces. Thus, Teflon, carbon, plastic gold tips, and titanium curettes are recommended. Ultrasonic systems fitted with plastic tips and used in conjunction with air polishing have proved more beneficial.

Re-osseointegration after peri-implantitis demands a clean, biocompatible surface with high surface energy [14]. Air powder machines use soft abrasives to clean and polish natural tooth surfaces by removing deposits or smoothing the tooth surface. This method is an alternative to curettes or sonic/ultrasonic scalers. The downside is that the remnant particles disturb the cell response in the pocket, which can prevent re-ossointegration.

However, using bioactive and osteoconductive powders as cleaning powders is beneficial for SLA surfaces because they leave a protected surface to which the remnant particles adhere.

HA, HA + TCP and the amino acid glycine are highly effective at cleaning the biofilm from titanium surfaces. TiO_2 and phosphoric acid are not as efficient [15].

Another treatment strategy is medicament therapy. This can encompass antiseptic rinses or local application of antibiotics/antiseptics. Local antibiotic and chlorhexidine application significantly reduce pocket depth because resorbable doxycycline releases nanospheres [16,17].

The bactericidal effect of laser therapy can be beneficial, whether it be via CO_2, Diode-, Er: YAG- (erbium-doped: yttrium-aluminium-garnet) or Er, Cr: YSGG- (erbium, chromium-doped: yttrium scandium-gallium-garnet). The last two types, with a wavelength of 3 microns, reduce biofilm by 90%, but they are recommended as an adjunctive treatment option, as photodynamic therapy. Laser wavelengths of 580-1400 nm and 10-50 ug/ml toluidine blue concentrations generate a bactericidal effect against aerobic and anaerobic bacteria. It is expensive and recommended only as an adjunctive therapy.

AKUT protocol:

The modification of Cumulative Interceptive Supportive Therapy (CIST) [18].

The regenerative approach has been pursued using various types of bone substitutes and barrier membranes. Bone fill has been observed, but complete re-osteointegration has been limited. A higher success rate can be achieved by combining different bone graft materials and different barrier membranes. The author cannot recommend any particular regenerative therapy at present and believes that research is still needed, not just in the aspects covered above but also in a more holistic manner. This means that while the surgical, materials, and implant surface problems will be studied, so will new approaches to disease control, host response, genetic predispositions, enhanced home care, and reparative nutrition. In fact, it may turn out that an undiscovered combination of any of these factors may be the most fruitful. Success will prove to be the sum of its parts.

A new surface is needed to increase the success rate and minimise the number of microbes before augmentation; augmentation and re-osseointegration are possible only in space-making defects, and autogenous bone, especially cortical bone, is the best option.

Stage	Result	Therapy
	PD (< 3mm) Plaque (no) Bleeding (no)	None
A	PD (< 3mm) Plaque (yes) Bleeding (no)	Mechanical cleaning, polishing, oral hygiene instructions
B	PD (4-5 mm) Xray (no bone loss)	Mechanical cleaning, polishing, oral hygiene instructions and local anti-infective therapy
C	PD (> 5mm) Xray (bone loss < 2mm)	Mechanical cleaning, polishing, oral hygiene instructions, systemic and local anti-infective therapy
D	PD (> 5mm) Xray (bone loss > 2mm)	Resective and regenerative surgery

PD= pocket depth

Resective surgery eliminates the peri-implant osseous defect by osteotomy and osteoplasty, smoothing and polishing the supracrestal implant surface (called implantoplasty). Post-operative recession is expected, and the patient should be warned, but it is the most predictable treatment.

Caution should be taken with implantoplasty due to the limited thickness of the conventional implant with an internal connection. Greater thickness is available for removal when an external connection is present, but the one-piece implant is the most convenient. The micro threads or threads at the crestal region, which are exposed due to bone loss, need to be reduced or removed. The implants without threads in the crest region provide a favourable surface as implantoplasty and polishing the surface is more efficient.

As any type of remedy is not 100 per cent effective, the patient's expectation should be warranted, and written consent is necessary.

11.4. Explantation

A dental implant will need to be extracted when there is total bone loss around it. The extraction will be easily carried out using a Periotome, straight elevator and root forceps. The forceps should be used without any force - simply to remove the implant. Vigorous curettage with different sizes of sharp curette is needed here, and the dentist must make sure to remove all the soft tissue inside the bone. Before any operative intervention, survey the local soft tissue anatomy to ensure that structures like the mental nerve, for instance, or sinus, are not invaded. The extraction of an osseointegrated implant is needed when clinical signs like active pus with a defect more than 50% of the remaining length of the implant and when it cannot be remediated. Usually, the apical part of the implant is well well-seointegrated, so different types of extractors are available to deal with the implant in question. Those extractors will have different diameters and lengths, and the dentist must make sure that the instrument selected is compatible with the implant system being used. A word of warning, though - applying too much pressure may fracture the dental implant and complicate matters. Trephine drills are recommended for the removal of the bone around the implant, but it is invasive, and there is an increased chance of removing both the buccal and/or lingual cortex.

The piezo Periotome is the instrument of choice for removing bone around implants due for extraction. After the bone around the implant has been released, the loosened implant now needs to be removed. There are now three removal instruments and techniques to choose from: root forceps, implant insertion adaptors, which are unique for each system, and screwdrivers to unscrew the implant.

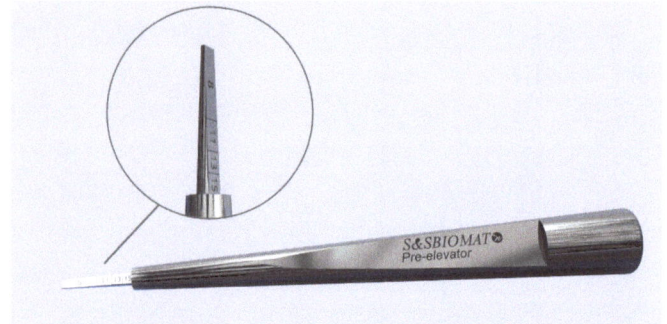

Figure 11.2 The pre-elevator designed by the author is a hybrid of a small chisel and periotome.

If the dentist does not have a piezo kit, a ¼ or ½ round drill, with good irrigation, can be used to drill multiple bone tunnels around the implant. A pre-elevator is then used sequentially to connect adjacent tunnels to allow the dental implant to be luxated. The pre-elevator the author designs is a type of chisel/Periotome designed by the author. The head of the handle can be tapped by a surgical mallet with gentle tapping to dislodge the bone from the implant surface without too much bone destruction, especially preserving the height of the remaining bone.

If the buccal or lingual bone has cracks, the best approach is not to do anything but wait for it to heal. A rigid, non-resorbable membrane should be placed if the cortex is damaged to prevent soft tissue invasion into the socket.

If the cavity is intact and its diameter and anatomy accept the placement of a dental implant, another dental implant immediately can be placed, if required.

It has been suggested that, after explantation, a healing period of 3 months is necessary, but it is not, and if the volume of the remaining bone permits, a wider and/or longer dental implant can be placed.

The dentist must bear in mind that if the risk factors have not been identified, the survival chances of the new dental implant may be lower than those of the previous one.

The use of short-span prostheses may be an alternative treatment plan in full-mouth rehabilitation cases and the reconstruction of 20 teeth in older adults.

References:

1.Louropoulou A, Slot DE, Van der Weijden F: Mechanical self-performed oral hygiene of implant supported restorations: A systemic review. J Evid Base Dent Pract 2014;14S:60-69.

2. Lee J, Kim YW. Bioelectric device for effective biofilm inflammation management of dental implants. Sci Rep. 2023 Dec 4;13(1):21372.

3. Heitz-Mayfield LJ. Peri-implant diseases: diagnosis and risk indicators. J Clin Periodontol 2008; 35: 292-304.

4. Spiekermann H: Implantologie. Stuttgart: Thieme; 1984.

5. Bollen CM, Papaioanno W, van Eldere J, Schepers E, Quirynen M, van Steenberghe D. The influence of abutment surface
roughness on plaque accumulation and peri-implant mucositis. Clin Oral Implants Res 1996;7:201–211.

6. Gruica B, Wang HY, Lang N, Buser D. Impact of IL-1 genotype and smoking status on the prognosis of osseointegrated implants. Clin Oral Implants Res. 2004;15:393-400.

7. Clementini M, Rossetti PH, Penarrocha D, Micarelli C, Bonachela WC, Canullo L: Systemic risk factors for peri-implant bone loss: a systematic review and meta-analysis. Int J Oral Maxillofac Surg 2014, 43:323–334.

8. García-Delaney C, Sánchez-Garcés MA, Figueiredo R, Sánchez-Torres A, Gay-Escoda C: Clinical significance of interleukin-1 genotype in smoking patients as a predictor of peri-implantitis: A case-control study. IL-1 genotype and peri-implantitis. Med Oral Patol Oral Cir Bucal. 2015 Nov 1;20 (6):e737-43.

9. Huynh-Ba G, Lang NP, Tonetti MS, Salvi GE. The association of the composite IL-1 genotype with periodontitis progression and/ or treatment outcomes: a systematic review. J Clin Periodontol. 2007;34:305-17.

10. Renvert S, Persson R. Periodontitis as a potential risk factor for peri-implantitis. J Clin Periodontol. 2009;36:9-14.

11. Vervaeke S, Collaert B, Cosyn J, Deschepper E, De Bruyn H: A multifactorial analysis to identify predictors of implant failure and peri-implant bone loss. Clin Implant Dent Relat Res 2013.

12. Linkevicius T, Puisys A, Vindasiute E, Linkeviciene L, Apse P: Does residual cement around implant-supported restorations cause peri-implant disease? A retrospective case analysis. Clin Oral Implants Res 2012, 24:1179–1184.

13. Hallström H, Persson GR, Lindgren S, Olofsson M, Renvert S: Systemic antibiotics and debridement of peri-implant mucositis. A randomized clinical trial. J Clin Periodontol 2012, 39:574–581.

14. Kubies, D., Himmlova´, L., Riedel, T., Cha´nova´, E., Balı´k, K., Doude˘rova´, M., Ba´rtova´, J. & Pes˘a´kova´ ,V. (2011) The interaction of osteoblasts with bone-implant materials: 1. The effect of physicochemical surface properties of implant materials. Physiological Research 60: 95–111.

15. Tastepe CS, van Waas R, Liu Y, Wismeijer D: Air powder abrasive treatment as an implant surface cleaning method: a literature review. Int J Oral Maxillofac Implants 2012, 27:1461–1473.

16. Javed F, Alghamdi AST, Ahmed A, Mikami T, Ahmed HB, Tenenbaum HC: Clinical efficacy of antibiotics in the treatment of peri-implantitis. Int Dent J 2013, 63:169–176.

17. Moura LA, Oliveira Giorgetti Bossolan AP, Rezende Duek EA, Sallum EA, Nociti FH, Casati MZ, Sallum AW: Treatment of peri-implantitis using nonsurgical debridement with bioresorbable nanospheres for controlled release of doxycycline: case report. Compend Contin Educ Dent (Jamesburg, NJ: 1995) 2012, 33:E145–E149.

18. Lang NP, Berglundh T, Heitz-Mayfield LJ, Pjetursson BE, Salvi GE, Sanz M: Consensus statements and recommended clinical procedures regarding implant survival and complications. Int J Oral Maxillofac Implants 2004, 19(Suppl):150–154.

CHAPTER TWELVE:

AUTHOR'S PROTOCOLS
(AUTHOR'S ALGORITHM)

12.   AUTHOR'S PROTOCOLS (Author's Algorithm)

High yield and high-risk treatment plan- to do or not to do

This chapter will concentrate on the author's basic protocols.

12.1. Management and Finance:

Patient safety, on the one hand, and extravagance, on the other, need balance. It is the patient who finally will pay for our expenses, and the increase in cost in vain will deprive some patients of life.

Any equipment we buy now maybe it will be a white elephant in a few years if it does not have the capability to grow with business.

12.2. Treatment planning

Patients' general health is classified as being in the ASA I; however, the class II group requires the dentist to consult with the patient's GP. An OPG is a prerequisite, and if there is doubt regarding the width or height of the remaining alveolar bone, CBCT is requested before giving the patient any promises.

12.3. Pre-operative:

On the day of implant placement surgery or graft, pre-operative antibiotics such as Amoxicillin 500 mg (if the patient is not allergic) and analgesics such as Ibuprofen 400 mg or Paracetamol 500 mg and Chlorhexidine mouthwash. Plain 3% Mepivacaine local anaesthetic is the material of choice. During surgeries under general anaesthetic, it is recommended to use a local anaesthetic to reduce post-operative pain [1].

12.4. Implant surgery:

For over 40 years, the one-piece dental implant placement was the standard implant. The major outcome of its failure rate was predictable primary stability and lack of access to titanium implants. Our understanding of primary stability has changed considerably, and implant design and surface treatment have greatly improved.

12.5. Pre-fabricated One-Piece Dental Implants:

Using a pre-fabricated one-piece dental implant is the first line of treatment, especially in the aesthetic region from premolar to premolar.

The one-piece implant comprises three parts: the rough surface, which contacts the bone; a polished surface, which contacts the soft tissue; and the abutment.

Three main questions need to be addressed: the available bone height, width, quality of the bone and thickness of the cortex, buccal, lingual and crestal.

When planning dental implant treatment, it is crucial to assess the thickness of the surrounding soft tissue and determine the appropriate provisional and permanent restorations needed, such as overdentures, single-tooth replacements, or implant-supported bridges.

The design of the implant and its abutment must cover the demands. The type of titanium affects the intra-oral preparation as titanium grades 1 and 2 are more friendly than types 3,4 or 5. As the number increases, carbide or diamond bur preparation would be challenging.

The angle of the abutment and the final crown can be adjusted depending on the dental implant system; thus, the dentist must bear in mind the limitations of the system used.

Does the one-piece implant have different types of gingival heights? In some cases, especially in the maxillae, the gingival thickness would be more than 2 mm, and there would be a need for a one-piece implant with the gingival height of the abutment more than 2 mm.

Some examples are Dentium, NSI, Cortex, Ziacom, Cowellmedi, Straumann, Z system, Ditron, Osteocare, S&S Biomat.

Even though the dentist must go through the treatment plan and ensure that placing a one-piece implant is possible, not all surgeries are predictable, which will be enhanced in complicated cases.

Ideally, the design of the master or final drill must be as if, for any reason, placing a one-piece implant is not possible; the dentist can place a conventional implant without any more modification in the prepared bone.

The dentist must ensure the patient fully understands that chewing hard food is forbidden during healing, even though placing a three-piece implant and removable provisional denture requires the same advice.

In patients who have suffered chronic periodontal disease, it has been noticed that they can display differing reactions to the placement of screw implants as opposed to that of cylinder implants.

It was found that, in a few cases where a screw implant has been used, the patient felt a degree of pain that could not be alleviated by infiltration of local anaesthetic. The patients involved had suffered advanced chronic periodontitis, hence the need for extractions and implants. What was noticed was that it was the placement of the screw implant that hurt, but not that of the cylindrical implant, which was placed like a nail in the wall instead of screwing. It is only a hypothesis, but could the nerve endings have been hypersensitised because of the chronic presence of advanced periodontal disease so that the cutting of the nerve endings by the tip of the screw produced pain? In contrast to the cutting effect of the non-screw implant, the cylindrical implants crush the bone debris onto the nerve endings, and the patient experiences less or no pain.

Usually, when dentists encounter poor-quality bone, they prefer to change their osteotomy technique to one involving the use of multiple osteotomies using a surgical mallet and osteotomes. This may be mildly unsettling for the patient. Instead of this, if the quality of the bone is soft, we recommend that after using the pilot drill, you immediately place a one-piece dental implant. It is essential to explain to the patient that osteotomy is an uncomfortable experience to undergo, but it is actually the best option.

The one-piece blade implant has been used in industry for centuries. The friction in elastic materials such as wood or bone may easily bind a narrow wedge. The elastic characteristics of bone with its double-sided cortex (buccal and lingual) will increase its frictional grip and, thus, the wedge's primary stability. Blade dental implants have a long, successful history, and recently, the FDA has reclassified the blade dental implant from class III to class II.

Using a 0.25 mm thick diamond disc to cut through the cortex and then continue with a pre-elevator is preferable. If the site is not easily accessed, then piezo Periotome tips can be useful. Even though, for reasons of access, it may be more practical to place the blade implant in the mandibular premolar region, if the patient is cooperative and can open the jaw widely enough, it can be placed distal to the mental nerve. It is important to note that to split the bone, we need a minimum thickness of 1.5 mm of cancellous bone between the buccal and lingual cortices. However, if an implant is to be placed, the minimum amount of bone required is 1.5 mm of bone on each side. However, bone tends to resorb preferentially on the buccal surface of all types of dental implants, so this dictates the need for at least 2mm of bone on the buccal surface and 1.5 mm on the lingual surface. As the thickness of the implants at the crestal level is 2.5 mm, less bone expansion is needed, so the chances of fracturing the reduced buccal plate. Also, as the cross-section of the required bone cavity is not round, the buccal cortex thinning in the middle will not be seen. This is because the thinned buccal cortex of the round implant may reduce vascularisation while the flat buccal cortex of the blade does not, reducing the probability of buccal bone resorption.

It is recommended only when the upper jaw has a removable denture and when there is insufficient bone height to place a dental implant in the distal mental foramina for a full mouth mandibular prosthesis. It is recommended that the bridge be a hybrid bridge or made of polymer like BIOHPP.

12.6. Conventional three/three-piece implants (implant- abutment- abutment screw):

The author recommends that the abutment be sterile and not removed again when placing the abutment. Even the use of a mounter reduces microbial contamination. Imagine sending the abutment to the laboratory many times [2].

12.7. Prosthesis:

If one-piece implants have been used, the abutments need to be prepared; but if conventional dental implants have been used, it is highly recommended at the second stage of surgery that the abutments be placed instead of the temporary healing screw or gingival former.

For an initial preparation of the titanium abutments, use a sound carbide bur, polished with black and red amalgam stones, with the green only for the last 1mm of the finishing margin. Provide the patient with a provisional crown and cement it with 50% zinc phosphate and 50% coconut oil; use a soft liner as the temporary cement for full-mouth bridges.

Ideally, the provisional fixed prosthesis should be cemented prior to suturing, as removing the excess cement and washing is a predictable method. If it is not feasible for any reason, the next week should not fit any provisional prosthesis. Leave the minor adjustment and polish for the next visit.

After healing of the gingivae, which may take 1-3 months, if there is some minor overgrowth of the soft tissue over the finishing margin, using a tissue trimmer without any irrigation at 30°-40° as the buccal finishing margin should be 1mm below the soft tissue, and the lingual finishing margin at the gingival margin. Clean and take a silicon medium wash and putty conventional dental impression using an addition-cured dental impression.

Usually, the subsequent sessions would be 1. controlling the frame, 2. porcelain (occlusion) and 2. glaze and cementation. However, the author recommends that a resin frame be fabricated and adjusted at the next impression session, and then the frame is requested. For every control session, a wash material should be placed inside them, and after polymerisation, they should proceed with the control, which, after removal, should cut through the finishing margin; if it is not, it is back to square one. The impression wash would be cut when the precision of the finishing margin is less than 0.04 mm (40 um).

It has been noted that the mean discrepancy of the marginal fit of a screw-retained prosthesis is 8.5 um and that cement-retained prosthesis as filler in the voids measured 57-67 um. This could be avoided with the use of the above technique [3].

A dental probe to gauge continuity between the crown margin and dental abutment is usually used but is not valid. The dimensions of the tips of dental probes are not calibrated and accurate; even the sharp one will be dull, yet it is used in a quality system for assessing potential leakage between the finishing margin of the crown and the abutment.

12.8. Direct Impression:

Do we need a shoulder finishing margin or a chamfer?

Inadequate marginal fit between tooth and crown, whether small or large, will have two immediate effects followed by a deterioration sequence. The first effect will be the dissolution of the cement-retained in the marginal gap. This will be followed immediately by progressive bacterial infiltration into that gap and plaque accumulation. This signals the start of gingivitis and the discolouration of the gingival margin. Advanced cases will develop increased pocket depth and loss of attached gingivae. There are arguments over which type of finishing margin is better - deep chamfer or shoulder. We believe they both work as long as the dentist and dental technician have the expertise and precision.

If the laboratory believes that minor adjustments to the preparation are needed, it should alter the preparation on the cast and provide a jig so that the dentist can copy it. So, when the jig sits entirely on the preparation in the mouth, the adjustment has been fully transferred to the patient's abutment. Using a transparent gig can be beneficial; however, a new impression is needed if 1mm of finishing margin needs to be prepared. Using wash material such as light body polyvinylsiloxane to cut the finishing margin of the resin frame, frame, porcelain, and glaze stages need to be applied.

The one-piece dental implant is designed to eliminate the built-in disadvantages of 2- and 3-piece implants – namely, their provision of a breeding ground for bacteria in the junction between implant and abutment, especially the movement-under-stress between the implant and the abutment.

Critics maintain that angulated abutments cannot be used even though some dental implant systems provide an angulated abutment within their one-piece cylindrical implant. This is designed specifically for use in the average-to-soft bone found in the maxillae. The best way to prepare the abutment is with a carbide or diamond bur. Some believe that a one-piece dental implant will not succeed, but the number of companies manufacturing one-piece dental implants is increasing. In cases presenting with limited interdental dimensions, the one-piece dental implant becomes a necessity in order to preserve the form of the dental papillae, especially in the lower Incisors replacement. Old habits and paradigms (default treatment) are hard to let go of.

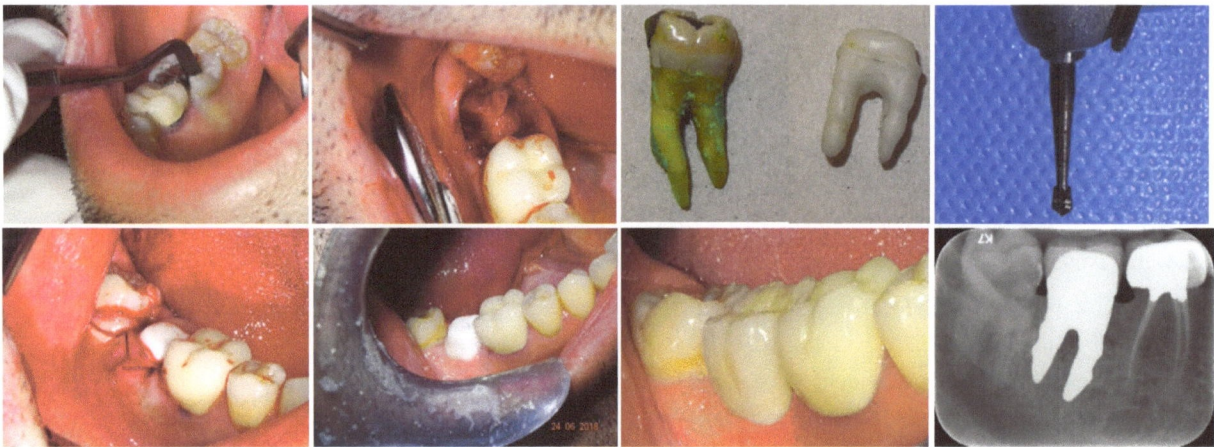

Figure 12.1 Customised dental implant placement. The lower right 6 has a vertical fracture, and the tooth cannot be saved. The tooth is extracted, the crown is prepared for the zirconia crown, scanned, and a copy is made. After accepting the final design, it is scanned, and the Zirconia dental implant is manufactured and sterilised. The customised implant is placed after curettage, and the inner surface of the alveolar bone is scratched to facilitate multiple bleeding points. After the healing period, a conventional impression is made, and the Zirconia crown is cemented.

Each generation of one-piece dental implants has been improved but does not yet provide a blanket solution for all cases, so conventional 3-piece implants still need to be available.

12.9. Customised Dental Implants

Personalized medicine has revolutionized the practice of medicine, and for implant designers, the ultimate goal is to tailor the implant to the needs of the individual patient. The advancing technologies of imaging and 3D printers herald the possibilities of made-to-measure implants, and, indeed, customised dental implants made of titanium, Zirconia or PEEK have already been introduced.

The author has experience with 2-rooted teeth (lower molars), (figure 12.1).

Extraction, Imaging, implant Manufacture

The procedure is as follows:

1 - extract the tooth,

2a - if it is intact, the tooth is ready for the next stage,

2b - if it is broken, the pieces are glued together,

3 - the tooth is scanned and studied,

4- a polymer of the prepared tooth is manufactured,

5a - the crown is prepared, and The prepared tooth should be 2.5mm off the occlusion, 5b - the undercuts of the roots are removed, their sharp tips are shortened,

6 – the dentist studies the polymer copy, and after confirmation,

8 - it is copied in medical-grade Zirconia,

9 - in the clean room, the surface is prepared and packed in 2 layers and sterilised by Eto.

The procedure must be completed within a maximum of 7 days. In the next session:

Clinical Placement of Customised Implant

10 - under local anaesthetics, vigorous soft tissue curettage within the socket is carried out. The author believes in using a round bur and, with good irrigation, just scratching the inner wall of the alveolar bone to initiate cancellous bleeding.

11 - The customised implant is removed from its containment and tapped into the socket. The proximal papillae are sutured. The prepared tooth should be 2.5mm off the occlusion.

12 - Antibiotics and analgesics are prescribed for five days, and the patient is instructed not to chew hard food for three months.

12.10. Postoperative Care and Crown Placement

13 - after three months, the finishing margin of the prepared tooth is analysed, and if the soft tissue is over-erupted, which is usually the case, the excess gingiva is removed by tissue trimmer without irrigation, but the finishing margin of the 180 degrees of the buccal side should be 0.5-1 mm below the gingival ridge.

14 - A conventional dental impression is taken.

12.11. Legal Responsibilities of Implant Manufacturer and Supervising Clinician

The manufacturer must comply with the requirements for the manufacture of custom-made implant medical devices, and it should be in accordance with a written prescription of a registered practitioner who is ultimately responsible. The sole design for a specific patient and its intended use must be registered and written in a prescription. The name of the person responsible should be provided in writing.

Preparation, prescription, implant adaptation, and placement do not fall within the scope of regulations, but the current degree of conformity needs to be assessed.

Even though the CE mark is not required, as the device falls within Class II (b), chemical, physical and biological properties, contamination, all relevant information must be supplied by the manufacturer, with labels containing the trade name, address of the manufacturer need to be provided and the protection against radiation must be addressed.

Description, serial number, order number and generic name should be registered. The patient data must be confidential, and the patient's name must be replaced with a number.

Conformity with the Annex I should be addressed as the grounds for believing it is safe for use.

The documents should be kept for 15 years from the date of manufacture.

Through an amendment to Article 2.3 of Directive 2007/47/EC, a requirement was introduced that the 'statement' detailed in Article 11.6 and Annex VIII of Directive 93/42/EC and Article 9(2) and Annex 6 of Directive 90/85 should be available to the named patient for whom the device has been manufactured. Previously, responsibility rested purely with the manufacturer of the custom-made device to provide a copy of the statement to the prescriber of the device. The amendment extends this duty by requiring that the statement is available to the patient. Whilst the technical document issued with the device should indicate if the manufacturer operates from more than one site, this need not be included in the statement.

We have examples of how each sector of custom-made medical devices has dealt with this requirement.

The Regulations, implementing Directive 2007/47/EC into UK law, simply require that patients are made aware that they can request a statement and that it should be made available on request. It does not go into detail about how this will be achieved.

This was left to member states to determine as a matter of implementation policy according to national systems for making custom-made devices available to patients.

Post-market surveillance, corrective action, and vigilance procedures are a necessity, and it is expected that regulation will be more complicated by the FDA and CE authorities.

The post-marketing vigilance system needs to be reported to the authorities. Any incidents which pose a severe risk to public health or any recall from the manufacturer must be reported.

Due to variations in medical regulations across different countries, it is imperative to consult local authorities for compliance and adherence to applicable guidelines and standards.

12.12. The Use of Dental Implants as Anchorage to Move Teeth

Dental implants have revolutionised modern dentistry, offering versatile applications beyond traditional tooth replacement. One innovative use of dental implants is as an anchorage device to facilitate orthodontic movements, such as pushing or pulling a tooth into the desired position. This technique can be particularly beneficial when conventional orthodontic methods are less practical or feasible. For example, we explore specific scenarios where dental implants are used to move teeth to close gaps or address impacted teeth.

Case Scenario 1: Moving a Second Molar Distally

Consider a patient with a missing lower first molar, resulting in a space between the second and third molars. After the dental implant has osseointegrated, a temporary crown is placed on the implant. This temporary crown is modified to contain a mechanism that allows controlled orthodontic movement (figure 12.2).

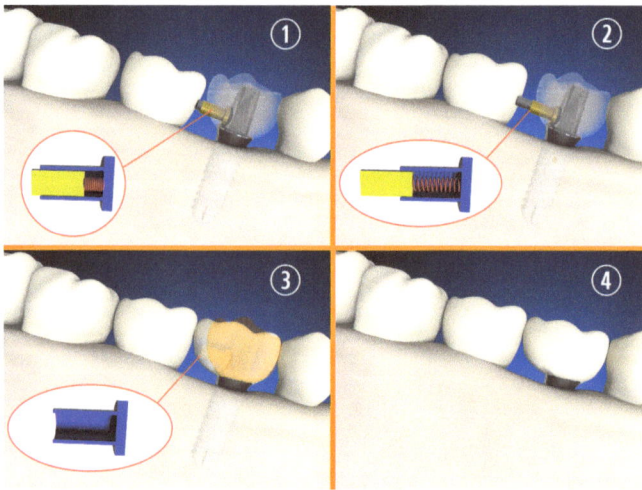

Figure 12.2 The orthotube mechanism facilitates controlled orthodontic tooth movement by using a spring-loaded system integrated into a temporary crown

Mechanism Description

Temporary Crown and Tube Assembly: The temporary crown cemented onto the implant includes a built-in tube. Inside this tube, a spring mechanism is installed. The spring's specifications, including type and length, are chosen based on the required force and distance for tooth movement.

Spring Protection and Piston Function: The spring is housed within a smaller protective tube, creating a piston-like mechanism where the smaller tube slides inside the larger fixed tube in the temporary crown. The purpose of this setup is to efficiently and safely direct the force applied by the spring onto the second molar.

Spring Positioning: The tip of the smaller protective tube is positioned as close as possible to the cementoenamel junction (CEJ) of the mesial side of the second molar. This proximity ensures that the force applied is directed appropriately to move the tooth with minimal tilting movement and should not damage the surrounding soft tissue.

Tooth Movement Process

Force Application: The spring applies a continuous and controlled force to the second molar, pushing it distally. The movement is monitored periodically to ensure proper alignment and prevent any complications. It usually takes 1-4 weeks, so the patient must revisit the clinic weekly.

Tilting Movement: This method can primarily induce a tilting movement of the second molar rather than a complete bodily shift. This tilting is sufficient to close small gaps and achieve the desired alignment.

Specific Use Case: This type of treatment is tailored for specific cases and is not a universal solution. It is particularly beneficial for patients who need minor adjustments and who prefer to avoid extensive orthodontic treatment.

Patient Demographics: The typical patients for this treatment are usually over 30 years old, working professionals who are reluctant to undergo complete orthodontic treatment with visible brackets. This discreet technique allows them to maintain their professional and social appearances without anyone knowing they are undergoing dental treatment.

Contact and Stop Mechanism: As the second molar moves distally, it eventually contacts the neighbouring tooth, which in this case is a third molar, acting as a natural stop. This ensures the second molar does not move beyond the desired position.

Removing the Force: The smaller tube (spring protector) and

spring are removed once the second molar is in the correct position. This cessation of force will not prevent the tooth from returning to its original position.

Retention Without a Traditional Retainer

To ensure the tooth remains in its new position without reverting, the space previously occupied by the spring and tube mechanism is filled with acrylic or composite material. This filling acts as a passive retainer, maintaining the new alignment of the second molar.

Advantages of This Method

Precision and Control: The use of a dental implant as an anchorage provides a stable and predictable force application, allowing for precise control over tooth movement.

Minimally Invasive: This method avoids the need for extensive orthodontic appliances, reducing patient discomfort and treatment complexity.

Aesthetic and Functional Benefits: The use of a temporary crown with an integrated movement mechanism ensures that the treatment remains aesthetically pleasing while being functionally effective.

Discreet Treatment: This technique is particularly advantageous for older patients who do not want to reveal that they are undergoing orthodontic treatment. It allows for tooth movement without the visibility of traditional braces.

Improved Outcomes: By leveraging the natural stopping point provided by the third molar, this technique ensures a stable and desirable final tooth position, enhancing overall treatment outcomes.

Potential Drawbacks

Limited Movement: This method only allows for a tilting movement of the tooth, which may not be suitable for all orthodontic needs.

Enamel Removal: If the occlusion does not permit the necessary movement, up to 1mm of enamel from the moving tooth may need to be removed. This option should be discussed with the patient, highlighting that although this technique is effective in specific cases, traditional full orthodontic treatment generally offers a more comprehensive solution.

Additional Considerations

This technique was originally developed with the anchorage provided by a molar. The pushback of the spring is stopped due to the presence of multiple posterior teeth, adhering to Newton's Third Law of Motion (action and reaction forces are equal and opposite). The traditional approach attaches the cylinder/piston/spring complex to the tooth via enamel etching and composite bonding. However, using a dental implant as the anchorage provides better results. Implants offer more space for maneuvering the cylinder/piston/spring complex and are more reliable for pushing the tooth. Furthermore, adding acrylic or composite to close the gap as a retainer results in a better and more controllable treatment outcome.

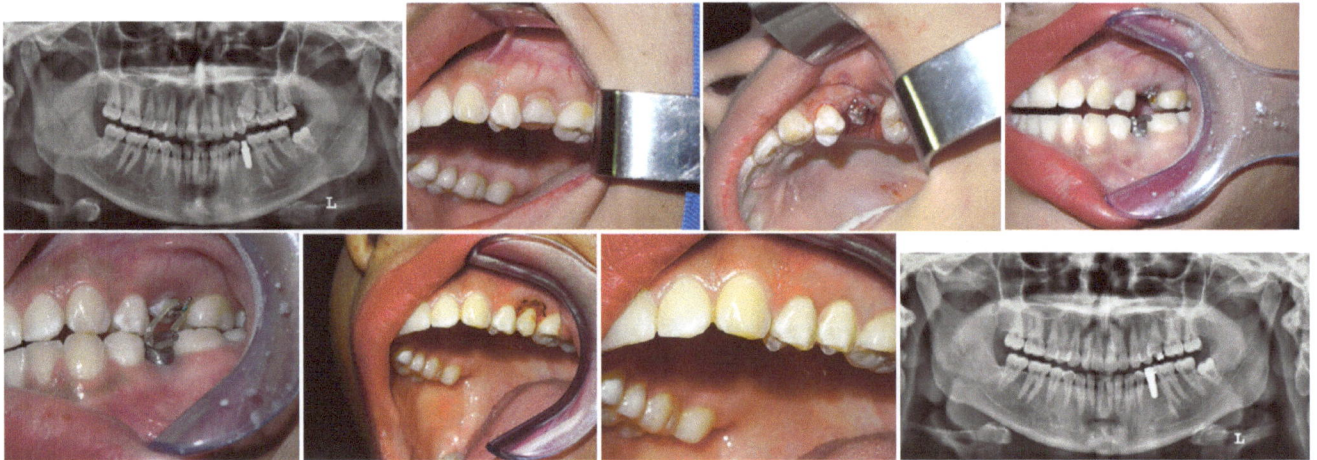

Figure 12.3 Orthodontic elastic bands and hooks are used to apply controlled force, with one side attached to the tooth being moved and the other side anchored to the immobile dental implant

Case Scenario 2: Addressing an Impacted Upper Premolar

Consider a patient with an impacted upper premolar and a deciduous molar with root resorption. After confirming that the mesiobuccal space is sufficient, the deciduous molar is extracted, and an envelope flap is created to expose the impacted premolar (figure 12.3).

Mechanism Description

Bracket Placement: Following the creation of a soft tissue flap, a bracket is affixed to the buccal surface of the impacted premolar using dental cement

Titanium Frame and Rod: A prefabricated titanium frame is secured to the dental implant, to which a titanium rod is welded. Alternatively, the laboratory can fabricate a custom frame with an orthodontic hook if a prefabricated option is unavailable.

Attachment and Force Application: The frame and rod assembly are cemented onto the implant using resin cement, and an orthodontic elastic band is used to pull the impacted premolar into the desired position.

Laser Soft Tissue Management: Laser treatment is utilised to contour the soft tissue for aesthetic purposes."

Advantages and Disadvantages

Advantages: This approach provides a stable and controlled means of addressing impacted teeth, with the dental implant offering a robust anchorage point. The use of customisable titanium frames and rods ensures precise force application and improved treatment outcomes.

Disadvantages: Standard orthodontic treatment remains the gold standard, and temporary anchorage devices (TADs) can also be used. TAD placement and removal after treatment can introduce potential complications. Additionally it may increase the cost and complexity of the procedure.

Conclusion

Utilising dental implants as anchorage for orthodontic tooth movement offers a sophisticated solution for complex dental cases. This method exemplifies the versatility and potential of dental implants beyond their traditional role, providing innovative approaches to enhance patient care and treatment success. As dental technology and techniques continue to evolve, such applications will likely become more refined and widespread, offering even greater benefits in orthodontic and restorative dentistry.

References:

1. Namjo Nik S, Drake D, Rood JP: The effects of pre-operative blockade with 4% prilocaine on the post-operative pain experienced by patients undergoing removal of impacted mandibular third molars, Ambulatory Surgery 1998,6:35-7.

2. Penarrocha-Oltra D, Rossetti PH, Covani U, Galluccio F, Canullo L: Microbial leakage at the implant-abutment connection due to implant insertion maneuvers: Cross-sectional study 5 years postloading in healthy patients.J Oral Implantol 2015;41(6):e292-6.

3. Keith SE, Miller BH, Woody RD, Higginbottom FL, Marginal discrepancy of screw-retained and cement retained metal-ceramic crowns on implant abutments. Int J Oral Maxillofac Implants 1999;14:369-378.